Thyroid Diseases in Pregnancy

Fereidoun Azizi • Fahimeh Ramezani Tehrani
Editors

Thyroid Diseases in Pregnancy

Springer

Editors
Fereidoun Azizi
Endocrine Research Center
Research Institute for Endocrine Sciences
Shahid Beheshti University of Medical Sciences
Tehran, Iran

Fahimeh Ramezani Tehrani
Reproductive Endocrinology Research Center
Research Institute for Endocrine Sciences
Shahid Beheshti University of Medical Sciences
Tehran, Iran

ISBN 978-3-030-98776-3   ISBN 978-3-030-98777-0 (eBook)
https://doi.org/10.1007/978-3-030-98777-0

This Springer imprint is published by the registered company Springer Nature Switzerland AG
The registered company address is: Gewerbestrasse 11, 6330 Cham, Switzerland

Preface

Pregnancy is a critical time for women, during which large physiological changes occur. Today, it has been found that the effects of fetal programming extend beyond fetal development, and thus, impaired prenatal programming has a profound effect on the emergence of the majority of chronic diseases that threaten human life.

Thyroid disorders are one of the most common endocrine abnormalities during pregnancy. Over the last two decades, the link between maternal thyroid dysfunction during pregnancy and adverse pregnancy outcomes, as well as the long-term health consequences, has been a subject of considerable interest. Given the importance of thyroid hormones for normal pregnancy and fetal development, understanding changes in thyroid function and the consequences of thyroid disease during pregnancy is very crucial. Overt thyroid disorders are linked to a variety of short- and long-term adverse impacts on maternal and fetal health. The majority of these complications can be avoided when diagnosed and treated early enough. Whether maternal subclinical hypothyroidism has adverse effects on pregnancy or the subsequent neuropsychological development of their offspring still remains uncertain.

For the purpose of authoring this book, we made a concerted effort to enlist the contribution of experts in the field of thyroid and pregnancy. In this regard, we wish to express our deep gratitude to Dr. Fatemeh Mahboobifard for having been the administrative manager of this book. Her role was designed to invite and get approval from expert scholars in the field of thyroid and pregnancy, implement regular project-in-progress administrative activities, and provide project updates on our behalf to reduce our workload. In addition, we are highly grateful to Ms. Smitha Diveshan, as the Project Coordinator of this book, who made the manuscript development process more efficient.

We hope that the information in this book will be helpful for physicians in the diagnosis and effective management of thyroid disease in pregnant women in order to promote the health of the mother, fetus, and infant.

Tehran, Iran

Fereidoun Azizi
Fahimeh Ramezani Tehrani

Contents

Contributors

Erik K. Alexander Thyroid Section, Division of Endocrinology, Diabetes and Hypertension, Brigham and Women's Hospital, Boston, MA, USA

Atieh Amouzegar Endocrine Research Center, Research Institute for Endocrine Sciences, Shahid Beheshti University, Tehran, Iran

Trevor E. Angell Division of Endocrinology and Diabetes, Keck School of Medicine of the University of Southern California, Los Angeles, CA, USA

Fereidoun Azizi Endocrine Research Center, Research Institute for Endocrine Sciences, Shahid Beheshti University of Medical Sciences, Tehran, Iran

Samira Behboudi-Gandevani Faculty of Nursing and Health Sciences, Nord University, Bodø, Norway

Norman J. Blumenthal Consultant Obstetrician and Gynaecologist Blacktown Hospital and Notre Dame University, Sydney, NSW, Australia

Giampiero Capobianco Gynecologic and Obstetric Clinic, Department of Medical, Surgical and Experimental Sciences, University of Sassari, Sassari, Italy

Alessandro Delitala Department of Medical, Surgical and Experimental Sciences, Institute of Internal Medicine, University of Sassari, Sassari, Italy

Hossein Delshad Micronutrient Research Office, Endocrine Research Center, Research Institute for Endocrine Sciences, Shahid Beheshti University of Medical Sciences, Tehran, Iran

Francesco Dessole Gynecologic and Obstetric Clinic, Department of Medical, Surgical and Experimental Sciences, University of Sassari, Sassari, Italy

Creswell J. Eastman Faculty of Medicine and Health Sydney Medical School, The University of Sydney NSW Australia and Consultant Emeritus Westmead Hospital, Westmead, NSW, Australia

K. Gkastaris Royal United Hospitals Bath NHS, Bath, UK

Spyridon N. Karras National Scholarship Foundation, Thessaloniki, Greece

G. E. Krassas IASEIO, Medical Center, Thessaloniki, Greece

Angela M. Leung Division of Endocrinology, Diabetes, and Metabolism, Department of Medicine, University of California Los Angeles David Geffen School of Medicine, VA Greater Los Angeles Healthcare System, Los Angeles, CA, USA

Eunice López-Muñoz Medical Research Unit in Reproductive Medicine, Unidad Médica de Alta Especialidad Hospital de Gineco Obstetricia No. 4 "Luis Castelazo Ayala", Instituto Mexicano del Seguro Social, Río Magdalena 289, Colonia Tizapan San Angel, Alcaldía Álvaro Obregón, Mexico City, Mexico

Margherita Maioli Department of Biochemical Science, University of Sassari, Sassari, Italy

Gesthimani Mintziori Medical School, Aristotle University of Thessaloniki, Thessaloniki, Greece

Pantea Nazeri Family Health Institute, Breastfeeding Research Center, Tehran University of Medical Sciences, Tehran, Iran

Caroline T. Nguyen Division of Endocrinology, Diabetes, and Metabolism, Keck School of Medicine, University of Southern California, Los Angeles, CA, USA

Onyebuchi E. Okosieme Diabetes Department, Prince Charles Hospital, Merthyr Tydfil, UK

Theodora Pappa Thyroid Section, Division of Endocrinology, Diabetes and Hypertension, Brigham and Women's Hospital, Boston, MA, USA

Marco Petrillo Gynecologic and Obstetric Clinic, Department of Medical, Surgical and Experimental Sciences, University of Sassari, Sassari, Italy

Jennifer B. Plotkin Department of Medicine, University of California Los Angeles David Geffen School of Medicine, Los Angeles, CA, USA

Fahimeh Ramezani Tehrani Reproductive Endocrinology Research Center, Research Institute for Endocrine Sciences, Shahid Beheshti University of Medical Sciences, Tehran, Iran

Themistoklis Tzotzas Department of Endocrinology, Diabetes, and Metabolism, St Luke's General Hospital, Thessaloniki, Greece

Inés Velasco Department of Obstetrics and Gynecology, Hospital Universitari Germans Trias i Pujol, Badalona, España

Thyroid Function in Pregnancy

Alessandro Delitala, Margherita Maioli, Francesco Dessole, Marco Petrillo, and Giampiero Capobianco

Normal Thyroid, Anatomy, Physiology

In normal adults the entire gland is 6–7 cm wide and 3–4 cm long and its weight ranges between 15 and 25 g. The isthmus usually is 20 mm wide and cross the trachea between the first and second rings. The gland is usually asymmetrical, with the right lobe larger than the left. The thyroid is enclosed by a thin connective capsule which penetrates the parenchyma to produce incomplete lobulation. The gland is highly vascularized by an arteriolar network which enters into the parenchyma, where capillaries are fenestrated and are localized in the interfollicular connective tissue. Both sympathetic and parasympathetic fibers innervate the gland in close proximity of capillaries and the follicular cells, where they regulate blood flow and, possibly, thyrocyte function. Peptidergic fibers are also present within the gland, regulating follicular cell function via a paracrine mechanism [1].

Anatomic variants are mainly represented by the presence of an accessory lobe (pyramidal lobe) which derives from the caudal part of the thyroglossal duct. Other rare variants include the absence of the isthmus or of an entire lobe. Another rare condition is the presence of a lingual thyroid in the posterior part of the tongue which is caused by a persistent part of the thyroglossal duct. The basic structure of

A. Delitala (✉)
Department of Medical, Surgical and Experimental Sciences,
Institute of Internal Medicine, University of Sassari, Sassari, Italy
e-mail: aledelitala@uniss.it

M. Maioli
Department of Biochemical Science, University of Sassari, Sassari, Italy
e-mail: mmaioli@uniss.it

F. Dessole · M. Petrillo · G. Capobianco
Gynecologic and Obstetric Clinic, Department of Medical,
Surgical and Experimental Sciences, University of Sassari, Sassari, Italy
e-mail: capobia@uniss.it

F. Azizi, F. Ramezani Tehrani (eds.), *Thyroid Diseases in Pregnancy*,
https://doi.org/10.1007/978-3-030-98777-0_1

the thyroid consists of spheroidal structures called follicles of varying size that contain colloid produced by the follicular cells. Follicles are composed of a single layer of epithelial cells surrounding a closed cavity filled with colloid, which is a concentrated solution of thyroglobulin (TG). They represent the morpho-functional unit of the thyroid gland [2]. The luminar surfaces of follicular cells protrude into the follicular lumen and are characterized by the presence of numerous microvilli and pseudopods that greatly increase the surface area in contact with colloid. Thyrotropin (TSH) receptors and Na+/I− symporter (NIS) are located in the basal domain. The rough endoplasmic reticulum and the Golgi apparatus are the dominant organelles in the cells [3]. Several vesicles are also present in the apical and subapical part of the cytoplasm. Smaller vesicles contain newly synthesized TG which, through a fusion with the apical membrane of the cell, where iodination occurs, is delivered into the follicle lumen. Larger vesicles (colloid droplets) contain iodinated TG which is reabsorbed from the follicular lumen through a macropinocytosis mechanism. This aspect of thyroid cell function is greatly stimulated by TSH [4]. The major regulators of biosynthesis and secretion process of thyroid hormones are the action of TSH, which controls most of the steps within thyroid cells, and the amount of iodide available for hormone synthesis. TSH, a glycoprotein hormone, is synthesized and secreted by pituitary thyrotrophs in the anterior pituitary gland, which are controlled by hypothalamic thyrotropin-releasing hormone (TRH) and other neurotransmitters and/or neuromodulators. TRH is tripeptide produced by hypothalamic neurons and transported in the median eminence of the hypothalamus, where it is released into hypophyseal portal vessels to reach and directly stimulate synthesis and secretion of TSH [5]. Hypothalamic lesions and hypothalamic-pituitary disconnection cause decreased TRH release and central hypothyroidism [6]. TSH controls thyroid function upon its interaction with the G protein-coupled TSH receptor, with predominantly stimulation of cyclic adenosine monophosphate (cAMP) and, in high concentrations, of inositol 1,4,5-triphosphate and diacylglycerol. The physiologic roles of TSH on the thyroid gland are complex. TSH stimulates multiple steps of hormone synthesis, including iodine uptake, organification, TG synthesis, as well synthesis and secretion of thyroid hormones from the gland. Moreover, TSH can induce hypertrophy and hyperplasia of thyrocytes in various clinical conditions [7]. The other major component of the hypothalamic-pituitary-thyroid unit is the inhibitory role of circulating thyroid hormones. This negative feedback control of thyroid hormones is exerted on thyrotrophs, via local intrapituitary conversion of thyroxine (T4) to triiodothyronine (T3), but it is also exerted, to a lesser extent, on TRH-producing neurons of the hypothalamus [8].

Other regulators of TSH secretion are represented by classical neurotransmitters and neuropeptides. In humans many data support an inhibitory role of dopamine on TSH secretion. This inhibition is probably mediated through a pituitary and/or median eminence site of action, since dopamine antagonists that do not cross the blood-brain barrier stimulate TSH secretion in humans. A small stimulatory effect of adrenergic pathways has been also suggested. Other modulators of TSH secretion in humans are endogenous opioids and somatostatin, the latter having an inhibitory action.

Transport of iodide across the thyroid cell membrane is linked to transport of sodium. This cotransport of Na^+ and I^- involves Na^+-K^+-ATPase which serves as a driving force by maintaining the Na^+ ion gradient [9, 10]. TG is a large dimeric protein with a molecular weight of 660 kDa. TG contains iodine in its native state: about 30% of TG's iodine is in T4 and T3, the rest being in the precursors monoiodothyronine (MIT) or diiodothyronine (DIT). TG is synthesized in endoplasmic reticulum, and then, properly folded and partly glycosylated, moves to the Golgi for further attachment of carbohydrates [11–13]. From the Golgi, glycosylated TG moves to the apical membrane, where it is iodinated. In the apical membrane thyroperoxidase (TPO) is the enzyme that catalyzes both the iodination of TG and the consequent formation of thyroid hormones.

Iodide, the form in which iodine enters the thyroid gland, must first be oxidized to a high oxidation state before being an effective iodinating agent. Hydrogen peroxide is sufficiently potent to oxidize I− and it represents the substrate for TPO activity. H_2O_2 generation requires reduced nicotinamide-dinucleotide phosphate (NADPH). TSH stimulates NADPH oxidase activity and H_2O_2 production [14]. The degree of TG iodination directly depends on the amount of available iodine. When the iodine supply is low, less T4 is synthesized and secreted. The pituitary increases TSH secretion which stimulates thyroid hormone synthesis, thus producing more T3 relative to T4, since T3 requires one less atom of iodine per iodothyronine molecule. The next step in thyroid hormone synthesis is the coupling of two DIT residues to form T4 and one DIT and one MIT to form T3, a process which is regulated by TPO. Thyroid hormones are stored in the follicular lumen as colloid, which forms a storage depot of thyroid hormones. When required, stored TG comes back from the follicular lumen into the cells, where, after passing through enzymatic digestive systems, free hormones are delivered to the basal membrane and secreted into the circulation.

The major thyroid hormone secreted by the thyroid gland is T4 whereas about 10% of circulating T3 is directly produced by the thyroid. T4 is considered to be a reservoir for the production of T3, since the majority of T3, which is considered to be the biological active form of thyroid hormones, is produced by T4 conversion by type 1 iodothyronine deiodinases (D1), which is distributed in all tissues [15]. Both deiodinase 2 (D2) and deiodinase 3 (D3) are expressed in the brain. D3 inactivates T4 by converting it into reverse T3, a metabolically inactive compound, and converts T3 to DIT whereas D2 functions to convert T4 to T3. D2 is primarily expressed in glial cells of various regions of the central nervous system and plays an important role in its development and function. In particular, D3 is expressed in high amounts in the placenta, where it protects the fetus from toxic levels of thyroid hormones by converting T4 to biologically inactive reverse T3 in the periphery [16].

One of the most important physiological mechanisms to keep the fetus euthyroid is the presence of uteroplacental barrier, which transfers thyroid hormone from the mother to the fetus. The delivery system of T4 and T3 is mediated by a series of circulating transport proteins with different concentration, affinity, and dissociation rates. The net result is that more than 99% of the circulating hormones is bound. Thyroxine-binding globulin (TBG), by virtue of its high affinity for T4 and T3, binds about 70% of the circulating thyroid hormones, whereas transthyretin (TTR) and thyroxine-binding pre-albumin bind only about 10–15% of the hormones. Binding to plasma proteins is noncovalent and rapidly reversible and hormone-bound has also a reservoir function. They represent an important aspect of thyroid physiology since they modulate the action of thyroid hormones in various tissues, since it is the free or unbound concentration of a hormone that determines its biologic activity. In particular, no evidence exists indicating that binding proteins facilitate tissue uptake of thyroid hormones. In recent years, it has become clear that circulating T4 and T3 do not passively cross cell membranes and several T4 and T3 transport proteins have been identified, including (a) the monocarboxylate transporters (MCT) 8 and MCT10; (b) the organic anion transporter (OATP)1 and OATP3; and (c) L-type amino acid transporter (LAT). MCT8 has preference for T3, whereas T4 and rT3 are preferentially transported by OATP1. LAT transports both T4 and T3 but with relative lower affinity [17, 18].

The complex actions of thyroid hormones are initiated by the intracellular binding of T3 to nuclear receptor where they cause alterations in gene expression. This nuclear genomic effect of thyroid hormones is exerted by either inducing or repressing the expression of target genes. Thyroid hormones also affect cell function through a non-genomic action, which is independent of nuclear receptor. This action is exerted at the cellular membrane with the generation of second intracellular second messengers, such as calcium and cAMP [19]. Both mechanisms are physiologically important in regulating cell differentiation and function. Thus, thyroid hormones play an important role in the regulation of many physiologic processes such as heart rate, blood pressure and arterial stiffening, lipid metabolism and atherosclerosis, and neural development [20–22].

Thyroid Physiology and Function in Pregnancy

Pregnancy has profound effects on thyroid function (Table 1). There are alterations in iodine metabolism, thyroid gland activity, thyroid hormone transport in serum, as well as peripheral metabolism of thyroid hormones. These alterations have profound consequences relating to the diagnosis and management of thyroid disorders in pregnant women.

Table 1 Physiologic changes in pregnancy that influence thyroid function tests

Change during pregnancy	Effect		
	Thyroxine (T4)	Triiodothyronine (T3)	Thyrotropin
Increased thyroxine-binding globulin	Increased total T4	Increased total T3	–
Increased hCG in the first trimester	Increased free T4	–	Reduction
Increased renal iodine clearance	Reduction in iodine-deficient areas	Reduction in iodine-deficient areas	Increase in iodine-deficient areas
Increased type 3 deiodinase	Increased degradation	Increased degradation	–

Iodine Metabolism

Iodine is a trace element present in the human body in small amount and is essential in the synthesis of thyroid hormones. Consequently, severe iodine deficiency will impair thyroid hormone synthesis. When the physiological requirements of iodine are not met during pregnancy, a series of functional and development alterations occur, including severe neurologic and psychological deficit in children; when iodine deficiency is severe, endemic goiter, intrauterine growth retardation (IUGR), increased pregnancy loss, and infant mortality occur [23–25]. These adverse effects are driven by the role of thyroid hormones in brain development, since their physiological concentrations are required for normal neuronal migration, myelin action, and synaptic transmission during fetal and postnatal life [26].

The World Health Organization recommends that pregnant (and lactating) women should have an iodine intake of 250 mcg per day, which is 100 mcg above that recommended dose for nonpregnant women. The critical role of iodine on thyroid function during pregnancy is clearly documented in iodine-deficient areas, where maternal iodine supplementation with iodized salt has demonstrated reduction in the rates of fetal death, endemic cretinism, and decreased thyroid volume as well as improvements in infants' neurocognitive functions [23].

Iodide is rapidly and fully absorbed through the stomach and duodenum and then transported through the circulation where it is taken up by the thyroid in different amounts, depending on the functional state of the thyroid. Iodide is renally excreted. The kidney represents the primary route of iodine excretion, which accounts for more than 90% of ingested iodine [27]. When evaluating adequacy of iodine supply in pregnant women, urinary iodine concentration, as a measure of iodine supply, should be measured.

Thyroid inorganic iodine is derived from two distinct sources: iodide transported from the serum and iodide produced by deiodination of organic iodine compounds within the thyroid gland.

During pregnancy, there is an increase in iodine demand. In early gestation, maternal thyroid hormone production normally increases by approximately 50% in response to the increased metabolic demands of the fetal–maternal unit. An adequate iodine supply, usually obtained from the diet or with supplemental iodine, is essential for this increased thyroid hormone demand. Moreover, when fetal thyroid hormone production physiologically increases during the second half of pregnancy, there is an additional maternal iodine requirement owing to transplacental passage of iodide to the fetus and placental metabolism of iodothyronines. The increase in iodine demand and thyroid hormone production is due to several factors, including alterations in circulating transport proteins, increased human chorionic gonadotropin level, presence of type 2 and type 3 deiodinases in the placenta, and increased maternal renal iodide excretion [28, 29].

The delivery mechanism for the thyroid hormones is mediated by a set of circulating transport proteins that bind more than 99% of the circulating hormones. TBG binds circulating thyroid hormones with high affinity, which is lower for TTR and thyroxine-binding pre-albumin, as they dissociate from them more rapidly. Serum TBG levels increase about 2.5-fold in pregnancy, reaching peak concentrations at about the 21st week [30]. The high levels of TBG in pregnancy cause a higher binding of thyroid hormones, leading to a fall in the levels of the free hormones available. This biochemical alteration leads to stimulation of pituitary TSH production with an overall increase in total thyroid hormone levels. The increase in TBG plasma levels is caused by the large amounts of estrogen that are secreted by the placenta. TBG synthesis in response to increased estrogen secretion is rich in triantennary oligosaccharide chains of N-acetylgalactosamine type, which cause a more slowly TBG clearance from the circulation than TBG of nonpregnant women. Serum TTR and albumin variations have little effect on overall binding of thyroid hormones.

In the first trimester, there is a transient inhibition of TSH that coincides with peak human chorionic gonadotropin (hCG) concentration. Due to the structural homology between TSH and hCG molecule, since the hormone-specific B subunits and the extracellular receptor-binding domains of hCG and TSH share multiple similarities [31], hCG exerts a stimulatory effect on thyroid hormone synthesis and secretion by binding to the TSH receptor on thyrocytes, which results in lowering TSH levels during the first trimester of pregnancy via the negative feedback system [28], as shown in Fig. 1.

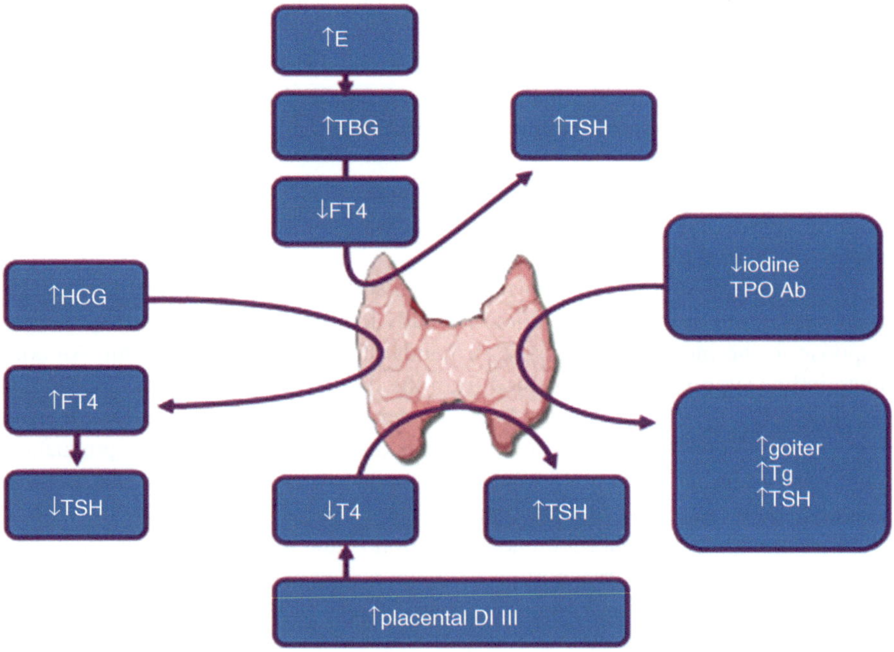

Fig. 1 Modification of thyroid function in pregnancy

Iodide metabolism rapidly changes during early pregnancy, because the glomerular filtration rate increases in pregnancy, resulting in increased renal clearance of iodide of 30–40% [32], thereby further decreasing the circulating pool of plasma iodine. However, the increased urinary excretion of iodine in pregnancy has not been consistent among different studies because some reported no difference, others reported an increase or even a decrease [29]. Furthermore, transplacental passage of iodide to the fetus and placental metabolism of iodothyronines later in gestation is an additional component to relative maternal iodine deprivation. A reduction of maternal urinary iodine has been associated with increased frequency of pregnancy outcomes [33].

All these physiological mechanisms are aimed to counterbalance changes that occur during pregnancy. A normal thyroid gland may carry out all these physiological mechanisms, aiming to counterbalance changes that occur during pregnancy. However, this delicate balance can fail in case of any disorder of the thyroid gland, such as iodine deficiency and autoimmune disease [34–36].

Thyroid Function Tests

The possibility of thyroid disease is suggested by signs or symptoms consistent with alterations in its function or physical abnormalities of the gland. Apart from a detailed history, a systematic examination of the thyroid should be part of every physical examination in clinical practice. A simple physical palpation may detect certain alteration of the gland, including the size, consistency, tenderness, or nodularity. Since most thyroid diseases require appropriate treatment, a number of diagnostic procedures, both in vivo and in vitro, have been proposed to provide a firm diagnosis.

Evaluation of thyroid function includes measurements of TSH, free T4 (fT4) and free T3 (fT3). TSH is the most sensitive measurement for detection of mild thyroid dysfunction, since abnormal TSH levels always proceed abnormal thyroid hormone concentrations. For instance, in subclinical thyroid diseases, TSH is outside the reference range in the presence of normal thyroid hormone concentrations.

In normal subjects, serum TSH levels vary as a result of pulsatile and diurnal secretion, with maximum concentrations at about 24.00 h, and nadir values in the afternoon. Cortisol exerts a small inhibitory influence on TSH secretion, whereas pharmacological doses of glucocorticoids inhibit TSH secretion and its circadian variations [37]. Serum TSH levels are also reduced in patients with depression, anorexia nervosa, after major surgery, and in nonthyroidal illness [38, 39]. Aging itself causes a slight decrease in TSH secretion possibly as a result of increased pituitary conversion of T4–T3.

The routine measurements of TSH in clinical practice initially used radioimmunoassay (RIA) techniques. These first-generation assays had a sensitivity level of about 1 mU/L. Newer techniques, such as immunoradiometric or chemiluminescent assay, result in greater sensitivity, with a sensitivity limit of 0.001 mU/L.

As an initial test, serum total T4 measurement gives a frequent rate of abnormal results, due to the frequency of alterations in serum thyroid hormone-binding proteins. The determination of free hormones by equilibrium dialysis has been the gold standard for estimation of fT4 and fT3. However, this method is cumbersome and technically demanding. Many laboratories have used the fT4 index which is derived from the product of total T4 (measured by immunoassay) and the value of an in vitro uptake test [33]. Commercial methods (two-step immunoassay, analog immunoassay) are being increasingly adopted in the routine evaluation of serum free hormones with good correlation over a broad range of free hormone levels. However, automated immunoassays for free hormones are tricky due to the estrogen-related increase of TBG and the decrease of albumin concentration [40, 41], which is frequently found after the first trimester of pregnancy and may be related to the plasma volume expansion [42]. Indicative normal reference ranges in a normal adult population for 0.7–2.1 ng/dL for fT4 and, respectively, 0.5–5.6 ng/dL for fT3.

In clinical practice, the thyroid antibodies most commonly used are directed against TG and thyroid cell microsomal proteins, the latter being principally represented by TPO. The concentration of these autoantibodies in absolute terms can be measured with sensitive enzyme-linked immunoassay. TPO antibodies are detectable in about 95% of patients with Hashimoto's thyroiditis whereas TG antibodies are present in 60% of adult patients with Hashimoto's thyroiditis. Positive antibody titers, although with a less frequency, can be found in patients with Graves's disease.

Thyroid-stimulating immunoglobulins are usually measured in patients with Graves' disease where they have a diagnostic value. The interaction of these immunoglobulins with thyroid follicular cells results in global stimulation of thyroid gland. The routine assay used in clinical practice is a radioreceptor assay, which is based on competition of the abnormal immunoglobulins and TSH on TSH receptor. The assay does not measure only thyroid-stimulating activity, inhibitory antibodies for TSH receptors can be measured, although the presence of these inhibitory antibodies is less sensitive.

Sonography is currently used to elucidate cryptic findings on physical examination and to complete morphological evaluation of the gland. The normal thyroid gland has a homogeneous pattern like ground glass. The surrounding muscles are of lower echogenicity. Trachea, carotid artery, and jugular vein are easily detected during the examination. Although an ultrasound image may confirm physical examination data, this procedure is very useful to detect small non-palpable thyroid nodules of few millimeters. Sonography can show alterations of the size and alteration of the echo pattern of the gland. Cysts or hemorrhagic degeneration are frequent findings particular in nodular goiter. The prevalence of thyroid nodules in the general population who is screened by ultrasonography is about 50% in older adults, although the risk of malignancy is between 5 and 10%. Among several ultrasound characteristics, hypo-echogenicity, spot microcalcifications, and the absence of halo sign have been suggested as useful markers of thyroid nodule malignancy [43]. Furthermore, the presence of chaotic vascularization pattern showed by color Doppler might rise the suspicion of malignancy [44]. Patients with autoimmune thyroiditis can have diffuse or focal hypo-echogenicity. Thyroid hypo-echogenicity is present in subacute thyroiditis which tend to return to a normal pattern. In Graves' disease color Doppler and duplex Doppler techniques can detect diffuse vascularization with increased flow velocity of the gland.

Recently, ultrasound elastosonography has been shown to represent a highly valuable tool in the diagnostic approach to thyroid nodules. Tissue elasticity may be studied by measuring the degree of distortion of the ultrasound beam under the application of an external force and transferring it into an image by a color scale. Indeterminate nodules, i.e., nodules with a nondiagnostic fine needle cytology results, but with high elasticity, have a low probability of malignancy. Thus, by adding ultrasound elastosonography, the sensitivity of ultrasound findings for malignancy is markedly increased [45].

Nuclear medicine techniques and 18F-fluorodeoxyglucose PET scan are used for diagnosing thyroid diseases in clinical practice, but are not suitable for diagnosis during pregnancy.

Assessment of Thyroid Function in Pregnancy: Gestation-Specific Reference Intervals for Thyroid Function Tests in Pregnancy

In pregnancy, a number of factors linked to the specific physiological changes that occur in thyroid function affect thyroid parameters, thus rendering the interpretation of maternal thyroid function test difficult. Thyroid function tests are frequently performed during pregnancy. These include TSH, fT4 and to a lesser extent, thyroid autoimmunity and fT3. They are similar to the nonpregnant state and represent the complete biochemical approach for the diagnosis of thyroid diseases. The most important clinical aspect is the definition of euthyroidism. Serum TSH and thyroid hormones are usually measured using several immunoanalytical systems with potential variations between the immunoassay used. This aspect, together with clinical heterogeneity of populations, and quality features of the studies contributed to the heterogeneity of results [46, 47]. In nonpregnant women, a normal serum TSH concentration generally rules out thyroid dysfunction. The diagnosis of thyroid disease in pregnancy is still based upon serum TSH concentration, although using trimester-specific TSH reference intervals for pregnant women [48]. Due to the physiological changes occurring during pregnancy, including the increase in hCG and TBG levels, TSH normal levels are lower in pregnancy than in nonpregnant women. Therefore, nonpregnant TSH reference intervals, if applied to pregnant women, would lead to overdiagnosis of hyperthyroidism or underdiagnosis of hypothyroidism. For this reason, in 2011 The American Thyroid Association (ATA) suggested that each Centre calculate its own reference range [49]. But for those who are unable, international guidelines provided fixed reference's range for TSH, specific for each trimester of pregnancy. This cutoff should be maintained at 0.1–2.5 mU/L in the first trimester and at 0.2–3.0 mU/L in the second trimester and 0.3–3.0 mU/L in the third trimester as per ATA [49], as well as for European Thyroid Association (ETA), which increased the upper limit in the third trimester to 3–5 mU/L [50]. However, a number of other studies published after release of ATA guidelines showed that the use of recommended upper limit of TSH's reference range resulted in overdiagnosis and, consequently, overtreatment [51, 52]. For this reason, in 2017 ATA updated guidelines and still advocates the use of reference range specific for pregnancy. If internal pregnancy-specific TSH reference ranges are not available, a simple clinical way for TSH reference interval in the first trimester of pregnancy could be calculated as the reference interval for the nonpregnant population decreased by 0.5 mU/L in the upper limit (for most centers ~4 mU/L). In patients with primary hypothyroidism taking levothyroxine, lowering TSH to <2.5 mU/L has been recommended not only to pregnant women but also for women planning to become pregnant [53].

The gold standard of serum fT4 measurements is solid phase extraction liquid chromatography tandem mass spectrometry [54, 55]. However, these techniques are expensive and are non-easily available in routine laboratories. fT4 is currently measured by immunoanalytical methods in clinical practice. The fT4 reference intervals in pregnancy may vary within the immunoassay techniques used, but they are generally comprised between 9 and 18 pmol/L in the first trimester of pregnancy. Total T4 can also be measured during pregnancy, but the variability in the plasma concentration of the binding protein TBG makes this measurement less useful in clinical practice [56]. Some authors have suggested that the reference values for TT4 in pregnancy might be obtained by multiplying the reference value of nonpregnant women by 1.5 [57].

Antibodies against (TPOAb) and against Tg (TGAb), which are the marker of thyroid autoimmunity, are the most important risk factor for thyroid dysfunction during pregnancy. TPOAb positivity is often associated with a risk of premature delivery and miscarriage [58, 59] since TPOAb positivity could lead to thyroid dysfunction and a subsequent risk of adverse pregnancy outcome. There are no TPOAb and TGAb reference intervals in pregnancy, although their concentrations tend to change throughout the pregnancy. TPOAb-positive pregnant women screened during the first trimester have a high titer of antibodies that tends to decrease in the second and third trimesters of pregnancy, but with an increase in postpartum. In the presence of elevated TSH and negative autoimmunity, thyroid ultrasonography may detect abnormal thyroid hypo-echogenicity and establish the diagnosis of autoimmune serum-negative thyroiditis.

Fetal Thyroid Gland (Embryology; Anatomy, Physiology)

The thyroid gland is a derivative of the primitive buccopharyngeal cavity and is composed of two sets of anlagen, a median anlage derived from the pharyngeal floor and two lateral anlagen from the fourth pharyngeal pouch [60].

The thyroid gland originates from the median anlage and from two lateral anlagen. The median anlage appears first during gestational days 16 and 17 and gives rise to the vast majority of thyroid follicle cells. The thyroid diverticulum evolves from the floor of the pharynx and at the base of the tongue. As the thyroid develops, it continues to expand ventrally, but it remains attached to the pharyngeal floor by the thyroglossal duct, which generally becomes entirely obliterated during gestational weeks 8–10. The thyroid rudiment then begins to expand laterally, which leads to the formation of a bilobed structure. The two lateral anlagen fuse with the median anlage. They give rise to a few thyroid follicular cells but are the main source of parafollicular C cells (calcitonin-secreting cells). These cells derive from cells associated with the fourth or fifth pharyngeal pouch and originate from the neural crest. The histologic differentiation of the follicular cells starts from the precolloid stage and then reaches the follicular stage after 14 weeks of pregnancy. During this phase, there is a progressive increase in diameter of the follicle with an increase in colloid content, while the number of lysosomes within the follicle cells significantly increase.

The function of fetal and adult thyroid gland is primarily regulated by the pituitary TSH and by the hypothalamic component. Fetal pituitary TSH can be detected by 13 weeks, but pituitary and serum TSH levels increase after the 18th week of gestation, and this increase is accompanied by increases in thyroid hormones, suggesting a progressive maturation of the hypothalamic-pituitary-thyroid axis mediated by a mature secretory response to TRH by the pituitary TSH producing cells. TRH is the main regulator of pituitary TSH synthesis and release. The tripeptide TRH is secreted by the supraoptic and paraventricular nuclei of the hypothalamus and is transported to the anterior pituitary through the hypophyseal portal system. The increase in circulating TSH and T4 levels represents progressive maturation of feedback mechanism of thyroid hormones. In contrast to T4, fetal serum T3 levels remain low until the final weeks of gestation. The low levels of circulating T3 are due to a limited conversion of T4 to active T3, whereas conversion of T4 to inactive reverse T3 is high [30, 61]. Although the fetal thyroid gland starts producing thyroid hormones at the end of the first trimester of gestation, the fetal thyroid is not fully active until approximately 20 weeks and therefore the fetus is very dependent on the maternal T4 supply during this period.

Placental Transfer and Metabolism of Thyroid Hormones

Thyroid hormones are transported from mother to the fetus in early fetal stages. Thyroid hormones of maternal origin can cross the placenta and reach the fetus whose receptors are expressed in the fetal brain before the onset of fetal thyroid function. There is now clear evidence of thyroid hormones in fetal serum, coelomic and amniotic fluid and brain in early pregnancy, a time when the fetal thyroid gland has not yet developed the capacity to secrete thyroid hormones [62].

There is also strong clinical evidence that, at least in the presence of a hypothyroid fetus, transfer of maternal T4 to the fetus continues throughout pregnancy. Different tissues modulate the impact of circulating THs according to their current needs via three iodothyronine deiodinases. They are membrane proteins, and differ in tissue distribution, substrate specificities, and physiological functions. By catalyzing removal of iodine from the T4 molecule, they either produce the potent thyroid hormone T3 or they generate the bio-inactive reverse T. There are three iodothyronine deiodinases involved in thyroid hormone metabolism: D1, D2, and D3. D1 is responsible for a large fraction of the circulating T3 and inactivates the sulfated conjugates of T4. D2 is responsible for the local conversion of T4 to active T3 in different tissues and one of the most important physiological mechanisms is to keep the fetus euthyroid. D3, which is expressed in particular in the brain and in the uteroplacental unit [63], mainly deactivates T3 and T4 to inactive iodothyronines, such as reverse T3, which is able to bind to TRs, thus blocking T3 action [64]. D2 and D3 are the major isoforms present in the fetus where they play a crucial role in maintaining sufficiently high brain T3 level to ensure normal brain development. In particular, D3 is expressed in high amounts in the placenta, which catalyzes the removal of an inner ring iodine atom from T4 to generate reverse T3, thus protecting the fetus from toxic levels of thyroid hormones. Moreover, D3 also represents an important source of iodine which is delivered to the fetus for fetal thyroid hormone synthesis. In the earlier stages of gestation D2 is crucial to guarantee appropriate intraplacental levels of T3, in particular during the trophoblast development and differentiation [65].

Two transporters carry out placental iodide transport from the maternal to the fetal circulation: the NIS and pendrin. In thyroid gland, NIS is localized at the basal membrane of thyrocytes and takes up iodide from the blood stream into the cells [66–68]. Pendrin is expressed on the apical membrane of thyrocytes and releases iodide into thyroid follicles for TH synthesis [69–71]. In placenta, NIS is localized to the apical membrane (maternal side) of syncytiotrophoblasts, which directly contacts with maternal blood and influxes iodide into the cells. Conversely, pendrin is located in the basal membrane (fetal side) of syncytiotrophoblasts and effluxes iodide into the extracellular space [72–74].

Excessive maternal iodide intake may, on the other hand, downregulate NIS expression in placenta and reduce iodide transport to the fetus, whereas maternal iodide deficiency upregulated placental NIS expression and increased materno-fetal placental iodide transport may allow the fetus to maintain normal TH levels.

Summary

Thyroid gland carries out different changes during pregnancy, aiming to guarantee a normal concentration of thyroid hormones for the mother and for the fetus. However, this delicate balance can fail in case of any disorder of the thyroid gland, such as iodine deficiency and autoimmune disease. Guidelines advocate the use of reference range specific for each trimester of the pregnancy and, if not available, a simple clinical way for TSH reference interval in the first trimester of pregnancy could be calculated as the reference interval for the nonpregnant population decreased by 0.5 mU/L in the upper limit (for most centers ~4 mU/L). In patients with primary hypothyroidism taking levothyroxine, lowering TSH to <2.5 mU/L has been recommended not only to pregnant women but also for women planning to become pregnant.

References

1. Di Lauro R, De Felice M. Anatomy and development. In: DLaJ JL, editor. Endocrinology; 2001. p. 1268–1277.
2. Yap AS, Stevenson BR, Armstrong JW, Keast JR, Manley SW. Thyroid epithelial morphogenesis in vitro: a role for bumetanide-sensitive Cl− secretion during follicular lumen development. Exp Cell Res. 1994;213(2):319–26.
3. Fujita H. Fine structure of the thyroid gland. Int Rev Cytol. 1975;40:197–280.
4. Engstrom G, Ericson LE. Effect of graded doses of thyrotropin on exocytosis and early phase of endocytosis in the rat thyroid. Endocrinology. 1981;108(2):399–405.
5. Chiamolera MI, Wondisford FE. Minireview: thyrotropin-releasing hormone and the thyroid hormone feedback mechanism. Endocrinology. 2009;150(3):1091–6.
6. Mullur R, Liu YY, Brent GA. Thyroid hormone regulation of metabolism. Physiol Rev. 2014;94(2):355–82.
7. Brent GA, Koenig RJ. Thyroid and antithyroid drugs. In: Brunton LB, Knollman B, editors. Goodman & Gilman's the pharmacological basis of therapeutics. 12th ed. New York: McGraw-Hill Professional; 2010.
8. Hoftijzer HC, Heemstra KA, Visser TJ, le Cessie S, Peeters RP, Corssmit EP, et al. The type 2 deiodinase ORFa-Gly3Asp polymorphism (rs12885300) influences the set point of the hypothalamus-pituitary-thyroid axis in patients treated for differentiated thyroid carcinoma. J Clin Endocrinol Metab. 2011;96(9):E1527–33.
9. Saito K, Yamamoto K, Takai T, Yoshida S. The sodium-dependent iodide transport by phospholipid vesicles reconstituted with the thyroid plasma membrane. J Biochem. 1982;92(6):2001–7.
10. Kaminsky SM, Levy O, Salvador C, Dai G, Carrasco N. Na(+)-I− symport activity is present in membrane vesicles from thyrotropin-deprived non-I(−)-transporting cultured thyroid cells. Proc Natl Acad Sci U S A. 1994;91(9):3789–93.
11. Kim PS, Arvan P. Folding and assembly of newly synthesized thyroglobulin occurs in a pre-Golgi compartment. J Biol Chem. 1991;266(19):12412–8.
12. Muresan Z, Arvan P. Thyroglobulin transport along the secretory pathway. Investigation of the role of molecular chaperone, GRP94, in protein export from the endoplasmic reticulum. J Biol Chem. 1997;272(42):26095–102.
13. Kuznetsov G, Chen LB, Nigam SK. Multiple molecular chaperones complex with misfolded large oligomeric glycoproteins in the endoplasmic reticulum. J Biol Chem. 1997;272(5):3057–63.
14. Kimura T, Okajima F, Sho K, Kobayashi I, Kondo Y. Thyrotropin-induced hydrogen peroxide production in FRTL-5 thyroid cells is mediated not by adenosine 3′,5′-monophosphate, but by Ca2+ signaling followed by phospholipase-A2 activation and potentiated by an adenosine derivative. Endocrinology. 1995;136(1):116–23.
15. Bianco AC, Larsen PR. Cellular and structural biology of the deiodinases. Thyroid. 2005;15(8):777–86.

16. Gereben B, McAninch EA, Ribeiro MO, Bianco AC. Scope and limitations of iodothyronine deiodinases in hypothyroidism. Nat Rev Endocrinol. 2015;11(11):642–52.
17. Jayarama-Naidu R, Johannes J, Meyer F, Wirth EK, Schomburg L, Kohrle J, et al. A nonradioactive uptake assay for rapid analysis of thyroid hormone transporter function. Endocrinology. 2015;156(7):2739–45.
18. Mendoza A, Hollenberg AN. New insights into thyroid hormone action. Pharmacol Ther. 2017;173:135–45.
19. Zhang J, Lazar MA. The mechanism of action of thyroid hormones. Annu Rev Physiol. 2000;62:439–66.
20. Klein I, Ojamaa K. Thyroid hormone and the cardiovascular system. N Engl J Med. 2001;344(7):501–9.
21. Williams GR. Neurodevelopmental and neurophysiological actions of thyroid hormone. J Neuroendocrinol. 2008;20(6):784–94.
22. Carreon-Rodriguez A, Perez-Martinez L. Clinical implications of thyroid hormones effects on nervous system development. Pediatr Endocrinol Rev. 2012;9(3):644–9.
23. Leung AM, Pearce EN, Braverman LE. Iodine nutrition in pregnancy and lactation. Endocrinol Metab Clin N Am. 2011;40(4):765–77.
24. Boyages SC. Clinical review 49: iodine deficiency disorders. J Clin Endocrinol Metab. 1993;77(3):587–91.
25. de Escobar GM, Obregon MJ, del Rey FE. Iodine deficiency and brain development in the first half of pregnancy. Public Health Nutr. 2007;10(12A):1554–70.
26. Morreale de Escobar G, Obregon MJ, Escobar del Rey F. Role of thyroid hormone during early brain development. Eur J Endocrinol. 2004;151(Suppl 3):U25–37.
27. Zimmermann MB, Jooste PL, Pandav CS. Iodine-deficiency disorders. Lancet. 2008;372(9645):1251–62.
28. Glinoer D. The regulation of thyroid function in pregnancy: pathways of endocrine adaptation from physiology to pathology. Endocr Rev. 1997;18(3):404–33.
29. Moleti M, Trimarchi F, Vermiglio F. Thyroid physiology in pregnancy. Endocr Pract. 2014;20(6):589–96.
30. Burrow GN, Fisher DA, Larsen PR. Maternal and fetal thyroid function. N Engl J Med. 1994;331(16):1072–8.
31. Smits G, Govaerts C, Nubourgh I, Pardo L, Vassart G, Costagliola S. Lysine 183 and glutamic acid 157 of the TSH receptor: two interacting residues with a key role in determining specificity toward TSH and human CG. Mol Endocrinol. 2002;16(4):722–35.
32. Glinoer D. The importance of iodine nutrition during pregnancy. Public Health Nutr. 2007;10(12A):1542–6.
33. Azizi F, Mehran L, Amouzegar A, Delshad H, Tohidi M, Askari S, et al. Establishment of the trimester-specific reference range for free thyroxine index. Thyroid. 2013;23(3):354–9.
34. Nazarpour S, Ramezani Tehrani F, Simbar M, Azizi F. Thyroid dysfunction and pregnancy outcomes. Iran J Reprod Med. 2015;13(7):387–96.
35. Nazarpour S, Ramezani Tehrani F, Simbar M, Azizi F. Thyroid autoantibodies and the effect on pregnancy outcomes. J Obstet Gynaecol. 2016;36(1):3–9.
36. Nazarpour S, Ramezani Tehrani F, Amiri M, Simbar M, Tohidi M, Bidhendi Yarandi R, et al. Maternal urinary iodine concentration and pregnancy outcomes: Tehran thyroid and pregnancy study. Biol Trace Elem Res. 2020;194(2):348–59.
37. Brabant G, Ocran K, Ranft U, von zur Muhlen A, Hesch RD. Physiological regulation of thyrotropin. Biochimie. 1989;71(2):293–301.
38. Souetre E, Salvati E, Wehr TA, Sack DA, Krebs B, Darcourt G. Twenty-four-hour profiles of body temperature and plasma TSH in bipolar patients during depression and during remission and in normal control subjects. Am J Psychiatry. 1988;145(9):1133–7.
39. Bartalena L, Placidi GF, Martino E, Falcone M, Pellegrini L, Dell'Osso L, et al. Nocturnal serum thyrotropin (TSH) surge and the TSH response to TSH-releasing hormone: dissociated behavior in untreated depressives. J Clin Endocrinol Metab. 1990;71(3):650–5.

40. Roti E, Gardini E, Minelli R, Bianconi L, Flisi M. Thyroid function evaluation by different commercially available free thyroid hormone measurement kits in term pregnant women and their newborns. J Endocrinol Invest. 1991;14(1):1–9.
41. Sapin R, D'Herbomez M, Schlienger JL. Free thyroxine measured with equilibrium dialysis and nine immunoassays decreases in late pregnancy. Clin Lab. 2004;50(9–10):581–4.
42. Gomez-Cantarino S, Agullo-Ortuno MT, de Dios-Aguado M, Ugarte-Gurrutxaga MI, Bouzas-Mosquera C. Prevalence of hypoproteinemia and hypoalbuminemia in pregnant women from three different socioeconomic populations. Int J Environ Res Public Health. 2020;17(17):6275.
43. Rago T, Vitti P, Chiovato L, Mazzeo S, De Liperi A, Miccoli P, et al. Role of conventional ultrasonography and color flow-doppler sonography in predicting malignancy in 'cold' thyroid nodules. Eur J Endocrinol. 1998;138(1):41–6.
44. Papini E, Guglielmi R, Bianchini A, Crescenzi A, Taccogna S, Nardi F, et al. Risk of malignancy in nonpalpable thyroid nodules: predictive value of ultrasound and color-Doppler features. J Clin Endocrinol Metab. 2002;87(5):1941–6.
45. Rago T, Vitti P. Diagnostic role of ultrasound and elastosonography in nodular goiter. Best Pract Res Clin Endocrinol Metab. 2014;28(4):519–29.
46. Springer D, Jiskra J, Limanova Z, Zima T, Potlukova E. Thyroid in pregnancy: from physiology to screening. Crit Rev Clin Lab Sci. 2017;54(2):102–16.
47. Delitala AP, Capobianco G, Cherchi PL, Dessole S, Delitala G. Thyroid function and thyroid disorders during pregnancy: a review and care pathway. Arch Gynecol Obstet. 2019;299(2):327–38.
48. Mannisto T, Vaarasmaki M, Suvanto E. Pregnancy outcomes in women with thyroid peroxidase antibodies. Obstet Gynecol. 2011;117(1):174–5.
49. Stagnaro-Green A, Abalovich M, Alexander E, Azizi F, Mestman J, Negro R, et al. Guidelines of the American Thyroid Association for the diagnosis and management of thyroid disease during pregnancy and postpartum. Thyroid. 2011;21(10):1081–125.
50. Lazarus J, Brown RS, Daumerie C, Hubalewska-Dydejczyk A, Negro R, Vaidya B. 2014 European thyroid association guidelines for the management of subclinical hypothyroidism in pregnancy and in children. Eur Thyroid J. 2014;3(2):76–94.
51. Medici M, de Rijke YB, Peeters RP, Visser W, de Muinck Keizer-Schrama SM, Jaddoe VV, et al. Maternal early pregnancy and newborn thyroid hormone parameters: the Generation R study. J Clin Endocrinol Metab. 2012;97(2):646–52.
52. Li C, Shan Z, Mao J, Wang W, Xie X, Zhou W, et al. Assessment of thyroid function during first-trimester pregnancy: what is the rational upper limit of serum TSH during the first trimester in Chinese pregnant women? J Clin Endocrinol Metab. 2014;99(1):73–9.
53. Alexander EK, Pearce EN, Brent GA, Brown RS, Chen H, Dosiou C, et al. 2017 guidelines of the American Thyroid Association for the diagnosis and management of thyroid disease during pregnancy and the postpartum. Thyroid. 2017;27(3):315–89.
54. Anckaert E, Poppe K, Van Uytfanghe K, Schiettecatte J, Foulon W, Thienpont LM. FT4 immunoassays may display a pattern during pregnancy similar to the equilibrium dialysis ID-LC/tandem MS candidate reference measurement procedure in spite of susceptibility towards binding protein alterations. Clin Chim Acta. 2010;411(17–18):1348–53.
55. Soldin SJ, Soukhova N, Janicic N, Jonklaas J, Soldin OP. The measurement of free thyroxine by isotope dilution tandem mass spectrometry. Clin Chim Acta. 2005;358(1–2):113–8.
56. Midgley JE, Hoermann R. Measurement of total rather than free thyroxine in pregnancy: the diagnostic implications. Thyroid. 2013;23(3):259–61.
57. Mandel SJ, Spencer CA, Hollowell JG. Are detection and treatment of thyroid insufficiency in pregnancy feasible? Thyroid. 2005;15(1):44–53.
58. Thangaratinam S, Tan A, Knox E, Kilby MD, Franklyn J, Coomarasamy A. Association between thyroid autoantibodies and miscarriage and preterm birth: meta-analysis of evidence. BMJ. 2011;342:d2616.
59. He X, Wang P, Wang Z, He X, Xu D, Wang B. Thyroid antibodies and risk of preterm delivery: a meta-analysis of prospective cohort studies. Eur J Endocrinol. 2012;167(4):455–64.

60. Pintar JE. Normal development of the hypothalamic-pituitary-thyroid axis. In: Lippincott J, editor. The Thyroid; 1996. p. 6–18.
61. Polk DH, Fisher DA. Fetal and neonatal thyroid physiology. In: PRAaF WW, editor.
62. Calvo RM, Jauniaux E, Gulbis B, Asuncion M, Gervy C, Contempre B, et al. Fetal tissues are exposed to biologically relevant free thyroxine concentrations during early phases of development. J Clin Endocrinol Metab. 2002;87(4):1768–77.
63. Van der Geyten S, Segers I, Gereben B, Bartha T, Rudas P, Larsen PR, et al. Transcriptional regulation of iodothyronine deiodinases during embryonic development. Mol Cell Endocrinol. 2001;183(1–2):1–9.
64. Darras VM, Houbrechts AM, Van Herck SL. Intracellular thyroid hormone metabolism as a local regulator of nuclear thyroid hormone receptor-mediated impact on vertebrate development. Biochim Biophys Acta. 2015;1849(2):130–41.
65. Chan SY, Vasilopoulou E, Kilby MD. The role of the placenta in thyroid hormone delivery to the fetus. Nat Clin Pract Endocrinol Metab. 2009;5(1):45–54.
66. Caillou B, Troalen F, Baudin E, Talbot M, Filetti S, Schlumberger M, et al. Na+/I− symporter distribution in human thyroid tissues: an immunohistochemical study. J Clin Endocrinol Metab. 1998;83(11):4102–6.
67. Dai G, Levy O, Carrasco N. Cloning and characterization of the thyroid iodide transporter. Nature. 1996;379(6564):458–60.
68. Royaux IE, Suzuki K, Mori A, Katoh R, Everett LA, Kohn LD, et al. Pendrin, the protein encoded by the Pendred syndrome gene (PDS), is an apical porter of iodide in the thyroid and is regulated by thyroglobulin in FRTL-5 cells. Endocrinology. 2000;141(2):839–45.
69. Dohan O, Carrasco N. Advances in Na(+)/I(−) symporter (NIS) research in the thyroid and beyond. Mol Cell Endocrinol. 2003;213(1):59–70.
70. Mian C, Lacroix L, Bidart JM, Caillou B, Filetti S, Schlumberger M. Sodium/iodide symporter in thyroid cancer. Exp Clin Endocrinol Diabetes. 2001;109(1):47–51.
71. Spitzweg C, Heufelder AE, Morris JC. Thyroid iodine transport. Thyroid. 2000;10(4):321–30.
72. Bidart JM, Lacroix L, Evain-Brion D, Caillou B, Lazar V, Frydman R, et al. Expression of Na+/I− symporter and Pendred syndrome genes in trophoblast cells. J Clin Endocrinol Metab. 2000;85(11):4367–72.
73. Manley SW, Li H, Mortimer RH. The BeWo choriocarcinoma cell line as a model of iodide transport by placenta. Placenta. 2005;26(5):380–6.
74. Mitchell AM, Manley SW, Morris JC, Powell KA, Bergert ER, Mortimer RH. Sodium iodide symporter (NIS) gene expression in human placenta. Placenta. 2001;22(2–3):256–8.

Iodine Deficiency/Excess and Pregnancy Outcomes

Pantea Nazeri and Hossein Delshad

Iodine Metabolism

Iodine is ingested in several chemical forms. Iodide is rapidly and nearly all absorbed (>90%) in the stomach and duodenum [1]. Iodate, widely used in iodization of salt, is reduced in the gut and absorbed as iodide. The body of a healthy adult contains 15–20 mg of iodine, of which 70–80% is in the thyroid. Iodine is used by the thyroid gland to produce thyroid hormones. For women, iodine is necessary for optimal function of the reproductive system and for normal fetal growth and development [2]. In chronic iodine deficiency, the iodine content of the thyroid might fall to less than 20 μg. In iodine-sufficient areas, the adult thyroid traps about 60 μg of iodine per day to balance losses and maintain synthesis of thyroid hormone. The sodium/iodide symporter (NIS) transfers iodide into the thyroid at a concentration gradient 20–50 times that of plasma. Thyroid clearance of circulating iodine varies with iodine intake: in situations with adequate iodine supply, 10% or less of absorbed iodine is taken up by the thyroid. In chronic iodine deficiency, this percentage can exceed 80% [3]. Iodine consists of 65% and 59% of the weights of thyroxine (T4) and tri-iodothyronine (T3), respectively. The released iodine enters the plasma iodine pool and can be taken up again by the thyroid or excreted by the kidney. More than 90% of ingested iodine is ultimately excreted in the urine.

Pregnancy alters thyroid physiology [4, 5] and several major changes occur in thyroid physiology that result in higher iodine requirements in pregnant than non-pregnant women. Increased circulating estrogen during pregnancy increases

P. Nazeri
Family Health Institute, Breastfeeding Research Center, Tehran University of Medical Sciences, Tehran, Iran

H. Delshad (✉)
Micronutrient Research Office, Endocrine Research Center, Research Institute for Endocrine Sciences, Shahid Beheshti University of Medical Sciences, Tehran, Iran
e-mail: delshad@endocrine.ac.ir

F. Azizi, F. Ramezani Tehrani (eds.), *Thyroid Diseases in Pregnancy*,
https://doi.org/10.1007/978-3-030-98777-0_2

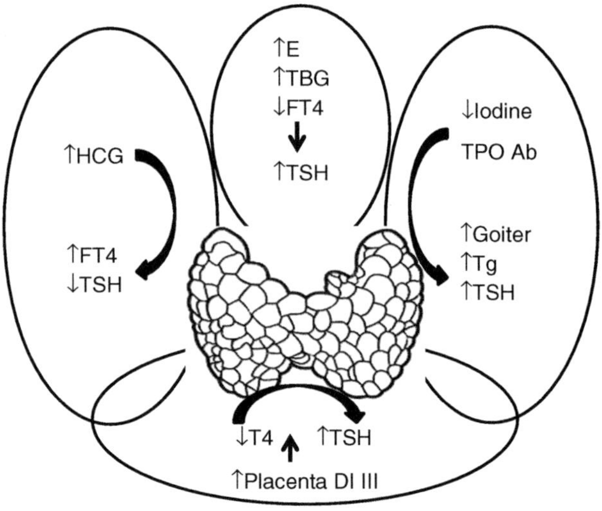

Fig. 1 Factors for thyroid stimulation during pregnancy

thyroid-binding globulin two- to threefold in response to this phenomenon. Also, because of thyroid stimulating hormone (TSH) receptor stimulation by human chorionic gonadotropin, thyroid hormone production increases by 50% during early gestation in pregnant women (Fig. 1). Another change during pregnancy is degradation of T4 to bio-inactive reverse tri-iodothyronine by the placental type 3 inner ring deiodinase [6]. On the other hand, the glomerular filtration rate of iodide increases by 30–50% in early pregnancy [7].

The placenta is a highly specialized organ whose primary function is to promote the exchange of nutrients and oxygen between maternal and fetal blood [8]. In 2006, Cosmo and co-workers for the first time described the presence of NIS in placental cells [9]. NIS expression in placenta is at lower levels than that in the thyroid, and it mediates the active uptake of iodide by the developing fetus for its proper thyroid hormone synthesis [10]. At the beginning of the second trimester, the fetal thyroid gland begins to synthesize thyroid hormones, and, at around 18–20 weeks of gestation, the pituitary-portal vascular system in the fetus completes its development [11]. Fetal and newborn neurogenesis and neurodevelopment are depicted in Fig. 2.

Altogether, these physiological changes, along with the need of the fetal thyroid gland for iodine to produce thyroid hormones during the second half of gestation, increase iodine requirements in normal pregnancy [12, 13]. Failure to meet this increased iodine demand results in an insufficient supply of thyroid hormones to the developing brain, leading to permanent brain damage and mental retardation in the newborn [14, 15]. Therefore, to meet the increased dietary iodine requirements during pregnancy, the World Health Organization (WHO) recommends ~ 250 μg iodine intake daily for pregnant and lactating women [16]. The United States Institute of Medicine's recommended daily allowance for iodine is 220 μg during pregnancy and 290 μg during lactation, higher than the 150 mg daily recommended for non-pregnant adults [17].

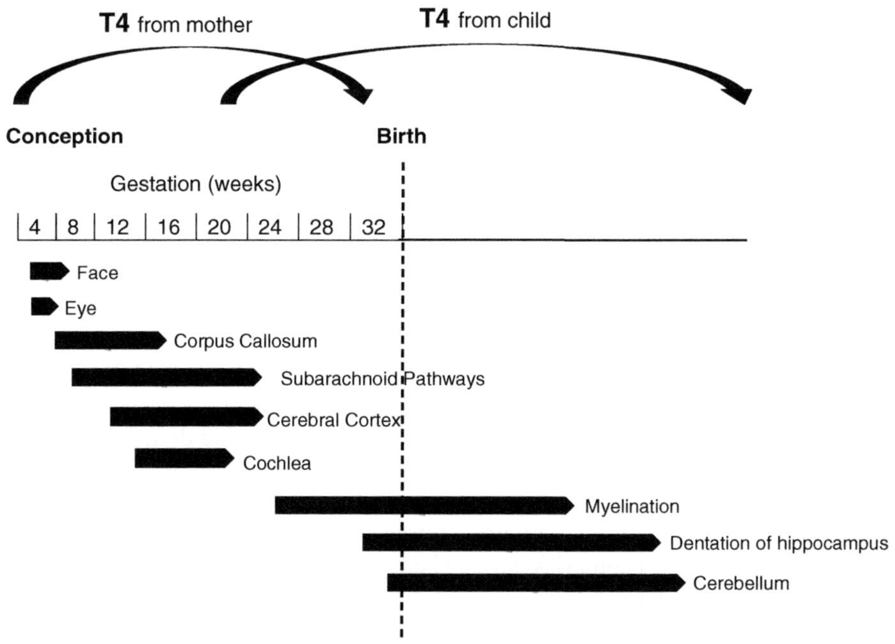

Fig. 2 Major events in fetal and neonatal central nervous system development. Developing brain needs normal level of circulation T4

Considering the importance of iodine deficiency in pregnant women and their fetuses, identifying a biomarker that accurately reflects iodine status during pregnancy is critical. According to the criteria of the WHO, the Iodine Global Network (IGN, formerly the International Council for the Control of Iodine Deficiency Disorders [ICCIDD]), and the United Nations Children's Fund (UNICEF), a median urinary iodine concentration (UIC) of 150–249 μg/L is represented for iodine sufficiency among pregnant women [16]. However, UIC is only considered to be a sensitive marker of recent iodine intake; it cannot be used to determine an individual's iodine status and thyroid function [18]. Recent studies propose that thyroglobulin (Tg), a thyroid-specific protein which plays an important role in the synthesis of thyroid hormones, may be a more reliable indicator for iodine status during pregnancy [19]. However, no consensus has been reached regarding the optimal cutoff value for Tg concentration to indicate iodine status during pregnancy. For instance, in Belgium, a mildly iodine-deficient country, a median Tg of <20 μg/L suggested iodine sufficiency in a population of pregnant women [20], whereas a review by Ma et al. used a median Tg of <13 μg/L to indicate adequate iodine status among populations of pregnant women [19], taken from the cutoff value proposed by Zimmermann et al. to indicate iodine status in school-aged children [21]. In a recent meta-analysis by Nazeri et al., the mean Tg concentration in populations of pregnant women with iodine deficiency and sufficiency was 10.73 μg/L and 7.34 μg/L, respectively, with overlapping of confidence intervals [22]. This finding was not entirely inconsistent with recent studies which proposed a cutoff Tg concentration of 10 μg/L measured in serum or dried blood spot as an indicator of iodine sufficiency during pregnancy [23–25]. It seems that Tg can provide a more reliable assessment than UIC alone; therefore, in pregnant women, iodine status should monitor using both UIC and Tg level.

World Status of Iodine Deficiency

It is well documented that universal salt iodization is still the most feasible and cost-effective approach for adequate dietary iodine intakes worldwide [16]. Data available from countries with mandatory salt iodization program reveals that they achieved great success in the control and elimination of iodine deficiency among general populations; however, where iodization of this type of salt is still voluntary, this can be a real constraint in achieving elimination of iodine deficiency [26]. Between 1942 and 2020, 123 countries introduced mandatory legislation on salt iodization. In 2021, 124 countries have legislation for mandatory salt iodization and at least 21 countries have legislation allowing voluntary salt iodization [26]. As a result, 88% of the global population uses iodized salt. For population surveys, the UIC should be measured and expressed as the median, in μg/L. As shown in Fig. 3, the number of countries with adequate iodine intake has increased from 67 in 2003 to 118 in 2020. However, 21 countries remain deficient, while 13 countries have excessive intakes, either due to excess groundwater iodine or over-iodized salt.

Recently, further studies have emphasized on surveying women of reproductive age and pregnant women. Number of countries according to their iodine status in women of reproductive age and pregnant women in 2017 is shown in Fig. 4. There

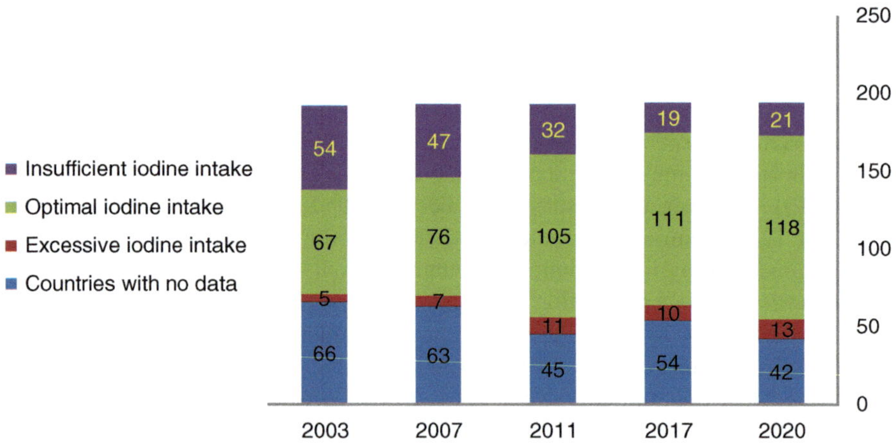

Fig. 3 Number of countries according to their iodine status in the general population between 2003 and 2020

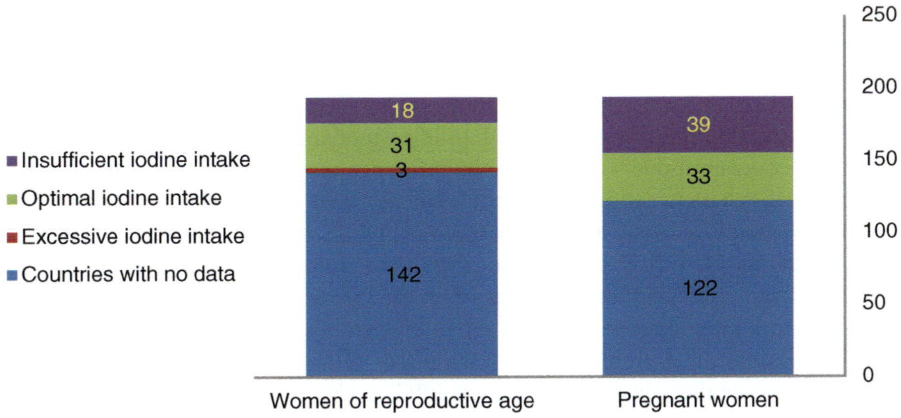

Fig. 4 Number of countries according to iodine status in women of reproductive age and pregnant women in 2017

is much evidence indicating suboptimal iodine status among pregnant and lactating women, despite iodine sufficiency among schoolchildren in countries designated as iodine sufficient [27]. Available data indicate that many pregnant women in both low- and high-income countries, including the USA [28] and several European countries [29], have low iodine intakes. Therefore, regular monitoring of both salt iodization programs and of population iodine status, specifically pregnant women, lactating mothers, and infants, remains crucially important.

Impact of Iodine Deficiency on Pregnancy Outcomes

Inadequate iodine intake has negative effects on the physical and mental development of millions of people living in iodine-deficient areas around the world [30]. The term iodine deficiency disorders (IDD), introduced by Basil Hetzel in 1983, has transformed the world's understanding of the problem from endemic goiter to a wide range of conditions [31]. The brain is particularly sensitive to iodine deficiency during its formation in early fetal and postnatal life [32, 33].

The most serious adverse effect of iodine deficiency occurs to the fetus. Severe maternal iodine deficiency in pregnancy increases the risk for stillbirth, miscarriage, perinatal and infant mortality, and congenital anomalies [34]. As normal amounts of thyroid hormones are needed for neuronal migration and myelination of fetal brain [35], in the most severely iodine-deficient regions infants may be born with cretinism, a syndrome of severe intellectual impairment, growth impairment, and sometimes deafness [36]. Iodine supplementation and fortification strategies in severely iodine-deficient regions have been shown to decrease the rates of cretinism [37], improve birth outcomes including birth weight [38], and increase offspring intelligence quotient (IQ) [39, 40].

Although severe iodine deficiency has been linked to maternal or neonatal thyroid dysfunction, mild-to-moderate iodine deficiency is not typically associated with thyroid function abnormalities. A few studies have reported the effect of iodine status on thyroid hormones in euthyroid pregnant women in areas with sufficient iodine intake. In pregnant women with mild-to-moderate iodine deficiency, thyroid hormone concentrations were within the reference range and did not reflect iodine status [41]. A recent study from Iran indicated that moderate iodine deficiency among pregnant women was not accompanied by alterations in serum TSH or FT4 concentrations [42]. It has been also shown that mid-to-moderate iodine insufficiency during pregnancy has minimal or no effects on birth weight or fetal growth [43–45]. In a systematic review and meta-analysis by Nazeri et al., there were no significant differences in birth weight, length, or head circumference between newborns whose mothers had UIC < 150 or UIC ≥ 150 μg/L during pregnancy [46]. Despite mild-to-moderate iodine deficiency remains prevalent in many parts of the world, defining its potential deleterious effects on fetal neurobehavioral development is not well documented. There are some studies reporting that maternal iodine deficiency in mild-to-moderate iodine-deficient areas can result in less sever, but measurable, long-lasting impacts, especially during the neonatal period, affecting the intellectual development of the child. For instance, a study from the UK indicated that mild maternal iodine deficiency during pregnancy was associated with lower child IQ [14]. Finding of a cohort study with 9 years follow-up demonstrated a reduction in spelling, grammar, and general English-literacy performance in children of mothers with mild iodine deficiency during pregnancy [47]. In the Norwegian Mother and Child Cohort Study, insufficient maternal iodine intake was linked with increased child attention-deficit/hyperactivity disorder (ADHD) symptom scores at 8 years of age, but not with ADHD diagnosis [48]. However, it is still unclear to what extent mild maternal iodine deficiency during pregnancy affects child neurobehavioral development.

Iodine Supplementation

In countries with effective salt iodization programs, although school children attain sufficient iodine status, abundant evidence indicates that pregnant women and lactating mothers have inadequate levels of iodine [42, 49, 50]. Iodized salt may not always be a sufficient source of iodine to meet the minimum requirements of the most vulnerable groups (i.e., pregnant and lactating women and infants). Therefore, leading international health authorities, such as the American Thyroid Association [51], the Endocrine Society [52], and the American Academy of Pediatrics [53], recommend that pregnant and lactating women or those who are planning for pregnancy should take supplements containing 150 μg of iodine to prevent deficiency. The correction of severe iodine deficiency through iodine supplementation or food fortification programs results in improved clinical outcomes [54]. As pointed out above, however, results of studies conducted on the impacts of iodine supplementation in mildly-to-moderately iodine-deficient pregnant women are inconsistent [55]. Observational cohorts reported significant positive consequences (both health and economic) of correcting iodine deficiency in pregnant women. Meanwhile, the findings of clinical trials are controversial [56]. Still, there are debates regarding the benefits of iodine supplementation, alone or in combination with other vitamins and minerals, in women before conception or during pregnancy.

Few studies have investigated the benefits of iodine supplementation before pregnancy. In Spain, pregnant women who consumed iodized salt for at least 1 year before pregnancy had significantly higher urinary iodine levels and smaller thyroid gland size in the third trimester than women who received 200 or 300 μg iodine during pregnancy [57]. Similarly, in Australia, urinary iodine levels in women who started iodine supplementation before conception did not decline throughout gestation period and were within the optimal range, compared with those who started supplementations following pregnancy confirmation [58]. These findings suggest that iodine supplementation during *preconception* provides satisfactory iodine status and improves thyroid storage during the pregnancy, with the need for thyroid hormones increasing substantially. A study by Delshad et al. showed that iodine supplementation with at least 150 μg of iodine per day improved the iodine intake of Iranian pregnant women. The prevalence of clinical hypothyroidism, clinical/subclinical thyrotoxicosis, TPO-Ab positivity, and isolated hypothyroxinemia decreased significantly [59]. However, in a study conducted among Chinese pregnant women, iodine supplementation in mildly iodine-deficient pregnant women increased the risk of subclinical hypothyroidism [24]. In recent systematic reviews and meta-analyses, no significant changes were observed in maternal and neonatal thyroid parameters (i.e., T4, FT4, T3, or FT3) following iodine supplementation *during pregnancy* [60, 61]. However, there was more consistent evidence regarding higher Tg concentration in non-supplemented women, which reflected thyroid stress to produce adequate thyroid hormone in response to limited iodine supply [62–67]. These observations agree with those of a previous meta-analysis, which found no difference in the likelihood of maternal or neonatal thyroid dysfunction between pregnant women who received iodine supplementation and those in the control group [68].

There is a large body of evidence indicating that severe iodine deficiency during pregnancy may lead to adverse effects on birth weight or fetal growth, and iodine repletion through the administration of iodized oil or salt significantly improves birth outcomes [38]. However, there is no definitive evidence that iodine repletion in pregnant women improves growth outcomes. In a meta-analysis performed by Farebrother et al., iodine supplementation to treat severe iodine deficiency in pregnant women, on average, resulted in a 200 g increase in weight and 0.4 cm greater head circumference at birth in infants born to supplemented women than those born to women in the control group, but no effect was found in mildly-to-moderately iodine-deficient pregnant women [69]. In a recent systematic review and meta-analysis by Nazeri et al. regardless of the degree of maternal iodine deficiency, there were no differences in birth weight, length, or head circumference between infants born to women who received iodine supplementation during pregnancy and those born to non-supplemented women [61].

Data on the benefits of iodine supplementation during pregnancy for child neurocognitive development are still inconclusive. For instance, a study conducted by Velasco et al. showed a positive effect on psychomotor scores that was observed in children of mothers who received 300 μg iodine starting 10 weeks before the gestation when compared with the control group [70]. Gowachirapant et al. did not report any beneficial effects but reported some indications of negative effects on the neurodevelopment of children following iodine supplementation 14 weeks before the gestation [64]. This discrepancy may be explained by the fact that the effect of iodine on the neurocognitive development of children varies at different stages of pregnancy. In a recent meta-analysis on individual-participants data from three cohorts, lower maternal iodine status during pregnancy was associated with lower child verbal IQ up until the start of the second trimester [71]. However, in two recent meta-analyses, iodine supplementation of mildly iodine-deficient pregnant women had no clear benefit on neurocognitive outcomes during infancy, which may be attributed to the physiological adaption of pregnant women to low intake of iodine to maintain fetal thyroid hormones at a normal level for in utero development [60, 61].

It is important to note that the lack of beneficial effects of iodine supplements can be related to many factors: (1) late administration of iodine supplementation, given the increasing evidence on the importance of preconception supplementation, (2) the physiologic response to iodine repletion, which may be different depending upon the degree of iodine deficiency before treatment, and (3) as evidence resulted from trials is not sufficient, drawing definitive conclusions may be difficult, particularly when considering trials on infant/child growth status and neurocognitive development.

Impact of Iodine Excess on Pregnancy Outcomes

Excess iodine intake may come from the consumption of excessive seaweed, dietary supplements, or over-iodized salt. In some countries, iodine-rich groundwater may be another cause of excess intake [72–74]. In normal individuals, high iodine intake induces a protective response in the thyroid gland known as the acute Wolff–Chaikoff effect [75]. Typically, the thyroid "escapes" from the acute Wolff–Chaikoff effect within a few days through downregulation of the iodide transporter in thyroid cells, and normal thyroid hormone synthesis resumes. Therefore, failure of the "escape" can result in alteration in thyroid hormones and function [76]. Pregnant women and the developing fetus are among vulnerable groups to iodine excess [77–80], though the consequences of iodine excess during pregnancy are poorly understood, and data are inconsistent. It has been shown that the fetal thyroid gland does not acquire the capacity to fully escape from the acute Wolff–Chaikoff effect until ~36 weeks gestation [81]. Therefore, a maternal iodine load may potentially cause fetal hypothyroidism, as reported in three infants of women ingesting 12.5 mg iodine daily during gestation [82]. The Institute of Medicine recommends an iodine upper limit of 1100 μg/day for pregnant women, whereas the WHO more conservatively recommends an upper limit of 500 μg/day [80].

Iodine supplementation is generally considered a safe intervention for pregnant women; however, some observational studies report that it might have risks. For instance, a cohort study conducted in Spain showed lower psychomotor development in infants whose mothers received ≥150 μg/day of iodine supplements [83, 84]. Another study on pregnant women who received excessive iodine reported an increased risk of developing thyroid disorders in both mothers and neonates [24]. In a study by Farebrother et al., chronic excess iodine intake during pregnancy was associated with maternal hypothyroxinemia [85]; it has been shown that hypothyroxinemia during pregnancy has been linked with adverse birth outcomes, including preterm delivery [86] and possibly irreversible low childhood IQ [35, 87–89]. However, only few clinical trials have investigated the adverse effect (s) of iodine supplementation during pregnancy. Some reported clinical complications, such as gastrointestinal side effects, gestational diabetes mellitus, pregnancy-induced hypertension, and preeclampsia, increased hospital admission, abortion, stillbirth, intrauterine death, cesarean section, and post-term induction following the iodine supplementation in pregnant women [62, 64, 65, 90]. Complications observed in neonates included premature, low birth weight, admission to neonatal intensive care unit, and death [64, 70, 90]. Notably, the frequency of the aforementioned outcomes in pregnant women and neonates did not show any differences between the two groups for various doses of iodine supplementation. More studies on long-term consequences of iodine excess on maternal and infant outcomes are still warranted.

Summary

Iodine, an essential component of thyroid hormones, plays a key role in the overall growth of the body and development of the central nervous system of the fetus and infant. During pregnancy, iodine requirements increase substantially to approximately 150% of those of non-pregnant women, due to increased thyroid hormone production, iodine transfer to the fetus, and increased urinary iodine excretion. Therefore, inadequate iodine intake during this critical period depending upon the timing and severity of the deficiency can cause cretinism, neonatal hypothyroidism, growth retardation, neurologic and cognitive deficits, increased risk of miscarriage, and infant mortality. Although the WHO does not recommend iodine supplementation for pregnant women, lactating mothers, or infants in countries with effective iodized salt programs, major medical societies such as the American Thyroid Association, the Endocrine Society, and the American Academy of Pediatrics recommend that pregnant women and lactating mothers should take daily supplements containing 150 μg of iodine. More consistent evidence reported that iodine supplementation could prevent the increase in Tg concentration during pregnancy.

However, there is no definitive evidence on the beneficial effects of iodine supplementation, specifically on infant growth or developmental outcomes, and further studies are required to clarify better these issues. More data are also needed to determine optimal and safe upper limits of iodine supplementation in pregnant women and assess the potential risks of chronic high iodine intake during pregnancy.

References

1. Zimmermann MB. Iodine deficiency. Endocr Rev. 2009;30(4):376–408.
2. Delange F. Iodine requirements during pregnancy, lactation and the neonatal period and indicators of optimal iodine nutrition. Public Health Nutr. 2007;10(12A):1571–80; discussion 81–3.
3. Zimmermann MB, Jooste PL, Pandav CS. Iodine-deficiency disorders. Lancet. 2008;372(9645):1251–62.
4. Glinoer D. The regulation of thyroid function in pregnancy: pathways of endocrine adaptation from physiology to pathology. Endocr Rev. 1997;18(3):404–33.
5. Krassas GE, Poppe K, Glinoer D. Thyroid function and human reproductive health. Endocr Rev. 2010;31(5):702–55.
6. Roti E, Fang SL, Emerson CH, Braverman LE. Placental inner ring iodothyronine deiodination: a mechanism for decreased passage of T4 and T3 from mother to fetus. Trans Assoc Am Phys. 1981;94:183–9.
7. Delshad H, Azizi F. Iodine nutrition in pregnant and breastfeeding women: sufficiency, deficiency, and supplementation. Hormones (Athens). 2020;19(2):179–86.
8. Gude NM, Roberts CT, Kalionis B, King RG. Growth and function of the normal human placenta. Thromb Res. 2004;114(5–6):397–407.
9. Di Cosmo C, Fanelli G, Tonacchera M, Ferrarini E, Dimida A, Agretti P, et al. The sodium-iodide symporter expression in placental tissue at different gestational age: an immunohistochemical study. Clin Endocrinol. 2006;65(4):544–8.
10. Bizhanova A, Kopp P. Minireview: the sodium-iodide symporter NIS and pendrin in iodide homeostasis of the thyroid. Endocrinology. 2009;150(3):1084–90.
11. Zoeller RT, Rovet J. Timing of thyroid hormone action in the developing brain: clinical observations and experimental findings. J Neuroendocrinol. 2004;16(10):809–18.
12. Glinoer D. The regulation of thyroid function during normal pregnancy: importance of the iodine nutrition status. Best Pract Res Clin Endocrinol Metab. 2004;18(2):133–52.
13. Smyth PP. Variation in iodine handling during normal pregnancy. Thyroid. 1999;9(7):637–42.
14. Bath SC, Steer CD, Golding J, Emmett P, Rayman MP. Effect of inadequate iodine status in UK pregnant women on cognitive outcomes in their children: results from the Avon Longitudinal Study of Parents and Children (ALSPAC). Lancet. 2013;382(9889):331–7.
15. Pop VJ, Kuijpens JL, van Baar AL, Verkerk G, van Son MM, de Vijlder JJ, et al. Low maternal free thyroxine concentrations during early pregnancy are associated with impaired psychomotor development in infancy. Clin Endocrinol. 1999;50(2):149–55.
16. World Health Organization. Assessment of iodine deficiency disorders and monitoring their elimination: a guide for programme managers. 2019. whqlibdoc.who.int/publications/2007/9789241595827_eng.pdf. Accessed October 2021.
17. Institute of Medicine (US) Panel on Micronutrients. Dietary reference intakes for vitamin A, Vitamin K, arsenic, boron, chromium, copper, iodine, iron, manganese, molybdenum, nickel, silicon, vanadium, and zinc. Washington, DC: National Academy Press; 2001.
18. Chen W, Wu Y, Lin L, Tan L, Shen J, Pearce EN, et al. 24-hour urine samples are more reproducible than spot urine samples for evaluation of iodine status in school-age children. J Nutr. 2016;146(1):142–6.

19. Ma ZF, Skeaff SA. Thyroglobulin as a biomarker of iodine deficiency: a review. Thyroid. 2014;24(8):1195–209.
20. Moreno-Reyes R, Glinoer D, Van Oyen H, Vandevijvere S. High prevalence of thyroid disorders in pregnant women in a mildly iodine-deficient country: a population-based study. J Clin Endocrinol Metab. 2013;98(9):3694–701.
21. Zimmermann MB, Aeberli I, Andersson M, Assey V, Yorg JA, Jooste P, et al. Thyroglobulin is a sensitive measure of both deficient and excess iodine intakes in children and indicates no adverse effects on thyroid function in the UIC range of 100-299 μg/L: a UNICEF/ICCIDD study group report. J Clin Endocrinol Metab. 2013;98(3):1271–80.
22. Nazeri P, Shab-Bidar S, Pearce EN, Shariat M. Thyroglobulin concentration and maternal iodine status during pregnancy: a systematic review and meta-analysis. Thyroid. 2020;30(5):767–79.
23. Katko M, Gazso AA, Hircsu I, Bhattoa HP, Molnar Z, Kovacs B, et al. Thyroglobulin level at week 16 of pregnancy is superior to urinary iodine concentration in revealing preconceptual and first trimester iodine supply. Matern Child Nutr. 2018;14(1):e12470.
24. Shi X, Han C, Li C, Mao J, Wang W, Xie X, et al. Optimal and safe upper limits of iodine intake for early pregnancy in iodine-sufficient regions: a cross-sectional study of 7190 pregnant women in China. J Clin Endocrinol Metab. 2015;100(4):1630–8.
25. Stinca S, Andersson M, Weibel S, Herter-Aeberli I, Fingerhut R, Gowachirapant S, et al. Dried blood spot thyroglobulin as a biomarker of iodine status in pregnant women. J Clin Endocrinol Metab. 2017;102(1):23–32.
26. Zimmermann MB, Andersson M. Global endocrinology: global perspectives in endocrinology: coverage of iodized salt programs and iodine status in 2020. Eur J Endocrinol. 2021;185(1):R13–21.
27. Pearce EN, Andersson M, Zimmermann MB. Global iodine nutrition: where do we stand in 2013? Thyroid. 2013;23(5):523–8.
28. Caldwell KL, Pan Y, Mortensen ME, Makhmudov A, Merrill L, Moye J. Iodine status in pregnant women in the National Children's Study and in U.S. women (15-44 years), National Health and Nutrition Examination Survey 2005-2010. Thyroid. 2013;23(8):927–37.
29. Zimmermann MB, Gizak M, Abbott K, Andersson M, Lazarus JH. Iodine deficiency in pregnant women in Europe. Lancet Diabetes Endocrinol. 2015;3(9):672–4.
30. Zimmermann MB, Andersson M. Update on iodine status worldwide. Curr Opin Endocrinol Diabetes Obes. 2012;19(5):382–7.
31. Hetzel BS. Iodine deficiency disorders (IDD) and their eradication. Lancet. 1983;2(8359):1126–9.
32. Glinoer D. The importance of iodine nutrition during pregnancy. Public Health Nutr. 2007;10(12A):1542–6.
33. Haddow JE, Palomaki GE, Allan WC, Williams JR, Knight GJ, Gagnon J, et al. Maternal thyroid deficiency during pregnancy and subsequent neuropsychological development of the child. N Engl J Med. 1999;341(8):549–55.
34. Pearce EN. Iodine nutrition: recent research and unanswered questions. Eur J Clin Nutr. 2018;72(9):1226–8.
35. Morreale de Escobar G, Obregón MJ, Escobar del Rey F. Is neuropsychological development related to maternal hypothyroidism or to maternal hypothyroxinemia? J Clin Endocrinol Metab. 2000;85(11):3975–87.
36. Zimmermann MB, Boelaert K. Iodine deficiency and thyroid disorders. Lancet Diabetes Endocrinol. 2015;3(4):286–95.
37. Pharoah PO, Buttfield IH, Hetzel BS. The effect of iodine prophylaxis on the incidence of endemic cretinism. Adv Exp Med Biol. 1972;30:201–21.
38. Krämer M, Kupka R, Subramanian SV, Vollmer S. Association between household unavailability of iodized salt and child growth: evidence from 89 demographic and health surveys. Am J Clin Nutr. 2016;104(4):1093–100.
39. Bougma K, Aboud FE, Harding KB, Marquis GS. Iodine and mental development of children 5 years old and under: a systematic review and meta-analysis. Nutrients. 2013;5(4):1384–416.

40. Qian M, Wang D, Watkins WE, Gebski V, Yan YQ, Li M, et al. The effects of iodine on intelligence in children: a meta-analysis of studies conducted in China. Asia Pac J Clin Nutr. 2005;14(1):32–42.
41. Amouzegar A, Khazan M, Hedayati M, Azizi F. An assessment of the iodine status and the correlation between iodine nutrition and thyroid function during pregnancy in an iodine sufficient area. Eur J Clin Nutr. 2014;68(3):397–400.
42. Delshad H, Touhidi M, Abdollahi Z, Hedayati M, Salehi F, Azizi F. Inadequate iodine nutrition of pregnant women in an area of iodine sufficiency. J Endocrinol Invest. 2016;39(7):755–62.
43. León G, Murcia M, Rebagliato M, Álvarez-Pedrerol M, Castilla AM, Basterrechea M, et al. Maternal thyroid dysfunction during gestation, preterm delivery, and birthweight. The Infancia y Medio Ambiente Cohort, Spain. Paediatr Perinat Epidemiol. 2015;29(2):113–22.
44. Olivares JL, Olivi GI, Verdasco C, Ortiz VA, Mayer MA, Cresto JC. Low iodine intake during pregnancy: relationship to placental development and head circumference in newborn. Endocrinol Nutr. 2012;59(5):326–30.
45. Torlinska B, Bath SC, Janjua A, Boelaert K, Chan SY. Iodine status during pregnancy in a region of mild-to-moderate iodine deficiency is not associated with adverse obstetric outcomes; results from the Avon Longitudinal Study of Parents and Children (ALSPAC). Nutrients. 2018;10(3):291.
46. Nazeri P, Shab-Bidar S, Pearce EN, Shariat M. Do maternal urinary iodine concentration or thyroid hormones within the normal range during pregnancy affect growth parameters at birth? A systematic review and meta-analysis. Nutr Rev. 2020;78(9):747–63.
47. Hynes KL, Otahal P, Hay I, Burgess JR. Mild iodine deficiency during pregnancy is associated with reduced educational outcomes in the offspring: 9-year follow-up of the gestational iodine cohort. J Clin Endocrinol Metab. 2013;98(5):1954–62.
48. Abel MH, Ystrom E, Caspersen IH, Meltzer HM, Aase H, Torheim LE, et al. Maternal iodine intake and offspring attention-deficit/hyperactivity disorder: results from a large prospective cohort study. Nutrients. 2017;9(11):1239.
49. Andersson M, Aeberli I, Wüst N, Piacenza AM, Bucher T, Henschen I, et al. The Swiss iodized salt program provides adequate iodine for school children and pregnant women, but weaning infants not receiving iodine-containing complementary foods as well as their mothers are iodine deficient. J Clin Endocrinol Metab. 2010;95(12):5217–24.
50. Zhang H, Lv S, Mu Z, Li W, Zhang X, Wang Y, et al. Iodised salt contribution to iodine nutrition status of pregnant and lactating women. Br J Nutr. 2015;114(1):126–33.
51. Stagnaro-Green A, Abalovich M, Alexander E, Azizi F, Mestman J, Negro R, et al. Guidelines of the American Thyroid Association for the diagnosis and management of thyroid disease during pregnancy and postpartum. Thyroid. 2011;21(10):1081–125.
52. De Groot L, Abalovich M, Alexander EK, Amino N, Barbour L, Cobin RH, et al. Management of thyroid dysfunction during pregnancy and postpartum: an Endocrine Society clinical practice guideline. J Clin Endocrinol Metab. 2012;97(8):2543–65.
53. Leung AM, Pearce EN, Braverman LE, Stagnaro-Green A. AAP recommendations on iodine nutrition during pregnancy and lactation. Pediatrics. 2014;134(4):e1282.
54. Chittimoju SB, Pearce EN. Iodine deficiency and supplementation in pregnancy. Clin Obstet Gynecol. 2019;62(2):330–8.
55. Taylor PN, Okosieme OE, Dayan CM, Lazarus JH. Therapy of endocrine disease: impact of iodine supplementation in mild-to-moderate iodine deficiency: systematic review and meta-analysis. Eur J Endocrinol. 2014;170(1):R1–R15.
56. Taylor PN, Vaidya B. Iodine supplementation in pregnancy—is it time? Clin Endocrinol. 2016;85(1):10–4.
57. Santiago P, Velasco I, Muela JA, Sánchez B, Martínez J, Rodriguez A, et al. Infant neurocognitive development is independent of the use of iodised salt or iodine supplements given during pregnancy. Br J Nutr. 2013;110(5):831–9.

58. Hynes KL, Seal JA, Otahal P, Oddy WH, Burgess JR. Women remain at risk of iodine deficiency during pregnancy: the importance of iodine supplementation before conception and throughout gestation. Nutrients. 2019;11(1):172.
59. Delshad H, Raeisi A, Abdollahi Z, Tohidi M, Hedayati M, Mirmiran P, et al. Iodine supplementation for pregnant women: a cross-sectional national interventional study. J Endocrinol Invest. 2021;44(10):2307–14.
60. Dineva M, Fishpool H, Rayman MP, Mendis J, Bath SC. Systematic review and meta-analysis of the effects of iodine supplementation on thyroid function and child neurodevelopment in mildly-to-moderately iodine-deficient pregnant women. Am J Clin Nutr. 2020;112(2):389–412.
61. Nazeri P, Shariat M, Azizi F. Effects of iodine supplementation during pregnancy on pregnant women and their offspring: a systematic review and meta-analysis of trials over the past 3 decades. Eur J Endocrinol. 2021;184(1):91–106.
62. Censi S, Watutantrige-Fernando S, Groccia G, Manso J, Plebani M, Faggian D, et al. The effects of iodine supplementation in pregnancy on iodine status, thyroglobulin levels and thyroid function parameters: results from a randomized controlled clinical trial in a mild-to-moderate iodine deficiency area. Nutrients. 2019;11(11):2639.
63. Glinoer D, De Nayer P, Delange F, Lemone M, Toppet V, Spehl M, et al. A randomized trial for the treatment of mild iodine deficiency during pregnancy: maternal and neonatal effects. J Clin Endocrinol Metab. 1995;80(1):258–69.
64. Gowachirapant S, Jaiswal N, Melse-Boonstra A, Galetti V, Stinca S, Mackenzie I, et al. Effect of iodine supplementation in pregnant women on child neurodevelopment: a randomised, double-blind, placebo-controlled trial. Lancet Diabetes Endocrinol. 2017;5(11):853–63.
65. Hiéronimus S, Ferrari P, Gal J, Berthier F, Azoulay S, Bongain A, et al. Relative impact of iodine supplementation and maternal smoking on cord blood thyroglobulin in pregnant women with normal thyroid function. Eur Thyroid J. 2013;1(4):264–73.
66. Nøhr SB, Jørgensen A, Pedersen KM, Laurberg P. Postpartum thyroid dysfunction in pregnant thyroid peroxidase antibody-positive women living in an area with mild to moderate iodine deficiency: is iodine supplementation safe? J Clin Endocrinol Metab. 2000;85(9):3191–8.
67. Pedersen KM, Laurberg P, Iversen E, Knudsen PR, Gregersen HE, Rasmussen OS, et al. Amelioration of some pregnancy-associated variations in thyroid function by iodine supplementation. J Clin Endocrinol Metab. 1993;77(4):1078–83.
68. Harding KB, Peña-Rosas JP, Webster AC, Yap CM, Payne BA, Ota E, et al. Iodine supplementation for women during the preconception, pregnancy and postpartum period. Cochrane Database Syst Rev. 2017;3(3):CD011761.
69. Farebrother J, Naude CE, Nicol L, Sang Z, Yang Z, Jooste PL, et al. Effects of iodized salt and iodine supplements on prenatal and postnatal growth: a systematic review. Adv Nutr. 2018;9(3):219–37.
70. Velasco I, Carreira M, Santiago P, Muela JA, García-Fuentes E, Sánchez-Muñoz B, et al. Effect of iodine prophylaxis during pregnancy on neurocognitive development of children during the first two years of life. J Clin Endocrinol Metab. 2009;94(9):3234–41.
71. Levie D, Korevaar TIM, Bath SC, Murcia M, Dineva M, Llop S, et al. Association of maternal iodine status with child IQ: a meta-analysis of individual participant data. J Clin Endocrinol Metab. 2019;104(12):5957–67.
72. Barikmo I, Henjum S, Dahl L, Oshaug A, Torheim LE. Environmental implication of iodine in water, milk and other foods used in Saharawi refugees camps in Tindouf, Algeria. J Food Compos Anal. 2011;24(4–5):637–41.
73. Kassim IA, Moloney G, Busili A, Nur AY, Paron P, Jooste P, et al. Iodine intake in Somalia is excessive and associated with the source of household drinking water. J Nutr. 2014;144(3):375–81.
74. Watts M, O'Reilly J, Maricelli A, Coleman A, Ander E, Ward N. A snapshot of environmental iodine and selenium in La Pampa and San Juan provinces of Argentina. J Geochem Explor. 2010;107(2):87–93.

75. Wolff J, Chaikoff IL, et al. The temporary nature of the inhibitory action of excess iodine on organic iodine synthesis in the normal thyroid. Endocrinology. 1949;45(5):504–13, illust.
76. Markou K, Georgopoulos N, Kyriazopoulou V, Vagenakis AG. Iodine-induced hypothyroidism. Thyroid. 2001;11(5):501–10.
77. Katagiri R, Yuan X, Kobayashi S, Sasaki S. Effect of excess iodine intake on thyroid diseases in different populations: a systematic review and meta-analyses including observational studies. PLoS One. 2017;12(3):e0173722.
78. Lee SY, Pearce EN. Reproductive endocrinology: iodine intake in pregnancy—even a little excess is too much. Nat Rev Endocrinol. 2015;11(5):260–1.
79. Leung AM, Braverman LE. Consequences of excess iodine. Nat Rev Endocrinol. 2014;10(3):136–42.
80. Pearce EN, Lazarus JH, Moreno-Reyes R, Zimmermann MB. Consequences of iodine deficiency and excess in pregnant women: an overview of current knowns and unknowns. Am J Clin Nutr. 2016;104 Suppl 3(Suppl 3):918S–23S.
81. Bartalena L, Bogazzi F, Braverman LE, Martino E. Effects of amiodarone administration during pregnancy on neonatal thyroid function and subsequent neurodevelopment. J Endocrinol Invest. 2001;24(2):116–30.
82. Connelly KJ, Boston BA, Pearce EN, Sesser D, Snyder D, Braverman LE, et al. Congenital hypothyroidism caused by excess prenatal maternal iodine ingestion. J Pediatr. 2012;161(4):760–2.
83. Murcia M, Rebagliato M, Iñiguez C, Lopez-Espinosa MJ, Estarlich M, Plaza B, et al. Effect of iodine supplementation during pregnancy on infant neurodevelopment at 1 year of age. Am J Epidemiol. 2011;173(7):804–12.
84. Rebagliato M, Murcia M, Alvarez-Pedrerol M, Espada M, Fernández-Somoano A, Lertxundi N, et al. Iodine supplementation during pregnancy and infant neuropsychological development. INMA Mother and Child Cohort Study. Am J Epidemiol. 2013;177(9):944–53.
85. Farebrother J, Zimmermann MB, Abdallah F, Assey V, Fingerhut R, Gichohi-Wainaina WN, et al. Effect of excess iodine intake from iodized salt and/or groundwater iodine on thyroid function in nonpregnant and pregnant women, infants, and children: a multicenter study in East Africa. Thyroid. 2018;28(9):1198–210.
86. Korevaar TI, Schalekamp-Timmermans S, de Rijke YB, Visser WE, Visser W, de Muinck Keizer-Schrama SM, et al. Hypothyroxinemia and TPO-antibody positivity are risk factors for premature delivery: the Generation R study. J Clin Endocrinol Metab. 2013;98(11):4382–90.
87. Henrichs J, Bongers-Schokking JJ, Schenk JJ, Ghassabian A, Schmidt HG, Visser TJ, et al. Maternal thyroid function during early pregnancy and cognitive functioning in early childhood: the Generation R study. J Clin Endocrinol Metab. 2010;95(9):4227–34.
88. Lavado-Autric R, Ausó E, García-Velasco JV, Arufe Mdel C, Escobar del Rey F, Berbel P, et al. Early maternal hypothyroxinemia alters histogenesis and cerebral cortex cytoarchitecture of the progeny. J Clin Invest. 2003;111(7):1073–82.
89. Yu X, Shan Z, Li C, Mao J, Wang W, Xie X, et al. Iron deficiency, an independent risk factor for isolated hypothyroxinemia in pregnant and nonpregnant women of childbearing age in China. J Clin Endocrinol Metab. 2015;100(4):1594–601.
90. Zhou SJ, Skeaff SA, Ryan P, Doyle LW, Anderson PJ, Kornman L, et al. The effect of iodine supplementation in pregnancy on early childhood neurodevelopment and clinical outcomes: results of an aborted randomised placebo-controlled trial. Trials. 2015;16:563.

Iodine Requirements in Pregnancy

Jennifer B. Plotkin and Angela M. Leung

Introduction

Adequate levels of iodine, a trace element variably distributed on the earth and found mostly in the soil and water of coastal areas, are required for the synthesis of the thyroid hormones that play key roles in various metabolic processes at tissues. The major concerns regarding the global burden of iodine deficiency are related to hypothyroidism resulting in adverse impacts on growth, the development of goiter, neurocognitive impairments, and in severe deficiency, cretinism [1].

Sources of Iodine

Iodine is a trace element that is found in the upper crust of the earth's surface. As a result of the atmospheric cycle, the iodine content of soils is diminished by exposure to rain, snow, and glaciation, which leach out the mineral and deposit it in the oceans, where most of the iodine on earth is found. Iodide ions in seawater are oxidized to form elemental iodine, which is volatile, evaporates into the atmosphere, from which iodine again returns to the soil through rainwater.

The diet is the primary method of achieving adequate iodine nutrition, with dairy products, some breads, seaweed and other seafood, and iodized salt as the most

J. B. Plotkin
Department of Medicine, University of California Los Angeles David Geffen School of Medicine, Los Angeles, CA, USA

A. M. Leung (✉)
Division of Endocrinology, Diabetes, and Metabolism, Department of Medicine, University of California Los Angeles David Geffen School of Medicine, VA Greater Los Angeles Healthcare System, Los Angeles, CA, USA
e-mail: AMLeung@mednet.ucla.edu

F. Azizi, F. Ramezani Tehrani (eds.), *Thyroid Diseases in Pregnancy*,
https://doi.org/10.1007/978-3-030-98777-0_3

common iodine-containing foods [2]. As table salt is easily found and consumed in virtually every country in the world, it represents an effective, inexpensive, and stable method for ensuring population-level access to adequate iodine nutrition [3]. Iodine-containing disinfectants used for cleaning milk cans and teats can additionally increase the iodine content of dairy products [4, 5]. Additional sources of iodine are breads and grain products made with iodine-containing dough oxidizers and iodine-containing conditioners, the latter of which are added to maintain freshness and prolong the shelf life of bread [5].

However, possible reductions in the iodine content of dairy products due to the removal of iodate conditioners in store-bought breads, recommendations for reducing salt intake toward improved blood pressure control, and the increase in dietary use of non-iodinated salts in processed and pre-packaged foods have been described as possible causes to the decrease in iodine intake in the USA in recent years [4]. Although substantial progress has been made over the past several decades by coordinated global public health efforts [6, 7], inadequate iodine nutrition remains one of the most important micronutrient deficiencies globally and is associated with substantial economic implications and increased healthcare costs [3, 8].

Furthermore, decreased thyroid hormone production can result not only from insufficient dietary iodine, but also from the ingestion of goitrogens which can interfere with thyroid hormone synthesis. Glucosinolates as goitrogens are found as a natural component of some foods commonly ingested in many parts of the world. Examples of goitrogenic cruciferous vegetables include cabbage, kale, cauliflower, broccoli, rutabaga, turnips, Brussels sprouts, and mustard greens [9].

Role of Iodine

The main function of iodine is the synthesis of the thyroid hormones, thyroxine (T4) and triiodothyronine (T3). The thyroid hormones have multiple effects on metabolism and are associated with direct or indirect effects on many systems and organs. The adult human body normally contains 15–20 mg of iodine, of which approximately 75% is found in the thyroid gland.

It is well established that following ingestion, dietary iodine is efficiently absorbed along the length of the gastrointestinal tract [10]. Circulating iodine is actively transported into the thyroid gland via the transmembrane sodium/iodide symporter (NIS). Under conditions of iodine sufficiency, iodine is concentrated into the thyroid gland at 20–50 times that of plasma; this gradient increases in situations of iodine deficiency [11]. The kidneys do not have a mechanism to conserve iodide, and thus represents the major route (over 90%) of iodide excretion [12]. Thus, urinary iodine levels are proportional to its plasma concentration and can be used as a convenient index of population-level iodine status [13]. Small amounts of iodine are also excreted from the body via feces and sweat [14].

Iodine Physiology During Pregnancy and Lactation

Thyroid hormone plays a particularly vital role in fetal and infant neurodevelopment in utero and in early life [15]. Beginning in early gestation, maternal thyroid hormone production normally increases by ~50% in response to increased levels of serum thyroxine binding globulin (resulting from the rise of estrogen levels) and due to stimulation of thyrotropin receptors by human chorionic gonadotropin [16]. The placenta is a rich source of the type 3 inner ring deiodinase, which enhances the degradation of T4 to bioinactive reverse T3 [17]. Additionally, although iodide readily crosses the placenta, fetal thyroid hormone production increases during the second half of pregnancy, further contributing to increased maternal iodine requirements [16]. Because of these alterations in iodine and thyroid physiology, dietary iodine requirements are higher among pregnant women than for nonpregnant adults [18, 19].

Adequate iodine status is also important for normal development in infants. During lactation, iodine is secreted into breastmilk at a concentration gradient 20–50 times that of plasma [20] through increased expression of NIS present on lactating breast cells [21], but thyroidal iodine turnover is also more rapid in early development than at any other age [22]. Studies have shown that breastmilk iodine concentration levels widely variable across populations are generally higher in colostrum and decrease gradually through later lactation periods, and that a breastmilk iodine concentration of approximately 150 mcg/L during the first 6 months of lactation are sufficient to prevent adverse consequences of iodine insufficiency [23]. As breastfed infants are reliant on maternal dietary iodine intake, recommendations for dietary iodine intake during lactation are also higher than in nonpregnant and non-lactating women [13]. However, supplementation may not be necessary in countries with effective salt iodization programs; one study of mother-infant pairs in Iran, a region with a sustained salt iodization program in place, revealed that all infants studied were iodine sufficient regardless of maternal iodine supplementation or whether infants were breast- or formula-fed, although this finding may not be universal [19, 24].

Studies of Iodine Status in Pregnancy

Due to substantial day-to-day variation of iodine intake, biological measurements of iodine status among individual persons are unreliable. This has resulted in the need to adopt a public health approach toward achieving iodine sufficiency across populations. Currently available and validated measures of iodine sufficiency in a population include median urinary iodine concentrations, the proportion of elevated serum thyroid stimulating hormone (TSH) concentrations among newborns and school-age children, the proportion of elevated serum thyroglobulin concentrations, and the prevalence of goiter [13].

Median urinary iodine concentrations have been widely used in the assessment of iodine status during pregnancy and lactation. Adequate iodine nutrition is represented by median urinary iodine concentrations of 150–249 mcg/L in pregnancy, higher than the range in lactation and in nonpregnant populations (100–199 mcg/L) [13]. The biomarkers denoting severe iodine deficiency in pregnancy have not been well-defined, but using the same thresholds median urinary iodine concentration thresholds as for nonpregnant individuals, available literature shows that very low iodine status is associated with irreversible adverse obstetric and offspring effects [25].

Universal salt iodization in most countries has improved inadequate iodine status among many groups, particularly over the past 2–3 decades [3]. However, despite this, studies assessing population-level iodine status show that iodine deficiency remains one of the most important public health issues globally, particularly among women of childbearing age, in certain regions [26]. In the USA, data from large population studies have shown that median urinary iodine levels decreased by approximately 50% between the early 1970s and the early 1990s, although the population overall has remained iodine sufficient [27]. Subsequent studies have shown that although this decrease has stabilized [28–30], some subsets of the population, such as women of childbearing age, may be at risk for mild to moderate iodine deficiency [31]. A systematic review of lactating mothers demonstrated that iodine deficiency was common worldwide, occurring in nearly all lactating mothers in countries with voluntary universal salt iodization and even in most women residing in countries with mandatory iodine fortification [32]. A nationwide Portuguese study of 3631 women showed that only 16.8% of pregnant women have sufficient urinary iodine levels [33], highlighting this continued global public health issue. A recent study in Iran, however, showed that if iodine supplementation of at least 150 mcg per day is taken throughout pregnancy, adequate median urinary iodine levels are achievable [34].

Studies Assessing the Effects of Maternal Iodine Status in Pregnancy

Insufficient iodine during pregnancy and the immediate post-partum period has been shown to be associated with neurological and psychological deficits in children [35], although the data are mixed. The prevalence of attention deficit and hyperactivity disorders (ADHD) is higher in the offspring of women living in iodine-deficient areas than in iodine-replete regions [36]. In Spain, a region of mild iodine deficiency, children with urinary iodine levels >100 mcg/L have significantly higher IQ levels than those with urinary iodine levels below this threshold [37]. Newer studies have followed children of iodine-insufficient mothers longitudinally. A study of over 30,000 mother-child pairs in Norway demonstrated language delay, behavior problems, and fine motor skill deficits in the 3-year-old children born to iodine-insufficient mothers, findings from which up to 5–16% may be potentially attributable to iodine deficiency [38]. Another study from Tasmania with 9-year follow-up showed long-term reductions in spelling among children born to mothers residing in a mildly iodine-deficient region, even when adjusted for biologic and socioeconomic factors [39]. In contrast, a Dutch birth cohort study found no relationship between maternal urinary iodine levels during early pregnancy and children's language comprehension at 6 years when controlled for confounders, a finding that may reflect the addition of iodinated salt to most processed foods in the Netherlands [40].

Prospective Studies of Maternal Iodine Supplementation in Pregnancy

The benefits of iodine supplementation may relate to the timing and severity of iodine deficiency during pregnancy. The most critical period is the first trimester of pregnancy, when a lack of maternal thyroid hormones during this critical window of fetal brain development may have irreversible consequences. Furthermore, data suggests that starting iodine supplementation prior to pregnancy is optimal; mothers who start 150 mcg of daily iodine supplementation before conception have higher median urinary iodine concentrations than those who start after pregnancy confirmation [41].

One of the earliest studies was a randomized controlled trial during the early 1970s from Papua New Guinea, in which severely iodine-deficient pregnant women who were administered injections of an iodinated poppy seed oil had decreased rates of fetal death and endemic cretinism, compared to untreated women [42]. There have since been additional longitudinal studies demonstrating favorable maternal and offspring thyroidal effects of iodine supplementation during pregnancy. In Italy, 18 iodine-untreated women had larger thyroid volumes than 17 women who received 120–180 mcg/day of iodine beginning during the first trimester [43]. Investigators in Denmark reported that iodine-supplemented women have decreased serum maternal TSH levels and increased cord blood TSH levels, compared to women who received no iodine supplementation [44]. In Belgium, infants of mothers who received iodine supplementation during pregnancy had decreased thyroid volumes [45]. In contrast, Antonangeli and colleagues reported that there were no differences in maternal serum thyroid function or thyroid gland size among 86 iodine-supplemented and unsupplemented women [46]. In a mildly iodine-deficient area of Italy, consumption of iodized salt in the 24 months preceding pregnancy, as compared to iodized salt ingestion upon becoming pregnant, decreased the risk of maternal thyroid dysfunction in women with negative serum thyroid autoantibody titers [47]. A recent study in Iranian pregnant women similarly found that 150 mcg of daily iodine supplementation decreased the prevalence of thyroid dysfunction in this group [34].

Insufficient iodine during pregnancy and the immediate post-partum period is thought to result in neurological and psychological deficits in children [22, 23], although the data are mixed. The prevalence of attention deficit and hyperactivity disorders (ADHD) is higher in the offspring of women living in iodine-deficient areas than in iodine-replete regions [36]. In Spain, a region of mild iodine deficiency, children with urinary iodine levels >100 mcg/L have significantly higher IQ levels than those with urinary iodine levels below this threshold [37].

Prospective studies of maternal iodine supplementation during pregnancy assessing neurocognitive outcomes in their offspring are summarized in Table 1 [48–56]. Berbel et al. reported that children of mildly hypothyroxinemic women from a mildly iodine-deficient region who were supplemented with 200 mcg potassium iodide/day beginning at 12–14 gestational weeks had delayed neurocognitive performance at 18 months of age, compared to children of women who received supplementation at 4–6 gestational weeks [48], strongly suggesting that adequate iodine intake during the first few weeks of gestation is essential. Similarly, Velasco and colleagues found that infants aged 3–18 months of mildly iodine-deficient mothers who received 300 mcg potassium iodide/day during the first trimester had higher neuropsychological assessment scores than those of mothers who received no iodine supplementation [49]. A randomized controlled trial conducted in Spain examining iodinized table salt use and two dosages of potassium iodide supplementation in pregnant women reported no differences in infants' neurocognitive development between the three groups, suggesting that the type of iodine supplementation may not be a crucial factor for these outcomes [56]. In contrast, a randomized, placebo-controlled, double-blinded trial of 832 women enrolled at a mean of 10.7 ± 2.7 (SD) gestational weeks in India and Thailand, 200 mcg daily iodine supplementation had no effect on childhood neurocognitive development at 5–6 years [51].

However, iodine supplementation does not ensure iodine sufficiency. A pilot study in the Netherlands measured urinary iodine levels at 20 and 36 gestational weeks and 4 weeks post-partum in women supplemented with 150 mcg of iodine daily starting at 20 weeks gestation [57]. Despite supplementation, substantial proportions of women (83%, 56%, and 40%, respectively) remained with suboptimal recommended iodine levels [57]. In another study, a representative sample of Belgian women was used to assess urinary iodine concentrations in pregnant women. Despite about 60% of women taking iodine supplements in pregnancy, 59.3% had with urinary iodine concentrations below 150 mcg/L and 37.8% below 100 mcg/L [58]. Further research is needed to better understand the risks and benefits of maternal iodine supplementation, particularly among mild to moderately iodine-deficient pregnant women [59].

Table 1 Prospective studies of maternal iodine supplementation in pregnancy assessing offspring neurocognition

Authors	Date	Study design	Country	*N*	Groups	Timing of iodine supplementation	Major findings
Berbel et al.	2009	Prospective cohort	Spain	345	200 mcg oral KI daily	Beginning at the first pregnancy visit	Delaying iodine supplementation by 6–10 weeks in hypothyroxinemic women increases the risk of neurodevelopmental delays in their offspring
Velasco et al.	2009	Prospective cohort	Spain	174	300 mcg oral KI daily versus no KI supplementation	First trimester	Higher neuropsychological assessment scores in offspring
Murcia et al.	2011	Prospective cohort	Spain	691	Mean estimated dietary iodine; and supplemental iodine intake classified as <100, 100–149, and ≥150 mcg/day	Enrolled at first prenatal visit	Maternal iodine intake ≥150 mcg/day, compared to <100 mcg/day, was associated with a 5.2 point decrease in Psychomotor Development Index at age 1 year
Rebagliato et al.	2013	Prospective cohort	Spain	1519	Mean estimated dietary iodine; and supplemental iodine intake classified as <100, 100–149, and ≥150 mcg/day	Enrolled at first prenatal visit	Maternal iodized salt intake and supplemental iodine use not associated with infant neuropsychological development at age 1 year
Santiago et al.	2013	Randomized prospective trial	Spain	131	Iodized salt use at least 1 year preconception, 200 mcg KI/day, versus 300 mcg/KI/day	Before 10 weeks gestation	No differences in neuropsychological tests at age 6–18 months

(continued)

Table 1 (continued)

Authors	Date	Study design	Country	*N*	Groups	Timing of iodine supplementation	Major findings
Brucker-Davis et al.	2015	Prospective cohort	France	44	Vitamins containing 150 mcg daily iodine versus vitamins without iodine	Before 12 weeks gestation	No significant differences in Bayley Infant and Toddler Development tests at age 2 years
Zhou et al.	2015	Randomized controlled trial	Australia	59	Placebo versus 150 mcg iodine daily	Before 20 weeks gestation	Trial aborted early due to funding termination
Gowachirapant et al.	2017	Randomized controlled trial	Thailand and India	832	Placebo versus 200 mcg oral iodine daily	At or before 14 weeks gestation	No significant differences at age 5–6 years
Verhagen et al.	2020	Randomized controlled trial examining only Thai subset of ***	Thailand	514	Placebo versus 200 mcg oral iodine daily	Before 14 weeks gestation	No significant differences at age 5.7 years

KI potassium iodide

Recommendations for Iodine Nutrition in Pregnancy and Lactation

The World Health Organization, United Nations Children's Fund (UNICEF), and the International Council for the Control of Iodine Deficiency Disorders (ICCIDD) [since renamed as the Iodine Global Network] recommend a daily iodine intake of 250 mcg for pregnant women and 150 mcg for lactating women [13]. In the USA, a Recommended Dietary Allowance (RDA) of 150 mcg/day iodine intake is recommended in nonpregnant, non-lactating adults, while pregnant women are advised 220 mcg/day and lactating women 290 mcg/day [18].

To achieve adequate iodine intake, guidelines by the American Thyroid Association (ATA), Endocrine Society, the American Pediatric Society, and the Neurobehavioral Teratology Society recommend that all women take a supplement containing 150 mcg iodine daily during preconception, pregnancy, and lactation [60–63]. However, data from the National Health and Nutrition Examination Survey (2001–2006) demonstrated that only 20.3% of US pregnant women routinely take an iodine-containing supplement [64]. Of the prenatal multivitamin formulations available in the USA, only approximately 60% list iodine (containing varying amounts), and measured levels can be discordant from labeled values [65, 66].

Finally, it is also important to recognize that excessive iodine exposure has the potential to also result in iodine-induced thyroid dysfunction [67]. Excess iodine exposure can result from iodine oversupplementation, the overconsumption of foods naturally high in iodine, and the use of iodine in some medical settings, such as iodine-containing antiseptics [68] and iodinated contrast media for radiologic imaging studies [69]. Additionally, saturated solution of potassium iodine may be indicated for the treatment of severe hyperthyroidism. The World Health Organization has proposed that an iodine intake of 500 mcg/day likely poses no excessive risk [13]. The European Food Safety Agency and the U.S. Institute of Medicine has recommended 600 mcg/day and 1100 mcg/day, respectively, as the Tolerable Upper Limit for iodine per day [18, 70], defined as the highest level of daily nutrient intake that is likely to pose no risk of adverse health effects in almost all individuals.

Conclusion

Adequate iodine intake is required for the synthesis of thyroid hormones that are important for normal fetal and infant neurodevelopment. In this review, we have discussed iodine physiology during pregnancy and lactation, the importance of adequate iodine nutrition in women of reproductive age, methods to assess population iodine sufficiency, and studies of iodine status and supplementation during pregnancy.

References

1. Vanderpump MP. Epidemiology of iodine deficiency. Minerva Med. 2017;108(2):116–23.
2. Knust K, Leung A. Iodine: basic nutritional aspects. In: Molecular, genetic, and nutritional aspects of major and trace minerals. Elsevier; 2017. p. 133–141.
3. Gorstein JL, Bagriansky J, Pearce EN, Kupka R, Zimmermann MB. Estimating the health and economic benefits of universal salt iodization programs to correct iodine deficiency disorders. Thyroid. 2020;30(12):1802–9.
4. Pearce EN, Pino S, He X, Bazrafshan HR, Lee SL, Braverman LE. Sources of dietary iodine: bread, cows' milk, and infant formula in the Boston area. J Clin Endocrinol Metab. 2004;89(7):3421.
5. Leung AM, Braverman LE, Pearce EN. History of U.S. iodine fortification and supplementation. Nutrients. 2012;4(11):1740.
6. Lazarus JH. Role of the iodine global network in elimination of iodine deficiency. Recent Pat Endocr Metab Immune Drug Discov. 2017;10(2):119–22.
7. Karwowska P, Breda J. The role of the World Health Organization in eliminating iodine deficiency worldwide. Recent Pat Endocr Metab Immune Drug Discov. 2017;10(2):138–42.
8. Rochau U, Qerimi Rushaj V, Schaffner M, Schönhensch M, Stojkov I, Jahn B, et al. Decision-analytic modeling studies in prevention and treatment of iodine deficiency and thyroid disorders: a systematic overview. Thyroid. 2020;30(5):746–58.
9. Felker P, Bunch R, Leung AM. Concentrations of thiocyanate and goitrin in human plasma, their precursor concentrations in brassica vegetables, and associated potential risk for hypothyroidism. Nutr Rev. 2016;74(4):248–58.
10. Nelson N, Palmes ED, Park CR, Weymouth PP, Bean WB. The absorption, excretion, and physiological effect of iodine in normal human subjects. J Clin Invest. 1947;26(2):301–10.
11. Zimmermann MB, Jooste PL, Pandav CS. Iodine-deficiency disorders. Lancet. 2008;372(9645):1251.
12. Johner SA, Shi L, Remer T. Higher urine volume results in additional renal iodine loss. Thyroid. 2010;20(12)
13. World Health Organization, United Nations International Children's Emergency Fund, and International Council for the Control of Iodine Deficiency Disorders. Assessment of the iodine deficiency disorders and monitoring their elimination. Geneva: World Health Organization; 2007. Report No.: WHO/NHD/01.1.
14. Oddie TH, Fisher DA, Long JM. Factors affecting the estimation of iodine entering the normal thyroid gland using short-term clearance studies. J Clin Endocrinol Metab. 1964;24:924–33.
15. Bernal J. Thyroid hormone receptors in brain development and function. Nat Clin Pract Endocrinol Metab. 2007;3(3):249–59.
16. Glinoer D. The importance of iodine nutrition during pregnancy. Public Health Nutr. 2007;10(12A):1542.
17. Roti E, Fang SL, Emerson CH, Braverman LE. Placental inner ring iodothyronine deiodination: a mechanism for decreased passage of T4 and T3 from mother to fetus. Trans Assoc Am Phys. 1981;94:183.
18. Food and Nutrition Board IoM. Dietary reference intakes. Washington, DC: National Academy Press; 2006. 320 p.
19. Delshad H, Azizi F. Iodine nutrition in pregnant and breastfeeding women: sufficiency, deficiency, and supplementation. Hormones (Athens). 2020;19(2):179–86.
20. Eskandari S, Loo DD, Dai G, Levy O, Wright EM, Carrasco N. Thyroid Na+/I− symporter. Mechanism, stoichiometry, and specificity. J Biol Chem. 1997;272(43):27230.
21. Tazebay UH, Wapnir IL, Levy O, Dohan O, Zuckier LS, Zhao QH, et al. The mammary gland iodide transporter is expressed during lactation and in breast cancer. Nat Med. 2000;6(8):871.
22. Stinca S, Andersson M, Herter-Aeberli I, Chabaa L, Cherkaoui M, El Ansari N, et al. Moderate-to-severe iodine deficiency in the "first 1000 days" causes more thyroid hypofunction in infants than in pregnant or lactating women. J Nutr. 2017;147(4):589–95.

23. Dror DK, Allen LH. Iodine in human milk: a systematic review. Adv Nutr. 2018;9(suppl_1):347S–57S.
24. Nazeri P, Tahmasebinejad Z, Mehrabi Y, Hedayati M, Mirmiran P, Azizi F. Lactating mothers and infants residing in an area with an effective salt iodization program have no need for iodine supplements: results from a double-blind, placebo-controlled, randomized controlled trial. Thyroid. 2018;28(11):1547–58.
25. Toloza FJK, Motahari H, Maraka S. Consequences of severe iodine deficiency in pregnancy: evidence in humans. Front Endocrinol (Lausanne). 2020;11:409.
26. Candido AC, Azevedo FM, Machamba AAL, Pinto CA, Lopes SO, Macedo MS, et al. Implications of iodine deficiency by gestational trimester: a systematic review. Arch Endocrinol Metab. 2021;64(5):507–13.
27. Hollowell JG, Staehling NW, Hannon WH, Flanders DW, Gunter EW, Maberly GF, et al. Iodine nutrition in the United States. Trends and public health implications: iodine excretion data from National Health and Nutrition Examination Surveys I and III (1971–1974 and 1988–1994). J Clin Endocrinol Metab. 1998;83(10):3401.
28. Caldwell KL, Makhmudov A, Ely E, Jones RL, Wang RY. Iodine status of the U.S. population, National Health and Nutrition Examination Survey, 2005–2006 and 2007–2008. Thyroid. 2011;21(4):427.
29. Caldwell KL, Miller GA, Wang RY, Jain RB, Jones RL. Iodine status of the U.S. population, National Health and Nutrition Examination Survey 2003–2004. Thyroid. 2008;18(11):1207.
30. Caldwell KL, Jones R, Hollowell JG. Urinary iodine concentration: United States National Health and Nutrition Examination Survey 2001-2002. Thyroid. 2005;15(7):692.
31. Panth P, Guerin G, DiMarco NM. A review of iodine status of women of reproductive age in the USA. Biol Trace Elem Res. 2019;188(1):208–20.
32. Nazeri P, Mirmiran P, Shiva N, Mehrabi Y, Mojarrad M, Azizi F. Iodine nutrition status in lactating mothers residing in countries with mandatory and voluntary iodine fortification programs: an updated systematic review. Thyroid. 2015;25(6):611–20.
33. Limbert E, Prazeres S, São Pedro M, Madureira D, Miranda A, Ribeiro M, et al. Iodine intake in Portuguese pregnant women: results of a countrywide study. Eur J Endocrinol. 2010;163(4):631–5.
34. Delshad H, Raeisi A, Abdollahi Z, Tohidi M, Hedayati M, Mirmiran P, et al. Iodine supplementation for pregnant women: a cross-sectional national interventional study. J Endocrinol Invest. 2021;44(10):2307–14.
35. Qian M, Wang D, Watkins WE, Gebski V, Yan YQ, Li M, et al. The effects of iodine on intelligence in children: a meta-analysis of studies conducted in China. Asia Pac J Clin Nutr. 2005;14(1):32.
36. Vermiglio F, Lo Presti VP, Moleti M, Sidoti M, Tortorella G, Scaffidi G, et al. Attention deficit and hyperactivity disorders in the offspring of mothers exposed to mild-moderate iodine deficiency: a possible novel iodine deficiency disorder in developed countries. J Clin Endocrinol Metab. 2004;89(12):6054.
37. Santiago-Fernandez P, Torres-Barahona R, Muela-Martinez JA, Rojo-Martinez G, Garcia-Fuentes E, Garriga MJ, et al. Intelligence quotient and iodine intake: a cross-sectional study in children. J Clin Endocrinol Metab. 2004;89(8):3851.
38. Abel MH, Caspersen IH, Meltzer HM, Haugen M, Brandlistuen RE, Aase H, et al. Suboptimal maternal iodine intake is associated with impaired child neurodevelopment at 3 years of age in the Norwegian mother and child cohort study. J Nutr. 2017;147(7):1314–24.
39. Hynes KL, Otahal P, Hay I, Burgess JR. Mild iodine deficiency during pregnancy is associated with reduced educational outcomes in the offspring: 9-year follow-up of the gestational iodine cohort. J Clin Endocrinol Metab. 2013;98(5):1954.
40. Ghassabian A, Steenweg-de Graaff J, Peeters RP, Ross HA, Jaddoe VW, Hofman A, et al. Maternal urinary iodine concentration in pregnancy and children's cognition: results from a population-based birth cohort in an iodine-sufficient area. BMJ Open. 2014;4(6):e005520.

41. Hynes KL, Seal JA, Otahal P, Oddy WH, Burgess JR. Women remain at risk of iodine deficiency during pregnancy: the importance of iodine supplementation before conception and throughout gestation. Nutrients. 2019;11(1):172.
42. Pharoah PO, Buttfield IH, Hetzel BS. Neurological damage to the fetus resulting from severe iodine deficiency during pregnancy. Lancet. 1971;1(7694):308.
43. Romano R, Jannini EA, Pepe M, Grimaldi A, Olivieri M, Spennati P, et al. The effects of iodoprophylaxis on thyroid size during pregnancy. Am J Obstet Gynecol. 1991;164(2):482.
44. Glinoer D, De Nayer P, Delange F, Lemone M, Toppet V, Spehl M, et al. A randomized trial for the treatment of mild iodine deficiency during pregnancy: maternal and neonatal effects. J Clin Endocrinol Metab. 1995;80(1):258.
45. Liesenkotter KP, Gopel W, Bogner U, Stach B, Gruters A. Earliest prevention of endemic goiter by iodine supplementation during pregnancy. Eur J Endocrinol. 1996;134(4):443.
46. Antonangeli L, Maccherini D, Cavaliere R, Di Giulio C, Reinhardt B, Pinchera A, et al. Comparison of two different doses of iodide in the prevention of gestational goiter in marginal iodine deficiency: a longitudinal study. Eur J Endocrinol. 2002;147(1):29.
47. Moleti M, Lo Presti VP, Campolo MC, Mattina F, Galletti M, Mandolfino M, et al. Iodine prophylaxis using iodized salt and risk of maternal thyroid failure in conditions of mild iodine deficiency. J Clin Endocrinol Metab. 2008;93(7):2616.
48. Berbel P, Mestre JL, Santamaria A, Palazon I, Franco A, Graells M, et al. Delayed neurobehavioral development in children born to pregnant women with mild hypothyroxinemia during the first month of gestation: the importance of early iodine supplementation. Thyroid. 2009;19(5):511.
49. Velasco I, Carreira M, Santiago P, Muela JA, Garcia-Fuentes E, Sanchez-Munoz B, et al. Effect of iodine prophylaxis during pregnancy on neurocognitive development of children during the first two years of life. J Clin Endocrinol Metab. 2009;94(9):3234.
50. Zhou SJ, Skeaff SA, Ryan P, Doyle LW, Anderson PJ, Kornman L, et al. The effect of iodine supplementation in pregnancy on early childhood neurodevelopment and clinical outcomes: results of an aborted randomised placebo-controlled trial. Trials. 2015;16:563.
51. Gowachirapant S, Jaiswal N, Melse-Boonstra A, Galetti V, Stinca S, Mackenzie I, et al. Effect of iodine supplementation in pregnant women on child neurodevelopment: a randomised, double-blind, placebo-controlled trial. Lancet Diabetes Endocrinol. 2017;5(11):853–63.
52. Verhagen NJE, Gowachirapant S, Winichagoon P, Andersson M, Melse-Boonstra A, Zimmermann MB. Iodine supplementation in mildly iodine-deficient pregnant women does not improve maternal thyroid function or child development: a secondary analysis of a randomized controlled trial. Front Endocrinol (Lausanne). 2020;11:572984.
53. Murcia M, Rebagliato M, Iniguez C, Lopez-Espinosa MJ, Estarlich M, Plaza B, et al. Effect of iodine supplementation during pregnancy on infant neurodevelopment at 1 year of age. Am J Epidemiol. 2011;173(7):804.
54. Brucker-Davis F, Ganier-Chauliac F, Gal J, Panaïa-Ferrari P, Pacini P, Fénichel P, et al. Neurotoxicant exposure during pregnancy is a confounder for assessment of iodine supplementation on neurodevelopment outcome. Neurotoxicol Teratol. 2015;51:45–51.
55. Rebagliato M, Murcia M, Alvarez-Pedrerol M, Espada M, Fernández-Somoano A, Lertxundi N, et al. Iodine supplementation during pregnancy and infant neuropsychological development. INMA Mother and Child Cohort Study. Am J Epidemiol. 2013;177(9):944–53.
56. Santiago P, Velasco I, Muela JA, Sánchez B, Martínez J, Rodriguez A, et al. Infant neurocognitive development is independent of the use of iodised salt or iodine supplements given during pregnancy. Br J Nutr. 2013;110(5):831–9.
57. Stoutjesdijk E, Schaafsma A, Dijck-Brouwer DAJ, Muskiet FAJ. Iodine status during pregnancy and lactation: a pilot study in the Netherlands. Neth J Med. 2018;76(5):210–7.
58. Vandevijvere S, Amsalkhir S, Mourri AB, Van Oyen H, Moreno-Reyes R. Iodine deficiency among Belgian pregnant women not fully corrected by iodine-containing multivitamins: a national cross-sectional survey. Br J Nutr. 2013;109(12):2276–84.

59. Ershow AG, Goodman G, Coates PM, Swanson CA. Research needs for assessing iodine intake, iodine status, and the effects of maternal iodine supplementation. Am J Clin Nutr. 2016;104 Suppl 3(Suppl 3):941S–9S.
60. Alexander EK, Pearce EN, Brent GA, Brown RS, Chen H, Dosiou C, et al. 2017 guidelines of the American Thyroid Association for the diagnosis and management of thyroid disease during pregnancy and the postpartum. Thyroid. 2017;27(3):315–89.
61. De Groot L, Abalovich M, Alexander EK, Amino N, Barbour L, Cobin RH, et al. Management of thyroid dysfunction during pregnancy and postpartum: an Endocrine Society clinical practice guideline. J Clin Endocrinol Metab. 2012;97(8):2543.
62. Rogan WJ, Paulson JA, Baum C, Brock-Utne AC, Brumberg HL, Campbell CC, et al. Iodine deficiency, pollutant chemicals, and the thyroid: new information on an old problem. Pediatrics. 2014;133(6):1163–6.
63. Obican SG, Jahnke GD, Soldin OP, Scialli AR. Teratology public affairs committee position paper: iodine deficiency in pregnancy. Birth Defects Res A Clin Mol Teratol. 2012;94(9):677–82.
64. Gregory CO, Serdula MK, Sullivan KM. Use of supplements with and without iodine in women of childbearing age in the United States. Thyroid. 2009;19(9):1019.
65. Leung AM, Pearce EN, Braverman LE. Iodine content of prenatal multivitamins in the United States. N Engl J Med. 2009;360(9):939.
66. Lee SY, Stagnaro-Green A, MacKay D, Wong AW, Pearce EN. Iodine contents in prenatal vitamins in the United States. Thyroid. 2017;27(8):1101–2.
67. Leung AM, Braverman LE. Consequences of excess iodine. Nat Rev Endocrinol. 2014;10(3):136.
68. Pramyothin P, Leung AM, Pearce EN, Malabanan AO, Braverman LE. Clinical problem-solving. A hidden solution. N Engl J Med. 2011;365(22):2123.
69. Rhee CM, Bhan I, Alexander EK, Brunelli SM. Association between iodinated contrast media exposure and incident hyperthyroidism and hypothyroidism. Arch Intern Med. 2012;172(2):153.
70. Scientific Committee on Food, European Commission Health and and Consumer Protection Directorate-General. Opinion of the Scientific Committee on Food on the tolerable upper intake level of iodine. Brussels: European Commission; 2002. http://ec.europa.eu/food/fs/sc/scf/out146_en.pdf.

Screening of Thyroid Function in Pregnancy

Fereidoun Azizi

Introduction

Thyroid dysfunction during pregnancy is accompanied with frequent adverse maternal and fetal outcomes [1]. Although screening for thyroid disease during pre-pregnancy and pregnancy states increases detection of various thyroid dysfunctions, no consensus has been reached whether physicians should screen all pregnant women for thyroid disease [2]. The major uncertainties exist in the beneficial effect of universal screening for detection of subclinical thyroid states and their treatment on pregnancy, fetal, and offspring outcomes [3, 4]. Therefore, majority of international medical societies do not recommend mandatory generalized screening for thyroid function in pregnancy [1, 4–6]. The American Thyroid Association (ATA) guidelines in 2011 recommended screening of high-risk groups in the pre-pregnancy and pregnancy periods [1]; this recommendation was not changed after 6 years in the 2017 ATA pregnancy guidelines [4]. Most recent studies have also demonstrated controversial conclusions for or against targeted screening [7–11].

The purpose of this review is to systematically evaluate various criterion for screening in relation to thyroid dysfunction during pregnancy and highlight the evidence-based controversies in regard to universal versus targeted screening.

Methods

A search of MEDLINE was consulted employing terms of screening, thyroid and pregnancy from January 2000 to December 2020. We excluded animal studies and used a combination of fast title search and filtering of abstract and used the

F. Azizi (✉)
Endocrine Research Center, Research Institute for Endocrine Sciences,
Shahid Beheshti University of Medical Sciences, Tehran, Iran
e-mail: azizi@endocrine.ac.ir

F. Azizi, F. Ramezani Tehrani (eds.), *Thyroid Diseases in Pregnancy*,
https://doi.org/10.1007/978-3-030-98777-0_4

reference of review articles for probable missing articles, in particular those published before year 2000. All types of observational and clinical studies, reviews, meta-analysis, and guidelines of major international societies were included.

Information regarding prevalence and occurrence of thyroid dysfunctions in pregnancy and their effects on pregnancy outcomes and fetal and offspring development were sought. In addition, the effect of treatment with levothyroxine in pregnancy and fetal outcomes were collected. Synthesis of the resources was mainly descriptive and focused on their value-added features that clarified the aim of this study.

Findings

Definitions of various thyroid dysfunctions are provided elsewhere in this comprehensive book. Overt hypo- and hyperthyroidism, subclinical hypo- and hyperthyroidism, and thyroid autoimmunity are common conditions during pregnancy.

In order to conclude if a medical condition or illness is suitable for screening, Wilson and Junger criteria published in 1968 [12] has been recommended by World Health Organization (WHO). Table 1 shows a summary of these criteria. Do thyroid dysfunction in pregnancy fulfill WHO recommended criteria for screening? Followings are systematic evaluation of each criterion for thyroid dysfunction in pregnancy.

The Condition Should Be an Important Health Problem

Prevalence rates of hypothyroidism, hyperthyroidism, and thyroid autoimmunity

Table 1 Major criteria for screening

The medical condition should have the following criteria:
(a) Important health problem
(b) Accepted treatment modality
(c) Available facilities for diagnosis and treatment
(d) Suitable test(s) or examination, acceptable to the population
(e) Recognizable latent or early symptomatic stage
(f) Clear natural history, from latent to declared disease
(g) Cost-benefit of case finding

are 2–3%, 0.1–0.4%, and 17%, respectively [13–15]. In population-based studies, the prevalence of subclinical hypothyroidism is 4–15% [16, 17]. Most studies report a prevalence of 2–3% for subclinical hypothyroidism during pregnancy [18].

Untreated overt hypo- and hypothyroidism are associated by serious maternal and fetal complications [4]. Preterm delivery, gestational hyperthyroidism, placenta abruption, low birth weight, gestational diabetes, cognitive delay, and abnormal neurobehavioral problems in offsprings have been reported [2, 4]. Although no prospective randomized clinical trial has been performed because of ethical issues, it is accepted that overt thyroid disorders must be treated prior to conception and during pregnancy.

There Should Be an Accepted Treatment

Accepted treatments have long been recognized for thyroid dysfunctions. Normal thyroid status would be reached by levothyroxine therapy in both overt and subclinical hypothyroidism. Treatment of overt hyperthyroidism during pregnancy is effectively performed by antithyroid drugs, while adverse effects should be carefully prevented. Gestational subclinical hyperthyroidism does not require treatment and may be a normal finding in the first trimester of pregnancy [4].

Availability of Facilities for Diagnosis and Treatment

The screening tools for detection of thyroid dysfunction, including measurements of serum TSH, T4, fT4, and T3, are available worldwide, mostly in affordable prices, although access to TPOAb measurement may be difficult in some parts of the world. Levothyroxine and antithyroid drugs are available worldwide for treatment of hypothyroidism and hyperthyroidism, respectively [2, 11].

Recognizable Latent or Early Symptomatic Stage

Overt thyroid dysfunction has symptomatic stages, mostly in early course of thyroid hypo- or hyperfunction. Subclinical dysfunctions of the thyroid and many subjects with thyroid autoimmunity are asymptomatic, of whom some patients may proceed to overt symptomatic stage [4, 5].

Suitable Test or Examination

The most suitable test for screening of thyroid dysfunction is the measurement of serum TSH, a reliable test that has high accuracy for subtle changes in thyroid function, even before any clinical presentation of the disease [2, 4]. Other tests for confirmation of the kind and etiology of thyroid disorders such as serum concentration of T4, fT4, T3, fT4, and thyroid antibodies have long been used in daily medical practice.

Acceptability of the Screening Test

Serum TSH measurement and other thyroid function tests and thyroid antibodies have long been used in clinical setting and they are acceptable to the population.

Natural History of the Condition

The pathophysiology and natural history of thyroid diseases during pregnancy have been vastly studied during last three decades and many clinical guidelines by international and national medical societies and reviews have been published [4, 6].

Agreed Policy on Whom to Treat as Patients

This criterion is a matter of controversy in thyroidology. There is no doubt that universal screening will detect unrecognized patients with overt hypo- and hyperthyroidism; however, most patients with overt disease are recognized before pregnancy and need no screening. In addition, unrecognized overt thyroid dysfunction is far less common that subclinical thyroid dysfunction. Since TSH suppression can be seen in the first trimester of normal pregnancy and subclinical hyperthyroidism is not associated with remarkable adverse events, the screening program will aim mostly to detect women with thyroid autoimmunity and subclinical hypothyroidism in pre-conception and pregnancy states [19].

Economical Reasoning of Screening

Since most of thyroid dysfunction in pregnant women is in the form of subclinical hypothyroidism, and given the lack of clear data for efficacy of treatment, ongoing debate regarding the need for universal screening for thyroid dysfunction during pregnancy versus risk-based screening continues. In addition, updated criteria for screening [20] have been presented to better suit the current technological advances in screening. Health authorities of each country should take into consideration all screening criteria and their gross national product (GNP) and the percentage for health budget before deciding universal versus risk-based screening for thyroid dysfunction in pregnancy for their own country. Many universal screening programs accepted for some conditions in high-income countries may not be suitable in underdeveloped or low-income countries. In fact, a 2014 Asian survey showed that 66% of responders performed targeted screening of only the high-risk group [21], while a 2012 European survey found that responders screened all pregnant women twice as many as Asian ones [22].

Continuity of Screening Program

Screening for thyroid dysfunction before conception and during pregnancy is usually accepted as country program; therefore case-finding is a continuing process and is adopted either by universal or targeted screening program.

The major controversies related to universal versus targeted screening have been focused on thyroid autoimmunity and subclinical hypothyroidism. Followings are discussions related to these two important issues in thyroid and pregnancy.

Thyroid Autoimmunity and Pregnancy

It has been reported that TPOAb positivity occurs in 12–18% of women [23–27] and that isolated increase in serum TPOAb in pregnant women with normal fT4 and TSH may have increased abortion and other pregnancy outcomes. However, treatment of such women with levothyroxine, even from pre-conception, did not alter maternal outcomes [28]. Therefore, the status of autoimmunity has been discussed together with issues of subclinical hypothyroidism.

Autoimmune thyroid disease is the most common autoimmune disorder in women of childbearing age [26, 27]. The prevalence of positive TPOAb ranges from 2 to 17% in pregnant women [24]. Serum TSH is higher during first trimester of pregnancy in TPOAb positive as compared to women without AITD. More than 40% of women with thyroid autoimmunity present with FT4 levels in the range of hypothyroidism during late pregnancy [23]. Therefore, TPOAb positivity at early gestation is considered as a good predictor of gestational hypothyroidism [25]. This failing thyroid activity is related to the inadequate maternal thyroid capacity for thyroid hormone production imposed by pregnancy [29]. This is caused in the first trimester, by stimulation of thyroid gland by chorionic gonadotropin (hCG); in addition, there is an increase in TBG which is responsible for increase in total T4 and T3 and contextual decrease in free T4 levels. Other changes in renal clearance and placental deiodination also add up to a demand for increase in thyroid hormone production in normal thyroid gland. However, in conditions with iodine deficiency and thyroid autoimmunity thyroid response is inadequate and serum TSH will increase.

Miscarriage, spontaneous pregnancy loss occurring before 20 weeks of pregnancy, and preterm delivery, birth before 37 weeks of gestation, are the most common complications in women with Hashimoto's thyroiditis. Prevalence of miscarriage is 2–3 times more in TPOAb-positive, as compared to TPOAb-negative, women [30, 31]. In a meta-analysis significant increase in the odds of preterm birth has been shown in TPOAb-positive women, OR 3.90 (2.48–6.12), $p < 0.001$ [31]. A few randomized clinical trials have shown decrease in the rate of miscarriages and premature deliveries after treatment of TPOAb-positive pregnant women with TSH > 2.5 mu/L women with LT4 [32–35]. No significant benefit has been reported in TPOAb-positive pregnant women with TSH <2.5 mu/L when levothyroxine therapy was undertaken [33, 34].

International guidelines have considered potential harmful effects of thyroid autoimmunity on pregnancy outcomes. The use of population-based trimester-specific serum TSH reference ranges has been recommended; however, when this local specific TSH range is not available, American Thyroid Association considers TSH of 4.0 mu/L as upper normal reference range in the first trimester [4]. In addition to TSH levels, TPOAb positivity is also considered as an important variable for treatment with levothyroxine before conception and during pregnancy. Accordingly, levothyroxine therapy is recommended for TPOAb-positive women with TSH greater than the upper limit of reference range (or TSH > 4.0 mU/L) and may be considered in women with serum TSH levels above 2.5 mU/L. While for TPOAb-negative pregnant women the recommendation for levothyroxine therapy is in women with TSH greater than 10.0 mU/L and may be considered in those with TSH of 4–9.9 mU/L. Table 2 shows a summary of recommendations for LT4 therapy during pregnancy.

Pregnancy Outcomes in Subclinical Hypothyroidism

There is no consensus regarding the impact of subclinical hypothyroidism on pregnancy outcomes. Some observational studies have reported that subclinical hypothyroidism increases adverse pregnancy outcomes such as preterm labor, placental abruption, miscarriage, gestational hypertension, preeclampsia, gestational diabetes, and fetal distress [19, 23], while others reported no important associations [13]. Many observational studies demonstrate an association between the presence of thyroid antibodies in euthyroid women in their first trimester with increased rates of spontaneous miscarriage and preterm delivery [36–39]. In general, obstetrical complications are more prominent in TPOAb-positive than TPOAb-negative pregnant women.

Studies have shown that euthyroid TPOAb-positive women treated with LT4 and euthyroid TPOAb-negative women showed a lower rate of preterm deliveries compared with euthyroid TPOAb-positive women who were not treated with levothyroxine. Both studies have shown that euthyroid TPOAb-positive women who received levothyroxine (LT4) had a significant reduction in preterm deliveries (from

Table 2 Indications for treatment with levothyroxine during pregnancy

TPOAb	Serum TSH (mU/L)	Levothyroxine therapy
Positive	>10	Strongly recommended
	4–10	Recommended
	2.5–4	May be considered
	<2.5	Not recommended
Negative	>10	Strongly recommended
	4–10	May be considered
	2.5–4	Should not be used
	<2.5	Not recommended

22 to 6%) and miscarriage rates (from 14 to 3.5%) [34, 40]. In a recent study, it was shown that LT4 could decrease preterm delivery in TPOAb-negative women with TSH values ≥4.0 mIU/L [41].

Subclinical Hypothyroidism and Fetal-Offspring Outcomes

A prospective observational study reported that the mean mental developmental index score at the age of 6 and 12 months was 16 points lower for infants who were born to mothers with subclinical hypothyroidism compared to controls born to euthyroid pregnant women [42]. Another study showed children aged 25–30 months of women with subclinical hypothyroidism during pregnancy had mean intelligence scores and mean motor scores lower than those the control group [43]. However, in a cohort study from Netherlands, maternal serum TSH levels in 9–18 weeks of pregnancy were not associated with child IQ evaluated at a median of 6 years of age [44].

Prospective randomized trials assessing the impact of levothyroxine on offspring IQ in women with subclinical hypothyroidism or isolated hypothyroxinemia found no significant effect [45]. Lazarus et al., conducted a well-designed randomized controlled trial of pregnant women with the aim of evaluating the treatment effect on intelligence quotient (IQ) at 3 years of age in children; all positive screening women were prescribed 150 μg of LT4 per day. It was found that antenatal screening and maternal treatment for hypothyroidism did not result in improved cognitive function in children at 3 years of age, as the mean IQ and the proportion of children with IQ levels of the mothers treated during pregnancy and the children of those who were not treated [46]. In follow-up of these children, IQ of children of 119 LT4-treated and 98 untreated mothers with subclinical thyroid dysfunction during their pregnancy was compared to that of children of 232 mothers with normal gestational thyroid function. Maternal LT4 treatment was not associated with neurocognitive improvement of offspring at age of 9.5 years [47].

Casey et al. also showed that treatment for subclinical hypothyroidism or hypothyroxinemia, initiated in 8–20 weeks of gestation, did not result in significantly better cognitive outcomes in children of mothers with levothyroxine-treated gestational subclinical hypothyroidism through 5 years of age, compared to outcomes in those who had received no treatment for the conditions [48]. Of course, the main shortcoming of most trials is that LT4 treatment were initiated at late first or in the second trimester of pregnancy when fetal thyroid development and thyroid hormone synthesis and secretion had nearly been completed [49].

Foregoing evidence-based studies may point to the fact that subclinical hypothyroidism is associated with some adverse pregnancy outcome but probably not an important fetal and offspring outcome.

What Would Be Missed During Targeted Screening?

A cross-sectional prospective study conducted on 1600 pregnant women in their first trimester of pregnancy found that the targeted high-risk case finding approach may miss one-third of pregnant women with thyroid dysfunction [50]. Another study showed that by using the targeted high-risk case finding approach, about 30% of women with hypothyroidism were overlooked [51]. A study of pregnant women also showed that 80.4% of pregnant women with TSH elevation would have been missed based on current high-risk screening guidelines [52].

In addition, 1–2% of pregnant women suffer from overt hypothyroidism that had been present before conception; in such cases, adverse pregnancy outcomes are almost inevitable and treatment of overt thyroid disease decreases maternal and fetal morbidity and mortality [53]. Targeted screening may not detect asymptomatic hypothyroid women before conception or during pregnancy.

Cost-Effectiveness of Various Screening Methods

Dosiou et al. have presented two articles related to cost-effectiveness and provided evidence about the cost-effectiveness of universal screening of pregnant women with both TSH and TPOAb compared to the risk-targeted screening, in the first trimester of pregnancy. Furthermore, a decision-analytic model that compared the incremental cost for quality-adjusted life-year (QALY) showed that even when the benefits of screening were focused on detection and management of overt hypothyroidism, screening was highly cost-effective [54, 55]. Similar findings have been reported by others [56, 57] and confirm that universal screening is more cost-effective than targeted screening for thyroid dysfunction in pregnancy.

Summary

Controversies continue regarding beneficial effect of universal screening for detection of subclinical thyroid dysfunction and its treatment during pregnancy. More evidence is needed for international consensus of universal or targeted screening of thyroid function in pregnancy. In addition, the criteria of screening along with GNP and health budget should be considered in each country for decision-making regarding the mode of screen of thyroid function in pregnancy.

References

1. Stagnaro-Green A, Roman H, Cobin RH, et al. Prospective study of lymphocyte-initiated immunosuppression in normal pregnancy: evidence of a T-cell etiology for postpartum thyroid dysfunction. J Clin Endorinol Metab. 1992;74:645–53.
2. Amouzegar A, Abdi H, Takyar M. Screening for thyroid dysfunction in pregnancy. Ann Thyroid. 2018;3:61–7.
3. Davies TF. The ATA, the Endocrine Society, and AACE confuse endocrinologists on thyroid disease in pregnancy. American Thyroid Association. American Association of Clinical Endocrinology. Thyroid. 2000;10:107.
4. Alexander EK, Pearce EN, Brent GA, et al. 2017 guidelines of the American Thyroid Association for the diagnosis and management of thyroid disease during pregnancy and the postpartum. Thyroid. 2017;27:315–89.
5. American College of Obstetrics and Gynecology. ACOG practice bulletin. Thyroid disease in pregnancy. Number 37, August 2002. American College of Obstetrics and Gynecology. Int J Gynaecol Obstet. 2002(79):171–80.
6. De Groot L, Abalovich M, Alexander EK, et al. Management of thyroid dysfunction during pregnancy and postpartum: an Endocrine Society clinical practice guideline. J Clin Endocrinol Metab. 2012;97:2543–65.
7. Hales C, Taylor PN, Channon S, et al. Controlled antenatal thyroid screening II: effect of treating maternal suboptimal thyroid function on child cognition. J Clin Endocrinol Metab. 2018;103:1583–91.
8. Sitoris G, Veltri F, Kleynen P, et al. Screening for thyroid dysfunction in pregnancy with targeted high-risk case finding: can it be improved? J Clin Endocrinol Metab. 2019;104:2346–54.
9. Hales C, Taylor PN, Chanon S, et al. Controlled antenatal thyroid screening II: effect of treating maternal suboptimal thyroid function on child behavior. J Clin Endocrinol Metab. 2020;105:e416–27.
10. Berbara TMBL, de Morais NS, Saraiva DA, et al. Selective case finding versus universal screening for detecting hypothyroidism in the first trimester of pregnancy: a comparative evaluation of a group of pregnant women from Rio de Janeiro. Arch Endocrinol Metab. 2020;64:159–64.
11. Van der Spek AH, Bisschop PH. Universal screening for thyroid disease should not be recommended before and during pregnancy. Best Pract Res Clin Endocrinol Metab. 2020;34:101429.
12. Wilson JM, Jungner YG. Principles and practice of mass screening for disease. Bol Oficina Sanit Panam. 1968;65:281–393.
13. Cleary-Goldman J, Malone FD, Lambert-Messerlian G, Sulivan L, Canick J, Luthy D, Gross S, Bianchi DW, D'Alton ME. Maternal thyroid hypofunction and pregnancy outcome. Obstet Gynecol. 2008;112:85–92.
14. Glinoer D. Thyroid hyperfunction during pregnancy. Thyroid. 1998;8:859–64.

15. Ashoor G, Maiz N, Rotas M, Jawdat F, Nicolaides KH. Maternal thyroid function at 11 to 13 weeks of gestation and subsequent fetal death. Thyroid. 2010;20:898–993.
16. Tunbridge WM, Evered DC, Hall R, et al. The spectrum of thyroid disease in a community: the Whickham survey. Clin Endocrinol. 1977;7:481–93.
17. Vanderpump MP, Tunbridge WM, French JM, et al. The incidence of thyroid disorders in the community: a twenty-year follow-up of the Whickham survey. Clin Endocrinol. 1995;43:55–68.
18. Krassas GE, Poppe K, Glinoer D. Thyroid function and human reproductive health. Endocr Rev. 2010;31:702–55.
19. Casey BM, Dashe JS, Wells CE, et al. Subclinical hypothyroidism and pregnancy outcomes. Obstet Gynecol. 2005;105:239–45.
20. Andermann A, Blancquaert I, Beauchamp S, et al. Revisiting Wilson and Jungner in the genomic age: a review of screening criteria over the past 40 years. Bull World Health Organ. 2008;86:317–9.
21. Azizi F, Amouzegar A, Mehran L, et al. Screening and management of hypothyroidism in pregnancy: results of an Asian survey. Endocr J. 2014;61:697–704.
22. Vaidya B, Hubalewska-Dydejczyk A, Laurberg P, Negro R, Vermiglio F, Poppe K. Treatment and screening of hypothyroidism in pregnancy: results of a European survey. Eur J Endocrinol. 2012;166:49–54.
23. Glinoer D, Riahi M, Grün JP, Kinthaert J. Risk of subclinical hypothyroidism in pregnant women with asymptomatic autoimmune thyroid disorders. J Clin Endocrinol Metab. 1994;79:197–204.
24. Vanderpump MP. The epidemiology of thyroid disease. Br Med Bull. 2011;99:39–51.
25. Moreno-Reyes R, Glinoer D, Van Oyen H, Vandevijvere S. High prevalence of thyroid disorders in pregnant women in a mildly iodine-deficient country: a population-based study. J Clin Endocrinol Metab. 2013;98:3694–701.
26. Nazarpour S, Ramezani Tehrani F, Simbar M, Azizi F. Thyroid autoantibodies and the effect on pregnancy outcomes. J Obstet Gynaecol. 2016;36:3–9.
27. Amouzegar A, Gharibzadeh S, Kazemian E, et al. The prevalence, incidence and natural course of positive antithyroperoxidase antibodies in a population based study: Tehran thyroid study. PLoS One. 2017;12:e0169283.
28. Dhillon-Smith RK, Middleton LJ, Sunner KK, et al. Levothyroxine in women with thyroid peroxidase antibodies before conception. N Engl J Med. 2019;380:1316–25.
29. Glinoer D. The regulation of thyroid function in pregnancy: pathways of endocrine adaptation from physiology to pathology. Endocr Rev. 1997;18:404–33.
30. Stagnaro-Green A, Roman SH, Cobin RH, et al. Detection of at-risk pregnancy by means of highly sensitive assays for thyroid autoantibodies. JAMA. 1990;264:1422–5.
31. Thangaratinam SH, Tan A, Knox E, et al. Association between thyroid autoantibodies and miscarriage and preterm birth: meta-analysis of evidence. BMJ. 2011;342:d2616.
32. Negro R, Schwartz A, Gismondi R, et al. Universal screening versus case finding for detection and treatment of thyroid hormonal dysfunction during pregnancy. J Clin Endocrinol Metab. 2010;95:1699–707.
33. Negro R, Greco G. Levothyroxine but not selenium increases endothelial progenitor cell counts in patients with hypothyroidism. Eur Thyroid J. 2016;5:100–5.
34. Nazarpour S, Ramezani Tehrani F, Simbar M, Tohidi M, Alavi Majd H, Azizi F. Effects of levothyroxine treatment on pregnancy outcomes in pregnant women with autoimmune thyroid disease. Eur J Endocrinol. 2017;176:253–65.
35. Nazarpour S, Ramezani Tehrani F, Amiri M, Bidhendi Yarandi R, Azizi F. Levothyroxine treatment and pregnancy outcomes in women with subclinical hypothyroidism: a systematic review and meta-analysis. Arch Gynecol Obstet. 2019;300:805–19.
36. Negro R, Schwartz A, Gismondi R, et al. Increased pregnancy loss rate in thyroid antibody negative women with TSH levels between 2.5 and 5.0 in the first trimester of pregnancy. J Clin Endocrinol Metab. 2010;95:E44–8.

37. Toulis KA, Goulis DG, Venetis CA, et al. Risk of spontaneous miscarriage in euthyroid women with thyroid autoimmunity undergoing IVF: a meta-analysis. Eur J Endocrinol. 2010;162:643–52.
38. Negro R. Thyroid autoimmunity and pre-term delivery: brief review and meta-analysis. J Endocrinol Invest. 2011;34:155–8.
39. Negro R, Schwartz A, Gismondi R, et al. Thyroid antibody positivity in the first trimester of pregnancy is associated with negative pregnancy outcomes. J Clin Endocrinol Metab. 2011;96:E920–4.
40. Negro R, Formoso G, Mangieri T, et al. Levothyroxine treatment in euthyroid pregnant women with autoimmune thyroid disease: effects on obstetrical complications. J Clin Endocrinol Metab. 2006;91:2587–91.
41. Nazarpour S, Ramezani Tehrani F, Simbar M, et al. Effects of levothyroxine on pregnant women with subclinical hypothyroidism, negative for thyroid peroxidase antibodies. J Clin Endocrinol Metab. 2018;103:926–35.
42. Smit BJ, Kok JH, Vulsma T, et al. Neurologic development of the newborn and young child in relation to maternal thyroid function. Acta Paediatr. 2000;89:291–5.
43. Li Y, Shan Z, Teng W, et al. Abnormalities of maternal thyroid function during pregnancy affect neuropsychological development of their children at 25–30 months. Clin Endocrinol. 2010;72:825–9.
44. Korevaar TI, Muetzel R, Medici M, et al. Association of maternal thyroid function during early pregnancy with offspring IQ and brain morphology in childhood: a population-based prospective cohort study. Lancet Diabetes Endocrinol. 2016;4:35–43.
45. Stagnaro-Green A. Second trimester levothyroxine treatment for subclinical hypothyroidism or hypothyroxinaemia of pregnancy does not improve cognitive outcomes of children. Evid Based Med. 2017;22:149.
46. Lazarus JH, Bestwick JP, Channon S, et al. Antenatal thyroid screening and childhood cognitive function. N Engl J Med. 2012;366:493–501.
47. Hales C, Taylor PN, Channon S, et al. Controlled antenatal thyroid screening II: effect of treating maternal sub-optimal thyroid function on child cognition. J Clin Endocrinol Metab. 2018;103:1583–91.
48. Casey BM, Thom EA, Peaceman AM, et al. Treatment of subclinical hypothyroidism or hypothyroxinemia in pregnancy. N Engl J Med. 2017;376:815–25.
49. Thorpe-Beeston JG, Nicolaides KH, Felton CV, et al. Maturation of the secretion of thyroid hormone and thyroid-stimulating hormone in the fetus. N Engl J Med. 1991;324:532–6.
50. Nazarpour S, Tehrani FR, Simbar M, et al. Comparison of universal screening with targeted high-risk case finding for diagnosis of thyroid disorders. Eur J Endocrinol. 2016;174:77–83.
51. Vaidya B, Anthony S, Bilous M, et al. Detection of thyroid dysfunction in early pregnancy: universal screening or targeted high-risk case finding? J Clin Endocrinol Metab. 2007;92:203–7.
52. Chang DL, Leung AM, Braverman LE, et al. Thyroid testing during pregnancy at an academic Boston Area Medical Center. J Clin Endocrinol Metab. 2011;96:E1452–6.
53. Taylor PN, Minassian C, Rehman A, et al. TSH levels and risk of miscarriage in women on long-term levothyroxine: a community-based study. J Clin Endocrinol Metab. 2014;99:3895–902.
54. Dosiou C, Sanders GD, Araki SS, et al. Screening pregnant women for autoimmune thyroid disease: a cost-effectiveness analysis. Eur J Endocrinol. 2008;158:841–51.
55. Dosiou C, Barnes J, Schwartz A, et al. Cost-effectiveness of universal and risk-based screening for autoimmune thyroid disease in pregnant women. J Clin Endocrinol Metab. 2012;97:1536–46.
56. Thung SF, Funai EF, Grobman WA. The cost-effectiveness of universal screening in pregnancy for subclinical hypothyroidism. Am J Obstet Gynecol. 2009;200(267):e1–7.
57. Cost Donnay Candil S, Balsa Barro JA, Álvarez Hernández J, et al. Cost-effectiveness analysis of universal screening for thyroid disease in pregnant women in Spain. Endocrinol Nutr. 2015;62:322–30.

Preconception Counseling

Theodora Pappa and Erik K. Alexander

Introduction

Preconception care consists of interventions that seek to identify and then modify risk factors or behaviors in any patient through either prevention or/and advanced management strategies. In order to optimize pregnancy outcome in a woman with (or at risk for) thyroid illness, certain steps are important before conception or early in pregnancy. This is certainly relevant with regard to thyroid health, as thyroid hormones (TH) are crucial for fetal development and the fetus depends on maternal supply of TH during early stages of intrauterine brain development. In terms of nutrition, iodine is an essential nutrient required for TH synthesis and iodine requirements substantially increase during pregnancy, thus optimizing iodine intake is an important preconception step, especially in areas with severe iodine deficiency [1]. Indeed, thyroid disease at the time of pregnancy is a common clinical problem and pregnancy itself significantly impacts maternal thyroid physiology most notably increasing hormone demand by approximately 40%. In this chapter, we will discuss the recommended preconception counseling for frequently encountered thyroid conditions in women of reproductive age, including iodine supplementation, hypothyroidism and autoimmune thyroid disease, hyperthyroidism, and thyroid nodules and cancer care, summarized in Fig. 1. Through proper prenatal counseling and subsequent antenatal care, we describe the reduction in risk that is accomplished as maternal and neonatal health are optimized.

For any discussion of preconception counseling, basic understanding of physiology and analytic test interpretation of thyroid function impacted by gestation should by emphasized. Pregnancy itself is a state characterized by increased demand for TH as the fetus depends on maternal supply of TH in early stages of intrauterine

T. Pappa · E. K. Alexander (✉)
Thyroid Section, Division of Endocrinology, Diabetes and Hypertension, Brigham and Women's Hospital, Boston, MA, USA
e-mail: theodora_pappa@dfci.harvard.edu; ekalexander@partners.org

F. Azizi, F. Ramezani Tehrani (eds.), *Thyroid Diseases in Pregnancy*,
https://doi.org/10.1007/978-3-030-98777-0_5

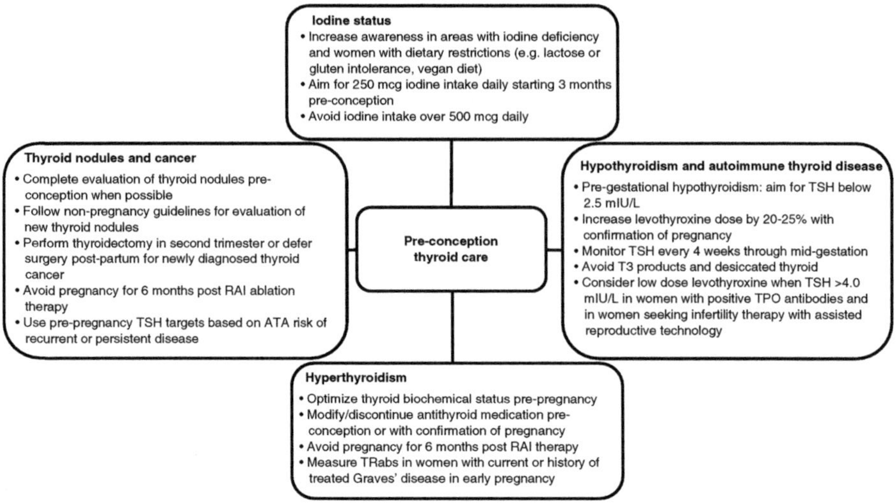

Fig. 1 Summary or preconception counseling recommendations for thyroid care. *TRabs* TSH receptor antibodies, *RAI* radioactive iodine, *TPO* thyroid peroxidase, *ATA* American Thyroid Association

development. On average, the fetal thyroid gland matures after week 18 of gestation. Furthermore, throughout pregnancy, iodine renal excretion increases, thyroxine binding globulin (TBG) concentrations rise in the presence of elevated estrogen concentrations, while placental type 3 deiodinase leads to degradation of maternal TH and human chorionic gonadotrophin (hCG) acts as a weak agonist to activate the TSH receptor. Through all of these changes, a healthy thyroidal axis responds by increasing TH production [2]. Analytically, serum free T4 (fT4) concentrations transiently increase during the first trimester, whereas TSH slightly decreases. But in cases with preexisting or subclinical thyroid dysfunction, pregnancy may therefore result in thyroid dysfunction progressing to a clinically overt state. Of note, interpretation of thyroid function tests during pregnancy can also be challenging given the many physiologic changes occurring in pregnancy, such as increased TBG, hCG rise, and increases in albumin. Quite frequently, these changes result in different reference ranges in comparison to nonpregnancy ones. For example, reference ranges for TSH change by trimester due to activation of the TSH receptor by hCG, whereas inaccurate determination of fT4 levels can be produced by several immunoassays due to the analytic impact of excess protein binding. Together, the physiologic changes and notable caveats above confirm that it is more relevant to screen for and treat thyroid conditions preconception whenever possible. This will allow time for intervention to be most effective, while analytical testing will prove more accurate and reliable. Finally, if needed, both medical and surgical management are safer and more easily managed.

Preconception Counseling Regarding Iodine Status

Adequate iodine supply is critical for maternal TH production, which then plays a critical role in fetal neurodevelopment. Severe iodine deficiency has been associated with increased risk of miscarriage, stillbirth, as well as increased perinatal and infant mortality. Iodine deficiency is among the leading causes of preventable intellectual deficit worldwide [3]. As an intervention, iodization of salt or other food sources is the most cost-effective way to provide adequate iodine stores and thus improve maternal-fetal health. Although in the last three decades there have been significant advances in correcting global iodine deficiency with salt supplementation, several countries remain iodine deficient. In the United States, approximately half of salt sold for household use is iodized, and major sources of dietary iodine include dairy foods, commercially baked bread, seafood, eggs, meat, and poultry, which are widely consumed [4, 5].

Preconception counseling regarding iodine status should first focus attention upon whether a woman resides in areas considered iodine sufficient or not. Separately, a dietary assessment should follow to better understand total daily iodine intake. The recommended dietary allowance by the US Institute of Medicine for total daily iodine intake (inclusive of both diet and supplements) is 150 mcg for women seeking pregnancy, 220 mcg for women currently pregnant, and 290 mcg during lactation. Notably however, the WHO recommends 250 mcg of daily iodine intake for both pregnant and lactating women [6]. The 2017 American Thyroid Association (ATA) thyroid and pregnancy guidelines raise attention to populations with certain dietary restrictions, such as women who are lactose or gluten intolerant, or those who follow low carbohydrate or vegan diets. Such individuals may have increased iodine needs. The American Thyroid Association recommends daily iodine supplementation with 150 mcg iodine in the form of potassium iodide, to optimally begin 3 months preconception and aim for total of 250 mcg iodine ingestion daily [7]. Of note, women on levothyroxine therapy do not require iodine supplementation because the substrate is not needed for thyroid hormone formation. On the other side of the spectrum, iodine excess is usually self-regulated through the Wolff–Chaikoff effect that transiently blocks thyroid hormone synthesis as a response to high iodine load, but escape occurs several days thereafter. Chronic excess iodine intake may have adverse outcomes on the mother and the fetus, when unable to escape from the Wolf–Chaikoff effect. Therefore, sustained iodine intake over 500 mcg daily should be avoided during pregnancy to minimize risk of fetal thyroid hypofunction [8]. In summary, preconception assessment of a woman's iodine intake is of great importance. When deficiency or excess iodine intake is identified, clear dietary interventions can be recommended which will optimize gestational health thereafter.

Preconception Counseling Regarding Hypothyroidism and Autoimmune Thyroid Disease

Primary overt hypothyroidism is characterized by identification of an elevated TSH and decreased fT4 concentration. As mentioned earlier, pregnancy is a state of increased T4 demand, though in the setting of any preexisting thyroid dysfunction the body is often unable to augment TH production without an adjustment in levothyroxine dose. Overt hypothyroidism affects 1–2% of women of reproductive age [9] and such maternal hypothyroidism has been associated with increased risk of complications for the maternal-fetal unit, such as pregnancy loss, low birth weight, or premature birth [10]. Thyroid hormones play a crucial role in fetal brain development, particularly in the first trimester when the fetus depends on maternal supply of thyroid hormones to regulate fetal neuronal cell proliferation, migration, and differentiation. Overt maternal hypothyroidism and cretinism have been associated with irreversible negative neurodevelopmental outcomes for the fetus including lower offspring IQ [11]. In recent years, there is growing evidence that even mild TH deficiency in early gestation may result in adverse neurocognitive outcomes including smaller gray matter volume [12, 13].

Beyond simply the impact of maternal hormonal status on the fetus, a positive association has separately been shown between the detection of elevated thyroid autoantibodies and increased risks of spontaneous pregnancy loss [14] or preterm delivery [15–17]. Prospective studies, however, have not demonstrated any benefit of levothyroxine supplementation preconception. In an UK randomized controlled trial of 19,589 euthyroid women with positive thyroid peroxidase (TPO) antibodies, supplementation with a low dose of levothyroxine (50 mcg daily) did not result in a higher rate of live births compared to placebo [18]. Thus, detection of an elevated TPO antibody titer should primarily convey an increased risk of maternal hypothyroidism during gestation ahead, allowing the practitioner to optimize a testing and intervention strategy when needed.

Taken together, the preconception period is a critical timepoint for assessment and counseling of a women with known or suspected hypothyroidism. Importantly, if and when any levothyroxine supplementation is required, a minimum of 3–4 weeks is then needed once therapy is initiated/adjusted before a new steady state of thyroid concentration is secured. This point becomes even more pertinent in hypothyroid women with minimal or no endogenous thyroid function [e.g., athyreotic patients, or those who have undergone radioactive iodine (RAI) ablation as treatment for Graves' disease or thyroid cancer].

It is important for women with pregestational hypothyroidism to be seen preconception where thyroid status can then be optimized before pregnancy. Notably, maternal TSH levels should be targeted below 2.5 mU/L. Equally important, women should be counseled to contact their endocrine provider upon suspicion of any pregnancy or a missed menstruation, allowing recommendations to empirically uptitrate their levothyroxine dose to mirror increasing demand. Indeed, more than half of levothyroxine-treated hypothyroid women can be expected to require higher doses during pregnancy. Two common approaches to address this clinically include either increasing the levothyroxine dose by two additional tablets weekly (nine tablets per week instead of seven, corresponding to a 29% increase) or to simply increase the daily dose by 25–30% as soon as pregnancy is confirmed [19]. Patients should then be counseled that during pregnancy serial monitoring with TSH evaluation every 4 weeks is recommended through mid-gestation. Thereafter, it is recommended that at least one more check of serum TSH occurs close to gestational week 30 as well.

The fetal brain is dependent on maternal T4 which is actively transported in the fetal central nervous system, whereas T3 is not. While the human thyroid gland secretes T4 to T3 at a ratio close to 14:1, the T4:T3 ratio in desiccated thyroid is significantly lower and approximately 4:1, with a relative T3 excess [20]. For the above reasons, women should be counseled against use of T3 products or desiccated thyroid during pregnancy. The recommended treatment should include administration of oral levothyroxine.

While preconception care is of paramount importance for women with known hypothyroidism, universal TSH screening in early pregnancy remains a controversial issue [21]. Based on the 2017 ATA guidelines, all pregnant women should be screened at the initial prenatal visit for any history of thyroid dysfunction, as well as the use of either thyroid hormone or antithyroid medication. If any other clinical risk factors are separately identified in a woman seeking pregnancy or newly pregnant, then testing for serum TSH is also recommended [7]. These include a known history or symptoms of hypothyroidism and TPO antibody positivity, as well as risk factors such as the presence of a goiter, history of head/neck irradiation or prior thyroid surgery, age over 30 years old, history of type 1 diabetes or other autoimmune disorders, any history of pregnancy loss, preterm delivery or infertility, family history of thyroid disease, morbid obesity, use of amiodarone or lithium or recent administration of iodinated radiologic contrast, multiple prior pregnancies, or if residing in area with moderate or severe iodine insufficiency. When maternal TSH is over 2.5 mU/L, reflex thyroid antibody testing should take place as well. For patients seeking pregnancy, consideration can be given to initiating levothyroxine therapy when maternal TSH is >4.0 mIU/L, especially in the setting of an elevated TPO antibody titer [7, 22]. In general, the administration of low-dose levothyroxine therapy (typically initiated at 50 mcg daily) is of minimal risk and may be considered in an attempt to prevent progression to overt hypothyroidism once pregnancy is attained [7]. For women seeking infertility therapy using assisted reproductive technology, existing evidence supports that treatment of subclinical hypothyroidism with levothyroxine may improve pregnancy and delivery rates [23, 24] and, thus, the 2017 ATA guidelines recommend treatment with levothyroxine in women with subclinical hypothyroidism undergoing fertility therapy aiming for TSH levels below 2.5 mU/L [7].

Preconception Counseling Regarding Hyperthyroidism

Thyrotoxicosis is a condition characterized by excess circulating thyroid hormone. The most frequent cause of thyrotoxicosis in women of reproductive age is Graves' disease, an autoimmune disorder triggered by antibodies activating the TSH receptor (TRabs) and thyroid stimulating immunoglobulins (TSI) and resulting in excess TH production by the thyroid gland. Preconception counseling is of great importance in hyperthyroid women of reproductive age, given the multiple complications and associated risks imparted by Graves' disease and its treatment with regard to the maternal-fetal unit. Several studies have demonstrated a clear association between thyrotoxicosis and poor maternal-fetal outcomes, which are positively impacted by the control of maternal thyroid hormone excess during pregnancy [25, 26]. Uncontrolled Graves' disease has been linked with higher rates of miscarriage, maternal congestive heart failure, premature birth, intrauterine growth restriction, and stillbirth. It has been suggested that intrauterine exposure to high thyroid hormone levels may predispose the offspring to increased risk of seizure or neurobehavioral disorders [27]. In addition, fetal risks associated with maternal Graves' disease include fetal and neonatal hyperthyroidism through the action of TRabs that cross the placenta and may remain elevated even after RAI ablation therapy, as well as fetal and neonatal hypothyroidism due to exposure to higher doses of antithyroid medication even when the mother is biochemically in a euthyroid state. Transient central neonatal hypothyroidism can also occur when control of maternal hyperthyroidism during pregnancy has been suboptimal [28, 29]. In addition, antithyroid medications commonly used for the treatment of Graves' disease [the mainstay being methimazole and propylthiouracil (PTU)] have been associated with several side effects as well as risk for birth defects in early pregnancy [30].

A primary goal of preconception counseling for the hyperthyroid women is to optimize thyroid biochemical status pre-pregnancy. Separate important goals are to align any time frame for RAI ablation therapy and modify or discontinue antithyroid medications to reduce the side effect profiles. Finally, monitoring of TRabs and TSI ahead must be strategically planned. In general, women with Graves' disease seeking future pregnancy should be counseled to consider delaying pregnancy and using contraception until a steady euthyroid state is achieved. This may be translated to having two sets of thyroid function tests within reference range at least 4 weeks apart without interim changes in thyroid therapy. Given the complexities in management of Graves' disease during pregnancy, it is reasonable to present patients desiring pregnancy all available options including antithyroid drugs (ATD), RAI ablation and thyroidectomy, reviewing their advantages and disadvantages and encouraging shared decision making toward a final solution [7].

If the patient elects to proceed with ATD therapy, preconception counseling regarding their potential side effects is critical. Such systemic side effects may occur in 3–5% of the general population who are taking thionamides and typically include allergic reactions such as a skin rash, whereas more severe side effects include agranulocytosis, vasculitis, and liver dysfunction [31]. Special attention should be given when using PTU, as PTU is linked to more severe, potentially fatal, liver injury especially in young individuals, and its use is recommended only in the first trimester of pregnancy. In contrast, methimazole has been associated more often with a cholestatic picture [32]. Yet, during pregnancy the greater risk regarding use of ATD involves their teratogenic potential. Methimazole use has been associated with congenital risks of aplasia cutis, choanal or esophageal atresia and various abdominal wall defects such as omphalocele and omphalomesenteric duct abnormalities [33]. Therefore, the ATA guidelines recommend switching from methimazole to PTU during the first trimester of pregnancy and when planning pregnancy, if antithyroid drugs are used. Studies from Danish national cohorts have indicated that PTU is also associated with some risk of birth defects, but often inclusive of only face and head defects and urinary system malformations. In general, these appear less severe compared to those related to methimazole use [34]. The possibility of withdrawal of antithyroid therapy may also be considered during the first trimester in cases with mild hyperthyroidism controlled on low-dose antithyroid drugs, as the goal is to avoid maternal biochemical euthyroidism which often translates to overtreatment of the fetus. Rather, the principle of ATD therapy during pregnancy is to reduce maternal hyperthyroid symptoms even if the mother remains biochemically hyperthyroid and use the lowest effective dose of ATD to achieve total T4 or fT4 levels at the upper or moderately above the reference range [7].

If the patient elects a definitive therapy before conceiving and proceeds with RAI therapy, a pregnancy test should be performed ~48 h prior to therapy and conception should be avoided for a minimum of 6 months thereafter, and until a stable euthyroid state is achieved. There is a small chance that patients with severe Graves' disease may not achieve euthyroidism within first year after RAI therapy [35]. In addition, TRabs titers may actually increase after RAI therapy and remain elevated, in which case continued monitoring is recommended during pregnancy. These factors may shift some patients with severe Graves' disease or high antibody titer to elect thyroidectomy instead of RAI therapy. Should thyroidectomy be indicated for the management of Graves' disease during pregnancy, the optimal time window is the second trimester to minimize peri-operative risks for the mother and the fetus.

Besides optimizing maternal thyroid function pre-pregnancy, another important issue is addressing the role of TRabs that cross the placenta and can have a direct impact on the fetus which at times induces fetal hyperthyroidism. Measuring TRAbs during early pregnancy is recommended not only in women with Graves' disease on antithyroid treatment, but also extends to those who have received definitive treatment for Graves' disease, such as RAI therapy or surgery in the past. If antibody titers are elevated, monitoring of their concentration is indicated again at weeks 18–22 of pregnancy and should be conveyed as part of preconception counseling.

Preconception Counseling Regarding Thyroid Nodules and Cancer

Preconception counseling in women with thyroid nodules and thyroid cancer poses a challenge in balancing the needs between effective and definitive diagnosis/treatment on one hand, versus minimizing risks for the maternal-fetal unit on the other hand. Much of the time, interventions may be safely postponed until after pregnancy, and in general avoiding surgery during pregnancy is preferrable because the peri-operative risks for pregnant patients are higher compared to non-pregnant ones [36].

Clinically relevant thyroid nodules are prevalent in 5–6% of adult women of childbearing age [37], and a few studies have suggested that the physiologic changes occurring in pregnancy may promote nodule formation and modest growth [38]. Biochemical and imaging workup for clinically relevant thyroid nodules should ideally be completed before pregnancy. There is no need to monitor cytologically benign thyroid nodules more closely during pregnancy, unless they demonstrate rapid growth in which case repeat fine needle aspiration (FNA) biopsy should be considered.

The evaluation of thyroid nodules during pregnancy follows the same guidelines as in the non-pregnant patient, including history, physical examination, thyroid ultrasound, and measurement of serum TSH levels. Thyroid ultrasound does not use ionizing radiation and can be safely used during pregnancy. When a thyroid nodule meets criteria for evaluation with FNA biopsy, this can be safely performed at any trimester. Pregnancy does not seem to change the cytologic interpretation of thyroid FNA results [39], although it could in theory affect gene expression markers and thus molecular testing is generally favored for cytologically indeterminate nodules in the preconception state as opposed to during pregnancy itself.

There is no convincing evidence that pregnancy itself may drive progression of thyroid cancer, and interventions for indeterminate cytologic results can often be deferred postpartum unless there are clinical indices of aggressive behavior (abnormal lymph nodes or signs of metastatic disease) [7]. Even when thyroid cancer is diagnosed during pregnancy, this should not be a reason to terminate pregnancy and management depends on gestational age and patient preferences [40]. With the exception of rare aggressive malignancies, such as anaplastic, poorly differentiated or medullary thyroid cancer and unless there is evidence of substantial growth or tracheal or vessel invasion, the timing of surgery either during pregnancy or deferred until postpartum has not been shown to affect the survival of women diagnosed with thyroid cancer during pregnancy [41]. When surgery during pregnancy is indicated or desired, the second trimester is the preferred time window to minimize complications to the mother and the fetus, as there is higher risk for altered organogenesis and spontaneous abortion during the first trimester and preterm labor and delivery in the third trimester.

For women with known thyroid cancer pre-pregnancy, it is important to counsel and optimize clinical status before conception. In specific, when RAI ablation is indicated, women should be counseled to defer pregnancy for 6 months post ablation therapy. There have been few reports associating RAI ablation therapy with transient amenorrhea and menstrual irregularities that however resolved within 1 year of therapy [42, 43]. For patients at low-intermediate risk, patients should be offered the option to delay RAI ablation therapy in order to fulfill plans for pregnancy first, taking into consideration the woman's age and desire to conceive. Regarding target TSH levels during pregnancy, the degree of TSH suppression ahead is guided by preexisting risk of recurrent or persistent disease, and the same goal for TSH levels should be set that would otherwise be recommended in the non-pregnant state [44, 45]. For example, in patients at high risk for recurrence, a TSH goal at or below 0.1 mU/L is generally recommended. One should again note that pregnancy is a type of thyroid stress test that increases T4 demand and patients must be counseled that an uptitration in levothyroxine dose 30–50% is usually required to maintain the same TSH concentration during pregnancy.

As a growing number of patients diagnosed with papillary micro-carcinoma elect to proceed with active surveillance rather than surgical intervention, it is worth noting that such patients require counseling to obtain thyroid ultrasound monitoring in each trimester in order to detect growth pattern changes [7, 46].

The use of tyrosine kinase inhibitors (TKI) (e.g., sorafenib, lenvatinib, cabozantinib) is an advanced medical option for patients with advanced metastatic differentiated thyroid cancer. All these agents have demonstrated teratogenicity in animal studies and in general pregnancy testing and contraception is recommended in patients prior to initiation of TKI treatment [44]. Lastly, women of reproductive age and interested to become pregnant that harbor a germline mutation of the *RET* oncogene with or without medullary thyroid cancer should be offered genetic counseling to discuss preimplantation and prenatal genetic diagnostic testing. If they opt out of prenatal *RET* mutation testing, counseling and genetic testing of the baby should be offered. The diagnosis of pheochromocytoma should be ruled out in women with multiple endocrine neoplasia type 2 seeking to become pregnant [47].

Summary

Preconception thyroid care plays an essential role toward improving the health of the maternal-fetal unit while also optimizing pregnancy outcomes. Most diagnostic and therapeutic interventions are more accurate and generally safer to perform pre-pregnancy. Optimizing the delivery of iodine, a key substrate of thyroid hormones, can easily be achieved through universal salt iodization on a population level and with daily supplementation of iodine intake on the individual level. It is important to counsel women with hypothyroidism to achieve desired TSH goals pre-pregnancy and be aware of need for higher levothyroxine doses through gestation to meet increased T4 demands. Screening of thyroid function in high-risk groups is also recommended before conception or at early pregnancy, in which cases levothyroxine supplementation may be considered at a lower TSH cutoff. Pregnant women on levothyroxine therapy require TSH monitoring every 4 weeks through mid-gestation. In contrast, women with Graves' disease should be counseled to achieve adequate control of hyperthyroidism before conception. When antithyroid therapy is continued during pregnancy, women should be counseled on ATD-associated birth defects, while the lowest effective dose of ATD should be used. Women with history of thyroid cancer should be optimized with regard to thyroid cancer status before conception. When RAI ablation is performed, pregnancy should be avoided for 6 months post therapy. The pre-pregnancy goal TSH based on the patient's recurrence risk remains the same during pregnancy. Finally, when thyroid cancer is identified early in pregnancy, surgical intervention can be safely deferred until postpartum in most cases, except for those with clinically aggressive cancers.

Additional high-quality, carefully designed studies will provide further insight on how to approach existing controversies related to the optimal care of the maternal-fetal unit.

References

1. O'Donnell KJ, Rakeman MA, Zhi-Hong D, Xue-Yi C, Mei ZY, DeLong N, et al. Effects of iodine supplementation during pregnancy on child growth and development at school age. Dev Med Child Neurol. 2002;44(2):76–81.
2. Korevaar TIM, Medici M, Visser TJ, Peeters RP. Thyroid disease in pregnancy: new insights in diagnosis and clinical management. Nat Rev Endocrinol. 2017;13(10):610–22.
3. de Escobar GM, Obregon MJ, del Rey FE. Iodine deficiency and brain development in the first half of pregnancy. Public Health Nutr. 2007;10(12A):1554–70.
4. Maalouf J, Barron J, Gunn JP, Yuan K, Perrine CG, Cogswell ME. Iodized salt sales in the United States. Nutrients. 2015;7(3):1691–5.
5. Pearce EN, Pino S, He X, Bazrafshan HR, Lee SL, Braverman LE. Sources of dietary iodine: bread, cows' milk, and infant formula in the Boston area. J Clin Endocrinol Metab. 2004;89(7):3421–4.
6. Trumbo P, Yates AA, Schlicker S, Poos M. Dietary reference intakes: vitamin A, vitamin K, arsenic, boron, chromium, copper, iodine, iron, manganese, molybdenum, nickel, silicon, vanadium, and zinc. J Am Diet Assoc. 2001;101(3):294–301.
7. Alexander EK, Pearce EN, Brent GA, Brown RS, Chen H, Dosiou C, et al. 2017 guidelines of the American Thyroid Association for the diagnosis and management of thyroid disease during pregnancy and the postpartum. Thyroid. 2017;27(3):315–89.
8. Theodoropoulos T, Braverman LE, Vagenakis AG. Iodide-induced hypothyroidism: a potential hazard during perinatal life. Science. 1979;205(4405):502–3.
9. Blatt AJ, Nakamoto JM, Kaufman HW. National status of testing for hypothyroidism during pregnancy and postpartum. J Clin Endocrinol Metab. 2012;97(3):777–84.
10. Abalovich M, Gutierrez S, Alcaraz G, Maccallini G, Garcia A, Levalle O. Overt and subclinical hypothyroidism complicating pregnancy. Thyroid. 2002;12(1):63–8.

11. Haddow JE, Palomaki GE, Allan WC, Williams JR, Knight GJ, Gagnon J, et al. Maternal thyroid deficiency during pregnancy and subsequent neuropsychological development of the child. N Engl J Med. 1999;341(8):549–55.
12. Jansen TA, Korevaar TIM, Mulder TA, White T, Muetzel RL, Peeters RP, et al. Maternal thyroid function during pregnancy and child brain morphology: a time window-specific analysis of a prospective cohort. Lancet Diabetes Endocrinol. 2019;7(8):629–37.
13. Korevaar TIM, Tiemeier H, Peeters RP. Clinical associations of maternal thyroid function with foetal brain development: epidemiological interpretation and overview of available evidence. Clin Endocrinol. 2018;89(2):129–38.
14. Chen L, Hu R. Thyroid autoimmunity and miscarriage: a meta-analysis. Clin Endocrinol. 2011;74(4):513–9.
15. Yuan N, Sun J, Li Z, Chai S, Zhang X, Ji L. Relationship between anti-thyroid peroxidase antibody positivity and pregnancy-related and fetal outcomes in euthyroid women: a single-center cohort study. BMC Pregnancy Childbirth. 2020;20(1):491.
16. Thangaratinam S, Tan A, Knox E, Kilby MD, Franklyn J, Coomarasamy A. Association between thyroid autoantibodies and miscarriage and preterm birth: meta-analysis of evidence. BMJ. 2011;342:d2616.
17. Dhillon-Smith RK, Coomarasamy A. TPO antibody positivity and adverse pregnancy outcomes. Best Pract Res Clin Endocrinol Metab. 2020;34(4):101433.
18. Dhillon-Smith RK, Middleton LJ, Sunner KK, Cheed V, Baker K, Farrell-Carver S, et al. Levothyroxine in women with thyroid peroxidase antibodies before conception. N Engl J Med. 2019;380(14):1316–25.
19. Alexander EK, Marqusee E, Lawrence J, Jarolim P, Fischer GA, Larsen PR. Timing and magnitude of increases in levothyroxine requirements during pregnancy in women with hypothyroidism. N Engl J Med. 2004;351(3):241–9.
20. Dayan C, Panicker V. Management of hypothyroidism with combination thyroxine (T4) and triiodothyronine (T3) hormone replacement in clinical practice: a review of suggested guidance. Thyroid Res. 2018;11:1.
21. Stagnaro-Green A, Dong A, Stephenson MD. Universal screening for thyroid disease during pregnancy should be performed. Best Pract Res Clin Endocrinol Metab. 2020;34(4):101320.
22. Taylor PN, Muller I, Nana M, Velasco I, Lazarus JH. Indications for treatment of subclinical hypothyroidism and isolated hypothyroxinaemia in pregnancy. Best Pract Res Clin Endocrinol Metab. 2020;34(4):101436.
23. Kim CH, Ahn JW, Kang SP, Kim SH, Chae HD, Kang BM. Effect of levothyroxine treatment on in vitro fertilization and pregnancy outcome in infertile women with subclinical hypothyroidism undergoing in vitro fertilization/intracytoplasmic sperm injection. Fertil Steril. 2011;95(5):1650–4.
24. Velkeniers B, Van Meerhaeghe A, Poppe K, Unuane D, Tournaye H, Haentjens P. Levothyroxine treatment and pregnancy outcome in women with subclinical hypothyroidism undergoing assisted reproduction technologies: systematic review and meta-analysis of RCTs. Hum Reprod Update. 2013;19(3):251–8.
25. Davis LE, Lucas MJ, Hankins GD, Roark ML, Cunningham FG. Thyrotoxicosis complicating pregnancy. Am J Obstet Gynecol. 1989;160(1):63–70.
26. Cooper DS, Laurberg P. Hyperthyroidism in pregnancy. Lancet Diabetes Endocrinol. 2013;1(3):238–49.
27. Andersen SL, Andersen S, Vestergaard P, Olsen J. Maternal thyroid function in early pregnancy and child neurodevelopmental disorders: a Danish nationwide case-cohort study. Thyroid. 2018;28(4):537–46.
28. McKenzie JM, Zakarija M. Fetal and neonatal hyperthyroidism and hypothyroidism due to maternal TSH receptor antibodies. Thyroid. 1992;2(2):155–9.
29. Kempers MJ, van Tijn DA, van Trotsenburg AS, de Vijlder JJ, Wiedijk BM, Vulsma T. Central congenital hypothyroidism due to gestational hyperthyroidism: detection where prevention failed. J Clin Endocrinol Metab. 2003;88(12):5851–7.

30. Andersen SL, Olsen J, Wu CS, Laurberg P. Birth defects after early pregnancy use of antithyroid drugs: a Danish nationwide study. J Clin Endocrinol Metab. 2013;98(11):4373–81.
31. Mandel SJ, Cooper DS. The use of antithyroid drugs in pregnancy and lactation. J Clin Endocrinol Metab. 2001;86(6):2354–9.
32. Suzuki N, Noh JY, Hiruma M, Kawaguchi A, Morisaki M, Ohye H, et al. Analysis of Antithyroid drug-induced severe liver injury in 18,558 newly diagnosed patients with Graves' disease in Japan. Thyroid. 2019;29(10):1390–8.
33. Andersen SL, Andersen S. Antithyroid drugs and birth defects. Thyroid Res. 2020;13:11.
34. Andersen SL, Knosgaard L, Olsen J, Vestergaard P, Andersen S. Maternal thyroid function, use of antithyroid drugs in early pregnancy, and birth defects. J Clin Endocrinol Metab. 2019;104(12):6040–8.
35. Moura-Neto A, Mosci C, Santos AO, Amorim BJ, de Lima MC, Etchebehere EC, et al. Predictive factors of failure in a fixed 15 mCi 131I-iodide therapy for Graves' disease. Clin Nucl Med. 2012;37(6):550–4.
36. Kuy S, Roman SA, Desai R, Sosa JA. Outcomes following thyroid and parathyroid surgery in pregnant women. Arch Surg. 2009;144(5):399–406; discussion.
37. Burman KD, Wartofsky L. Clinical practice. Thyroid nodules. N Engl J Med. 2015;373(24):2347–56.
38. Karger S, Schotz S, Stumvoll M, Berger F, Fuhrer D. Impact of pregnancy on prevalence of goitre and nodular thyroid disease in women living in a region of borderline sufficient iodine supply. Horm Metab Res. 2010;42(2):137–42.
39. Marley EF, Oertel YC. Fine-needle aspiration of thyroid lesions in 57 pregnant and postpartum women. Diagn Cytopathol. 1997;16(2):122–5.
40. Rakhlin L, Fish S. Pregnancy as a risk factor for thyroid cancer progression. Curr Opin Endocrinol Diabetes Obes. 2018;25(5):326–9.
41. Moosa M, Mazzaferri EL. Outcome of differentiated thyroid cancer diagnosed in pregnant women. J Clin Endocrinol Metab. 1997;82(9):2862–6.
42. Sioka C, Fotopoulos A. Effects of I-131 therapy on gonads and pregnancy outcome in patients with thyroid cancer. Fertil Steril. 2011;95(5):1552–9.
43. Acibucu F, Acibucu DO, Akkar OB, Dokmetas HS. Evaluation of ovarian reserve with AMH level in patients with well-differentiated thyroid cancer receiving radioactive iodine ablation treatment. Exp Clin Endocrinol Diabetes. 2016;124(10):593–6.
44. Haugen BR, Alexander EK, Bible KC, Doherty GM, Mandel SJ, Nikiforov YE, et al. 2015 American Thyroid Association management guidelines for adult patients with thyroid nodules and differentiated thyroid cancer: the American Thyroid Association guidelines task force on thyroid nodules and differentiated thyroid cancer. Thyroid. 2016;26(1):1–133.
45. Angell TE, Alexander EK. Thyroid nodules and thyroid cancer in the pregnant woman. Endocrinol Metab Clin N Am. 2019;48(3):557–67.
46. Shindo H, Amino N, Ito Y, Kihara M, Kobayashi K, Miya A, et al. Papillary thyroid microcarcinoma might progress during pregnancy. Thyroid. 2014;24(5):840–4.
47. Papaleontiou M, Haymart MR. Thyroid nodules and cancer during pregnancy, post-partum and preconception planning: addressing the uncertainties and challenges. Best Pract Res Clin Endocrinol Metab. 2020;34(4):101363.

Maternal Clinical Hypothyroidism

Inés Velasco and Onyebuchi E. Okosieme

Definition

Hypothyroidism is a condition characterized by insufficient production of thyroid hormones by the thyroid gland. This may arise from pathology within the thyroid gland itself (primary), or from reduction of the pituitary (secondary) or hypothalamic (tertiary) stimulus for thyroid hormone production [1]. Because of the large variation in clinical presentation and general absence of symptom specificity, the definition of hypothyroidism is predominantly biochemical, based on statistical reference ranges of the relevant biochemical parameters [2].

In the setting of pregnancy, maternal hypothyroidism is defined as a thyroid-stimulating hormone (TSH) concentration elevated beyond the upper limit of the pregnancy-specific reference range [3].

Primary overt hypothyroidism (OH) is defined as the presence of an elevated TSH and a decreased serum free thyroxine (FT4) concentration during gestation, with both concentrations outside the (trimester-specific) reference ranges [3]. Women with TSH levels of 10.0 mIU/L or above, irrespective of their FT4 levels, are also considered to have OH [4, 5].

I. Velasco (✉)
Department of Obstetrics and Gynecology, Hospital Universitari Germans Trias i Pujol, Badalona, España

O. E. Okosieme
Diabetes Department, Prince Charles Hospital, Merthyr Tydfil, UK
e-mail: OkosiemeOE@carfiff.ac.uk

F. Azizi, F. Ramezani Tehrani (eds.), *Thyroid Diseases in Pregnancy*,
https://doi.org/10.1007/978-3-030-98777-0_6

Prevalence

Primary hypothyroidism is up to 8–9 times more common in women than in men, and the prevalence increases with age, with a peak incidence between the ages of 30 and 50 years [6]. Overt hypothyroidism is a common endocrine disorder affecting 1–2% of women of reproductive age [7].

The prevalence of hypothyroidism varies according to diagnostic criteria [8], the method used to quantify TSH [9], the trimester of pregnancy [10, 11], and maternal nutritional iodine status [5]. Factors which may influence thyroid function parameters during pregnancy and, hence, affect the prevalence of hypothyroidism in pregnant women are summarized in Table 1.

A recent meta-analysis that calculated pooled-prevalence rates for overt hypothyroidism in pregnancy taking into account the impact of diagnostic methodology reported prevalence estimates ranging from 0.5 to 1.5% [8]. Since there are substantial differences in the upper reference limit for TSH between different populations, the diagnosis of hypothyroidism in pregnancy should ideally be defined using pregnancy- and population-specific reference ranges [3]. The use of non-pregnant

Table 1 Factors that modify thyroid function parameters during pregnancy

Biochemical measurement
• Thyroid immunoassay tests
• Upper limit cut-off values
• MacroTSH
• Measurements by LC/MS/MS
• Pitfalls (imported reference-ranges or results)
Population factors
• Geographical area
• Ethnicity
• Regional iodine nutritional variations
Physiological factors in pregnancy
• Dynamism of thyroid function across gestation (gestational age)
• Increased thyroxine-binding globulin
• Secretion of human chorionic gonadotrophin
• Increased iodine excretion
• Expanded plasma volume
• Increased type 3–5 deiodinase activity from the placenta
Individual factors
• Age
• BMI
• Smoking habit
• Iodine intake
• Thyroid autoimmunity
• Exposure to endocrine disruptors
• Drugs (amiodarone, glucocorticoids, iodinated antiseptics)

or arbitrary TSH diagnostic thresholds may underestimate or overestimate hypothyroidism depending on the cut-off applied [12].

The prevalence of overt hypothyroidism is much higher in regions of moderate and severe iodine deficiency [13]. In populations that shift from severe to mild iodine deficiency, the prevalence of hypothyroidism decreases; in populations shifting from mild deficiency to optimum or excessive intake of iodine, the prevalence of autoimmune hypothyroidism increases [14]. On the other hand, smoking decreases the risk of hypothyroidism [15, 16], and has a protective effect on the development of thyroid antibodies, i.e. thyroid peroxidase (TPO-Ab) and thyroglobulin (Tg-Ab) antibodies [17]. Maternal smoking during pregnancy has been associated with a subsequent decreased risk of developing hypothyroidism and an increased risk of hyperthyroidism [18].

In general, the prevalence of undiagnosed overt hypothyroidism in early pregnancy in an unselected pregnant population in iodine-replete and mildly-iodine deficient populations using conventional population-specific trimester-specific clinical thresholds for TSH and FT4 can vary substantially from 0.2 to 1% [19, 20].

Other factors that can affect the epidemiology of thyroid disease are the increasingly widespread use of thyroid function testing and lowering of treatment thresholds, particularly in pregnant women, resulting in an increased prevalence of hypothyroidism in the pregnant as well as non-pregnant population [8, 21].

Aetiology

Iodine deficiency and chronic autoimmune thyroiditis (known as Hashimoto's disease) account for the vast majority of cases of primary thyroid gland failure [21]. Hypothyroidism can also occur as a result of radioactive iodine treatment or thyroidectomy. Other causes include drug adverse effects (e.g. amiodarone and lithium), transient hypothyroidism due to silent thyroiditis, subacute thyroiditis, or post-partum thyroiditis [22].

Iodine deficiency is the most common cause of acquired hypothyroidism worldwide. In mild-to-moderate iodine deficiency, increased thyroid activity can compensate for low iodine intake and maintain euthyroidism in most individuals, but severe iodine deficiency causes goitre and hypothyroidism because, despite an increase in thyroid activity to maximize iodine uptake and recycling in this setting, iodine concentrations are still too low to enable production of thyroid hormone [14]. A third of the world's population lives in iodine-deficient areas. In addition, changes in diet and agricultural practices since the 1950s have led to the re-emergence of iodine deficiency in countries previously believed to be iodine sufficient, including several developed countries [21].

In iodine-sufficient areas, the most common cause of hypothyroidism is chronic autoimmune thyroiditis characterized by lymphocytic infiltration of the thyroid gland and the production of autoreactive antibodies, namely TPOAb and TgAb. In individuals with chronic thyroiditis, the transition from euthyroidism to autoimmune hypothyroidism is a gradual progress which may take several years [23]. The importance of thyroid antibodies in predicting progression from subclinical to overt hypothyroidism has been highlighted in different studies [24–26]. Hashimoto's disease will develop in a subject depending on the interplay between a particular genetic background involving multiple genes (a number of polymorphisms in susceptible genes) and a variety of environmental factors (especially ambient iodine intake and smoking).

In very rare cases, it is important to exclude other causes of abnormal thyroid function such as TSH-secreting pituitary tumours, thyroid hormone resistance, or central hypothyroidism with biologically inactive TSH [3].

Central hypothyroidism is rare (prevalence <1%) and affects both sexes equally. This condition is the consequence of anatomic or functional disorders of the pituitary gland (secondary hypothyroidism) or the hypothalamus (tertiary hypothyroidism) causing variable alterations of TSH secretion [27]. Biochemically, it is defined by low or low-to-normal TSH concentrations and a disproportionately low concentration of FT4 [2].

Even more exceptional are peripheral forms of hypothyroidism, due to aberrant expression of the deiodinase 3 enzyme (which inactivates thyroid hormone) in tumour tissues [28] or genetic syndromes with reduced sensitivity to thyroid hormone [29].

Clinical Features

Overt hypothyroidism may occur with highly non-specific symptoms and signs, such as weakness, lethargy, slurred speech, memory impairment, intolerance to cold, coarse hair, eyelid oedema, facial and peripheral oedema, macroglossia, goitre, cardiomegaly, bradycardia, constipation, decreased deep tendon reflexes, pallor, cold, dry, thick skin, decreased sweating and inappropriate weight gain for gestational age in pregnancy [30].

Hypothyroidism is also associated with decreased quality of life, most likely related to symptoms such as changes in body weight, fatigue, weakness and emotional susceptibility [1]. In women of childbearing age, hypothyroidism is associated with infertility and menstrual irregularities [6].

Although symptoms more accurately predict overt hypothyroidism in men than in women [31], it is accepted that neither the presence nor absence of any individual hypothyroidism symptom is particularly reliable in deciding who should have their thyroid function tested [32].

Pregnancy in general is a period where a woman undergoes a wide variation of bodily changes which are often accompanied by signs and symptoms such as concentration problems, general fatigue and mood changes. Thus, it is difficult to distinguish these non-specific features of pregnancy from those of thyroid disease per se and presents challenges to clinicians in detecting women at risk of thyroid function abnormalities that require immediate treatment [33]. However, the Billewicz

Scoring System has been proposed as an auxiliary diagnostic tool for detection of overt hypothyroidism during pregnancy in resource-constrained settings. This scale was developed based on seven symptoms and six signs, which were typically associated with hypothyroidism. According to this scale, higher positive scores indicate a higher level of clinical hypothyroidism [34].

Diagnosis

The 2017 American Thyroid Association (ATA) Guidelines on Thyroid and Pregnancy, based on an exhaustive review of the literature, concluded that there is insufficient evidence to recommend for or against universal screening of thyroid function during early gestation (ATA 2017). Instead, they advocate for a case-finding strategy in which all pregnant women should be verbally screened at the initial prenatal visit for any history of thyroid dysfunction, and prior or current use of either thyroid hormone (LT4) or anti-thyroid medications (methimazole, carbimazole, or propylthiouracil). (*Strong recommendation, high-quality evidence*) [3].

If any risk factors are identified, TSH concentrations are the principal first test to rule out thyroid disease [35]. Abnormal TSH concentrations should trigger the determination of FT4 concentrations [9].

However, previous studies have already shown that case-finding by means of the risk factors mentioned by the ATA will miss up, at least one-third of women with significant thyroid dysfunction, who need immediate treatment [20, 36]. Additionally, a meta-analysis showed poor sensitivity of "case-based screening" when using risk factors such as higher age, body mass index (BMI) and family history of thyroid dysfunction to predict unknown (overt) thyroid dysfunction: on average, 49% of the cases were missed [12].

It is important to recognize that assessment of thyroid function in pregnancy is more complex than in the general adult population. The well-known physiologic changes in pregnancy (simultaneous increases in thyroxine-biding globulin, placental deiodinase activity, and urinary iodine excretion as well as the increase in human chorionic gonadotrophin secretion) have a substantial effect on the interpretation of thyroid function tests and result in a downward shift of TSH reference intervals [37].

It is well established that normal thyroid status changes over the duration of pregnancy and accurate classification of thyroid function in pregnant women requires the use of gestational age-specific reference ranges [11]. There is also growing evidence that specific reference ranges may be considered based on ethnicity [38], body mass index [39] and parity [40]. In this regard, current ATA guidelines advocate the use of pregnancy-specific, local population-based reference ranges where possible although such data are not widely available [41].

Each laboratory or hospital should ideally seek to determine their own trimester-specific reference ranges, obtained from analysis of healthy, TPOAb negative pregnant women with optimal iodine intake and without thyroid illness [3]. When this is not feasible, pregnancy-specific TSH reference ranges obtained from similar patient populations and performed using similar TSH assay methods should be substituted (*Strong recommendation, High-quality evidence*). If internal or transferable pregnancy-specific TSH reference range is not available, an upper reference limit of ~4.0 mU/L may be used. For most assays, this represents a reduction in the non-pregnant TSH upper limit of ~0.5 mU/L. (*Strong recommendation, Moderate quality evidence*) [3].

Clinically, the complex inverse relationship between TSH and thyroid hormones results in small changes in thyroid hormone levels causing larger changes in TSH [37]. In order to differentiate between overt and subclinical thyroid disease, it is essential to measure, besides TSH, serum T4 concentration (free T4, total T4 or free thyroxine index). However, the current ATA guidelines only recommend testing for serum TSH in case of any risk factors for thyroid dysfunction are identified.

Adverse Outcomes (Maternal, Foetal and Child Risks)

Preconception

The frequency of menstrual disturbances in hypothyroidism is approximately three times greater than in the general population [42]. The thyroid disorders that are left untreated or in some cases undiagnosed can lead to subfertility or infertility, which may be due to high prolactin (PRL) levels, anovulatory cycles, and defects in luteal phase and sex hormones [43].

Until the late 1980s it was thought that pregnancy in hypothyroid patients was uncommon because most affected women were anovulatory [44, 45]. Nowadays, patients with overt thyroid failure are probably detected before referral to infertility clinics, thereby introducing a bias in the estimated prevalence of infertility disorders [46].

During Pregnancy

Overt maternal hypothyroidism has consistently been shown to be associated with an increased risk of adverse pregnancy complications [47, 48]) as well as detrimental effects upon foetal neurocognitive development [49]. Specific adverse outcomes associated with overt maternal hypothyroidism include increased risk of miscarriage [50, 51], anaemia in pregnancy [44, 52], arterial hypertension and pre-eclampsia [45, 53, 54], abruption placentae [53, 55], congenital malformations [50, 54], threatened preterm labour [56], preterm delivery [50, 51, 56], post-partum haemorrhage, cardiac insufficiency [44], low birthweight [57, 58], increased neonatal respiratory distress [59, 60], stillbirth [61, 62] as well as lower offspring intelligence quotient (IQ) [63, 64].

The initial studies which described the consequences of overt thyroid deficiency during pregnancy showed limited number of cases, as well as the proportion of adverse events [44, 45, 60]. Over the last decade, studies using large administrative datasets have offered more accurate estimations of the risk for potential foeto-maternal complications in cases of overt hypothyroidism (Table 2). The lower

Table 2 Studies reporting adverse maternal and foetal outcomes associated with maternal hypothyroidism in pregnancy

Study	Population	Results	Odd Ratio *(95% CI)*
Allan[c] [65]	*N* = 9403 pregnant women, 209 with TSH > 6 mU/L (USA) Prospective study	Foetal death	4.40 *(1.90–9.48)*
Idris[b] [57]	*N* = 167 pregnant women with TSH > 5.5 mU/L (UK) Retrospective study	Low birth weight	3.55 *(0.96–10.31)*
Wolfberg[b] [54]	*N* = 482 pregnant women treated with LT4 (USA) Retrospective study	Chronic HTA Pre-eclampsia	1.91 *(1.49–2.47)* 1.65 *(1.20–2.31)*
Wikner[b] [66]	*N* = 9.866 pregnant women treated with LT4 (Sweden) Retrospective, population-based register	Pre-eclampsia Pre-existing HTA Caesarean section Induction of labour Preterm birth Large-for-gestational age newborns Foetal congenital malformations	1.32 *(1.19–1.47)* 1.59 *(1,20–2.11)* 1.26 *(1.19–1.33)* 1.22 *(1.14–1.31)* 1.13 *(1.03–1.25)* 1.10 *(1.01–1.19)* 1.14 *(1.05–1.26)*
Männistö[a] [67]	*N* = 9247 pregnant women, 54 with OH (Finland) Prospective, population-based cohort	Preterm delivery (not significant) Higher placental weight Higher mean neonatal ponderal index (kg/m^3)	
Sahu[a] [58]	*N* = 633 pregnant women, 29 with OH (India) Prospective study	Gestational HTA Intrauterine growth restriction Intrauterine demise	3.60 *(1.5–8.7)* 3.50 *(1.1–11)* 7.60 *(2.7–21.6)*
Su[a] [62]	*N* = 1017 pregnant women, 9 with OH (China) Prospective, population-based study	Foetal loss Low birth weight Congenital circulation malformations	13.45 *(2.54–71.20)* 9.05 *(1.01–80.90)* 10.44 *(1.15–94.62)*
Männistö[b] [53]	*N* = 223,512 pregnant women, 3183 with primary hypothyroidism (USA) Retrospective, population-based cohort	Pre-eclampsia Superimposed pre-eclampsia Gestational diabetes Preterm birth Induction of labour Caesarean section prelabour Caesarean section after spontaneous labour Maternal ICU admission	1.47 *(1.20–1.81)* 2.25 *(1.53–3.29)* 1.57 *(1.33–1.86)* 1.34 *(1.17–1.53)* 1.15 *(1.04–1.28)* 1.31 *(1.11–1.54)* 1.38 *(1.14–1.66)* 2.08 *(1.04–4.15)*

(continued)

Table 2 (continued)

Study	Population	Results	Odd Ratio *(95% CI)*
Männistö[b] [68]	*N* = 223,512 pregnant women, 3183 with primary hypothyroidism (USA) Retrospective, population-based cohort	Neonate admitted to NICU Respiratory distress syndrome Apnea Transient tachypnea Sepsis Neonatal anemia	1.22 *(1.10–1.35)* 1.29 *(1.08–1.55)* 1.34 *(1.08–1.66)* 1.29 *(1.09–1.53)* 1.42 *(1.16–1.74)* 1.28 *(1.00–1.64)*
Andersen [69]	*N* = 1,605,529 pregnant women, 11,186 hypothyroid women (Denmark) Retrospective, population-based study	Preterm birth Large-for-gestational age new-borns	1.27 *(1.01–1.60)* 1.22 *(1.04–1.43)*
Hirsch[a] [51]	*N* = 101 pregnant women with TSH > 20 mU/L (Israel) Prospective study	Combined abortions + preterm birth All pregnancy related complications	2.50 *(95% CI not available)* 1.68 *(95% CI not available)*
Bryant[a] [19]	*N* = 26,518 pregnant women, 106 with TSH > 4.5 mU/L and 47 with OH treated with LT4 (USA) Prospective, population-based study	Severe preeclampsia (unconfirmed OH or SCH) Severe preeclampsia (treated OH)	2.53 *(1.41–4.54)* 1.69 *(0.06–4.71)*
Turunen[b] [59]	*N* = 16,364 pregnant women, treated with LT4 (Finland) Retrospective, population-based study	Gestational diabetes Gestational HTA Severe preeclampsia Cesarean section Preterm birth Large-for-gestational age new-borns Neonatal intensive care admission	1.19 *(1.13–1.25)* 1.20 *(1.10–1.30)* 1.38 *(1.15–1.65)* 1.22 *(1.17–1.27)* 1.25 *(1.16–1.34)* 1.30 *(1.19–1.42)* 1.23 *(1.17–1.29)*
Lee[c] [70]	*N* = 8413 pregnant women, 130 with TSH > 4 mU/L (USA) Prospective	Preterm birth Neonatal respiratory distress	2.17 *(1.15–4.07)* 2.83 *(1.02–7.86)*
Lai[a] [71]	*N* = 1226 pregnant women, 36 with OH (China) Prospective study	Gestational HTA	3.61 *(1.52–8.57)*

[a]Clinical or Overt Hypothyroidism defined by an increased TSH associated with low T4 levels
[b]Data obtained from national or institutional registers (pregnant women who were taken thyroid hormones)
[c]Cases above a TSH cut-off value (no distinction between subclinical and overt hypothyroidism)

prevalence rates of perinatal complications in more recent studies, compared with the older ones, may be attributed to delayed diagnosis and/or suboptimal treatment of hypothyroidism in the earlier studies, which would have resulted in a more severe clinical picture [42]. Additionally, the information obtained from national registers usually reported complications in pregnant women who were treated with levothyroxine, but does not include untreated or undiagnosed cases, which could potentially underestimate the true incidence of perinatal adverse events.

The association between overt hypothyroidism and preterm delivery has also been confirmed in two different meta-analyses [72, 73], and a recent meta-analysis has demonstrated that pregnancies with overt hypothyroidism have increased risk for anaemia [52].

Together, these data provide substantial evidence of multiple associations between overt maternal hypothyroidism and risk to the maternal-foetal unit [3].

Effects on Child Development

Thyroid hormones participate in multiple neurogenic processes including cell differentiation, neuronal activation and migration, axonal growth, dendritic arborisation, synaptogenesis and myelination. Insufficient maternal thyroid hormones in the early stages of pregnancy, especially before the foetal thyroid function is functionally mature at week 18–20, can lead to severe impairments in the development of the foetal central nervous system [74].

Untreated maternal hypothyroidism in pregnancy has been associated with delayed offspring psychomotor development, language and attention disorders, and a decrease of approximately seven points in the intellectual development of the offspring in comparison with children of euthyroid women [75]. Interestingly, these deficits were not observed in children born to mothers who reported receiving levothyroxine treatment later in pregnancy [75]. An inverse correlation between the severity of maternal hypothyroidism and IQs in the offspring was present at a mean age of 8 years [63].

Although TSH concentrations have always been considered as the best reflection of thyroid function during pregnancy, practically, all positive studies investigating child neurodevelopment outcomes find an association with maternal FT4 rather than TSH concentrations. Therefore, maternal FT4 more likely represents the availability of thyroid hormone for the foetal brain, since only maternal T4, but not TSH, passes the placental barrier [76].

More recently, maternal overt hypothyroidism has also been linked with other adverse neurocognitive outcomes, such as behavioural and psychiatric disorders in offspring, not only in early childhood but also in late adolescence and adulthood [77]. A very recent meta-analysis has provided evidence for the association between maternal hypothyroidism during pregnancy and an increased risk for attention deficit hyperactivity disorder (ADHD), autism spectrum disorder (ASD), and epilepsy in the progeny [78]. These epidemiological findings are supported by studies which have shown that both low and high maternal thyroxine levels impact foetal brain size and structure [79, 80].

Finally, a prospective population-based study in Finland demonstrated the association between maternal thyroid status during pregnancy and thyroid function parameters in adolescent offspring [81]. So, children of hypothyroid mothers will have a higher risk of being hypothyroid, although the long-term effects of these changes in thyroid function in adolescence is still unknown.

Treatment (Dosage, Goal, Outcomes)

Although no prospective, randomized investigation of levothyroxine intervention to improve obstetric outcomes or child development has occurred in pregnant women with overt hypothyroidism, such an investigation would be unethical to complete. Nonetheless, available data confirm the benefits of treating severe hypothyroidism during pregnancy [82, 83]. Hence, treatment of overt hypothyroidism is recommended during pregnancy (*strong recommendation, moderate quality evidence*) [3].

The ultimate goal in the management of overt hypothyroidism should be to ensure maintenance of maternal euthyroidism from preconception and throughout pregnancy and lactation. Hence, the ideal that of extending the window for monitoring of euthyroid maintenance both before and beyond pregnancy itself [7].

Preconception Management

Treatment of overt hypothyroidism with levothyroxine usually restores a normal menstrual pattern, reverses hormonal alterations, and improved fertility [84]. However, some women with treated hypothyroidism still fail to conceive and seek infertility treatment, including controlled ovarian hyperstimulation (COH) and/or in-vitro fertilization (IVF). Detailed information regarding the effect of hypothyroidism on COH and IVF outcomes (or vice versa) is limited, since no randomized controlled trials are available. It is unlikely that we will ever have these data since it would be unethical not to treat patients with clinical overt hypothyroidism [46].

The latest ATA guidelines recommend to evaluate serum TSH concentration in all pregnant women seeking care for infertility (*Weak recommendation, moderate*

Table 3 Preconception management of hypothyroidism

Preconception plan
Monitor FT4 and TSH
Adjust levothyroxine dose to target TSH between lower reference limit and 2.5 mU/L
Advise delay conception till FT4 and TSH within target
Emphasize treatment adherence
Provide specific conception advice
Conception advice
Seek medical advice once pregnancy is suspected, for example, positive pregnancy test or missed period
Obtain a blood test: FT4 and TSH
Increase levothyroxine dose according to the pre-specified regimen, before the blood test result is obtained. For example:
(a) Double the daily dose on 2 days each week, for example, 100 mcg Monday to Friday and 200 mcg Saturday and Sunday
or
(b) Increase the dose by 25 mcg daily if receiving ≤100 mcg daily and by 50 mcg if receiving >100 mcg
Avoid co-ingestion of levothyroxine with antenatal vitamin supplements, iron tablets or antacids

With permission from John Wiley and son Publishers (previously published in Okosieme OE, Khan I, Taylor PN. Preconception management of thyroid dysfunction. Clin Endocrinol (Oxf). 2018 Sep;89(3):269–279. https://doi.org/10.1111/cen.13731)

quality evidence) and endorse levothyroxine treatment for infertile women with overt hypothyroidism who desire pregnancy (*strong recommendation, moderate quality evidence*) [3].

Preconception care is paramount, not only to prevent hypothyroidism with the onset of pregnancy, but to optimize maternal well-being before and during pregnancy. Ideally, women should be seen preconception and educated about the importance of maintaining euthyroidism and how pregnancy can create challenges in doing so [7]. However, many patients taking long-term thyroxine had a thyroid-stimulating hormone above the reference range during pregnancy and especially during the first trimester of pregnancy. Thyroid-stimulating hormone declines during pregnancy reflecting active management. However, the decline in TSH occurs too late in pregnancy and it should be managed earlier in pregnancy or pre-pregnancy [85]. Table 3 offers a programmatic framework of preconception counselling [86].

During Pregnancy

Although universal screening in pregnancy remains contentious, there is universal agreement that overt hypothyroidism must be diagnosed and treated in pregnancy, and scientific societies endorse early and aggressive treatment in order to prevent significant negative harm to both the mother and the foetus [3, 35].

Table 4 Guidelines for management of overt hypothyroidism during pregnancy

Approach	
Newly diagnosed	Known before pregnancy
• Levothyroxine dosage should be titrated to rapidly restore euthyroidism (around 2 mcg/kg/day)	(a) *Adequately treated before pregnancy:* Increase their dosage of levothyroxine by 20–30% and urgently notify their caregiver for prompt testing and further evaluation
	(b) *Inadequately treated before and in early pregnancy:* Levothyroxine dosage should be increased to achieve euthyroidism as soon as possible (great increase) or gradually
Treatment	
• Adjust levothyroxine dosage to maintain serum TSH ≤ 2.5 mU/L	
• Separate the ingestion of levothyroxine from other vitamins or supplements containing iron or calcium	
• Reduce levothyroxine to pregestational dosage after delivery	
Monitoring	
• Check serum TSH level preconceptionally or as soon as gestation is diagnosed	
• Perform thyroid function test (TSH and T4 levels) every 4 weeks after each increase of dosage and during the first half of pregnancy	
• Monitor TSH levels (without T4) every 6 weeks once euthyroidism has been achieved and also after delivery	

The recommended treatment of maternal hypothyroidism is administration of oral levothyroxine. Other thyroid preparations such as T3 or desiccated thyroid should not be used in pregnancy (*Strong recommendation, low-quality evidence*) [3]. Levothyroxine therapy offers a safe, rational, and simplified approach to the correction of hypothyroidism [87].

In addition, pregnant women should be cautioned against simultaneous use of iron and calcium supplements (commonly recommended during pregnancy) with levothyroxine. A clinically significant reduction in levothyroxine efficacy can occur with use of these supplements, probably caused by binding of levothyroxine with iron or calcium. A time gap of 4–6 h between levothyroxine and these supplements should be maintained [88].

At this point, it is important to make a distinction between the cases of overt hypothyroidism detected for the first time during pregnancy and those hypothyroid patients already on replacement therapy who become pregnant. Table 4 contains the recommended programmatic actions in case of overt hypothyroidism during pregnancy.

Overt Hypothyroidism Newly Diagnosed in Pregnancy

It has been calculated that the prevalence of undiagnosed overt hypothyroidism in pregnant women is around 0.65% [89]. This population group, who definitely require treatment, can only be detected through a universal screening policy [90].

When overt hypothyroidism is detected for the first time during pregnancy, the subsequent challenge will be to rapidly restore euthyroidism with appropriate levothyroxine therapy. There is much variation in the way treatment is commenced and limited evidence on the optimal starting dose [7]. Different strategies have been proposed: employing a standard dose of either 100 or 150 mcg daily for all regardless of the degree of hypothyroidism [91]; and to decide the starting dose of levothyroxine according to TSH concentrations, or calculate it based on bodyweight with a mean dose of 2.33 mcg/kg bodyweight per day [85]. This latter approach could induce sub-normal TSH concentrations in some patients, whose potential of such effects upon conception and/or implantation are unknown [92].

Levothyroxine dosage should be titrated to rapidly reach, and thereafter maintain, serum TSH concentrations to trimester-specific normal TSH ranges [93]. Factors determining the appropriate dose for initiation of therapy are time of gestation, and the aetiology and severity of the disease. In patients with severe hypothyroidism, one approach is to initiate therapy for the first few days with a levothyroxine dose corresponding to two times the estimated final replacement daily dose, thereby expediting normalization of the extra-thyroidal thyroxine pool [94].

It is reasonable to target a TSH in the lower half of the trimester-specific range. When this is not available, it is reasonable to target maternal TSH concentrations below 2.5 mU/L [3].

Overt Hypothyroidism Known Before Pregnancy

In spite of the general consensus that overt hypothyroidism during pregnancy should be treated as early as possible and most of women are already being treated prior conception, there is a worrying discrepancy between published guidelines and clinical practices. The reasons for this are likely to be multifactorial including a lack of familiarity among clinicians with the current guidelines, high rates of unplanned pregnancies, noncompliance with levothyroxine and inconsistencies in management strategies among endocrinologists and obstetricians [95].

Treated hypothyroid women of reproductive age should be counselled regarding the likelihood of increased demand for levothyroxine during pregnancy. Such women should also be counselled to contact their caregiver immediately upon a confirmed or suspected pregnancy (*strong recommendation, high-quality evidence*) [3]. In this regard, the distinction between those hypothyroid pregnant women adequately and inadequately treated preconception and in early pregnancy should be emphasized.

Hypothyroid Patients Adequately Treated Before Pregnancy

Between 50 and 85% of LT4-treated hypothyroid women need to increase exogenous levothyroxine dosing during pregnancy [96]. This increase is probably due to a combination of factors: rapid rise in thyroxine-binding globulin (TBG) levels resulting from the physiological rise in oestrogen, increased distribution volume of thyroid hormones, and increased placental transport and metabolism of maternal T4 [88].

Clinical studies have confirmed that the increased requirement for thyroxine (or exogenous levothyroxine) occurs as early as 4–6 weeks of pregnancy [96]. The incremental increase largely depends on the underlying aetiology of the hypothyroidism [97] as well as the preconception level of TSH. Patients with overt hypothyroidism after thyroidectomy and radioiodine ablation therapy will be likely to require more levothyroxine than those with hypothyroidism due to autoimmune thyroiditis [98].

Hypothyroid patients receiving levothyroxine treatment with a suspected or confirmed pregnancy (e.g. positive home pregnancy test) should independently increase their dose of levothyroxine by ~20–30% and urgently notify their caregiver for prompt testing and further evaluation [99]. One means of accomplishing this is to administer two additional tablets weekly of the patient's current daily LT4 dosage (nine tablets per week instead of seven tablets per week, giving a 29% increase) can effectively mimic gestational physiology and thus prevent a worsening of maternal hypothyroidism during the first trimester (*strong recommendation, high-quality evidence*) [3].

In women who may be more at risk of worsening hypothyroidism in pregnancy such as those with no residual thyroid function or athyreosis and therefore unable to respond to hCG, a strategy of doubling the dose of levothyroxine three times a week (43% total increase) should be considered [7].

Such requirements gradually increase through 16–20 weeks of pregnancy and plateau thereafter until the time of delivery. These data provide the basis for recommending adjustments of levothyroxine dosage when affected women become pregnant and also for the timing of follow-up intervals for TSH in treated patients [3].

In clinical practice, titration of levothyroxine treatment during pregnancy may be performed in two ways: to adjust medication dose predictively or reactively. Predictive dose adjustment refers to a strategy of titrating the levothyroxine dose to maintain TSH levels within the trimester-specific reference ranges, while reactive dose adjustment refers to a strategy of changing the dose only when maternal TSH falls out of the reference ranges [7]. The predictive approach works better in practice by avoiding periods of hypothyroidism [99].

Hypothyroid Patients Inadequately Treated Before and In Early Pregnancy

There is no standard recommendation in this group of pregnant women, which include those who did not receive preconception advice and present once become pregnant, or did not accomplish an empirical dose increase, or even doing so, got worse to overtly hypothyroid [7].

A retrospective, population-based study in United Kingdom, demonstrated that the majority of levothyroxine-treated women have early gestational TSH level above the recommended targets, and the risk of pregnancy loss increased proportionally to the degree of TSH elevation, with no increased risk associated with TSH normalization [95]. Additionally, increasing levothyroxine dose for women with uncontrolled hypothyroidism in the first trimester of pregnancy was associated with a decreased risk of pregnancy loss [92].

There are mainly two schools of thought about how such cases should be approached. The first is to increase the levothyroxine dose by a greater magnitude to achieve euthyroidism as soon as possible in pregnancy, with the risk of transient mild hyperthyroidism, then titrate down the dose to a suitable maintenance level for the remainder of pregnancy. The second is to increase the levothyroxine dose more gradually with more frequent thyroid function testing of less than 4 weekly intervals, avoiding hyperthyroidism, until euthyroidism with a TSH target of <2.5 mU/L is reached [7]. So far, neither of these approaches had a good evidence base and were both clinically acceptable practice; however, recent findings have demonstrated that the risk to the pregnancy of transient hyperthyroidism and its potential consequences upon the developing foetal brain and infant behaviour are not negligible [80, 100].

No data suggest that women with adequately treated overt hypothyroidism have an increased risk of any obstetrical complication. Consequently, there is no indication for any additional obstetric testing or surveillance in pregnancies of women with overt hypothyroidism who are being monitored and treated appropriately [3].

At Post-partum

The increased levothyroxine dose requirements during gestation are a function of pregnancy itself. Therefore, following delivery, maternal levothyroxine dosing should be reduced to pre-pregnancy levels, and a serum TSH assessed 6 weeks thereafter [3]. However, this suggestion is also made on the assumption that pregnancy physiology returns to normal immediately post-partum.

Nowadays, due to an increased appreciation of the relationship between thyroid disease and maternal/foetal adverse outcomes, the number of women identified during pregnancy with overt thyroid dysfunction and initiated on levothyroxine therapy is increasing. The post-partum management of these women depends on multiple factors including the degree of hypothyroidism at diagnosis, the maximum dose of levothyroxine required to maintain the euthyroid state during pregnancy, the presence or absence of thyroid antibodies, and whether or not post-partum thyroiditis occurs, presumably due to an exacerbation of autoimmune thyroid dysfunction post-partum [101].

It is also plausible that in women with pre-existing hypothyroidism, immediate reversion of levothyroxine doses to pre-pregnancy levels could affect lactation; hence maintaining the pregnancy levothyroxine dose for two more weeks or a gradual dose reduction over 4 weeks post-partum may be more appropriate [7].

Monitoring

Preconception

The difficulties inherent to achieving rapid, postconceptional TSH normalization have also focused attention upon preconception TSH modulation. Different cut-off values for preconception TSH, ranging from <1.2 [102] to <2.5 mU/L, have been advocated. A maternal serum TSH concentration <2.5 mU/L is a reasonable goal for such women [3].

In hypothyroid women treated with levothyroxine who are planning pregnancy, serum TSH should be evaluated preconception, and levothyroxine dose adjusted to achieve a TSH value between the lower reference limit and 2.5 mU/L (*strong recommendation, moderate-quality evidence*) [3].

During Pregnancy

Treatment targets for titration of levothyroxine therapy need to be distinguished from the use of trimester-specific reference ranges to diagnose thyroid disease in an untreated individual. The 2017 ATA guidelines now recommend an upper reference limit of TSH around 4.0 mU/L for diagnostic purposes, meanwhile TSH should be kept in the lower-half of the trimester-specific reference range (<2.5 mU/L) when it comes to treatment targets for those on levothyroxine replacement [7].

Women with overt hypothyroidism should be monitored with a serum TSH measurement approximately every 4 weeks until mid-gestation and at least once near 30 weeks gestation (*strong recommendation, high-quality evidence*) [3].

In the care of women with adequately treated hypothyroidism, no other maternal or foetal testing (such as serial foetal ultrasounds, antenatal testing, and/or umbilical blood sampling) is recommended beyond measurement of maternal thyroid function unless needed due to other circumstances of pregnancy. An exception to this is women with Graves-Bassedow effectively treated with ^{131}I ablation or surgical resection, who require TSH receptor antibody (TRAb) monitoring (*strong recommendation, moderate-high quality evidence*) [3].

Women newly diagnosed with overt hypothyroidism or those women known to be hypothyroid but inadequately treated in early gestation will need more frequent thyroid function testing of less than 4 weekly intervals until the target TSH is reached. In women who are overtly hypothyroid in the first trimester, increased surveillance for maternal hypertension and pre-eclampsia as well as foetal growth restriction in the second half of pregnancy may be appropriate [7].

After Delivery

Following delivery, LT4 should be reduced to the patient's preconception dose. Additional thyroid function testing should be performed at approximately 6 weeks post-partum (*strong recommendation, moderate-quality evidence*) [3].

This thyroid function test performed 6 or 8 weeks post-partum will be necessary to confirm euthyroidism or to institute appropriate levothyroxine dose adjustments, particularly in those women who are breastfeeding, or required high dose of levothyroxine or even those who developed post-partum thyroiditis [101].

Summary

- Overt hypothyroidism is present in 1–2% of women of reproductive age.
- This endocrine disorder can have a profound effect on both the well-being of the mother and the foetus, and has been associated with a myriad of adverse perinatal outcomes, such as miscarriage, gestational hypertension, pre-eclampsia, preterm delivery, stillbirth or respiratory distress syndrome in new-borns.
- The long-term consequences of maternal overt hypothyroidism are related to disruption of early brain development: intellectual impairment, behavioural disturbances and other neurodevelopmental disorders in children.
- Treatment of overt hypothyroidism is mandatory, particularly in pregnant women and those who plan to become pregnant.
- Levothyroxine therapy should be closely monitored with a serum TSH measurement every 4 weeks until mid-gestation and at least once near 30-week gestation.
- The main goal in the management of overt hypothyroidism must be to achieve euthyroidism as soon as possible, as well as its maintenance from preconception and throughout pregnancy and post-partum.

References

1. Chiovato L, Magri F, Carlé A. Hypothyroidism in context: where we've been and where we're going. Adv Ther. 2019;36(Suppl 2):47–58. https://doi.org/10.1007/s12325-019-01080-8.
2. Chaker L, Bianco AC, Jonklaas J, Peeters RP. Hypothyroidism. Lancet. 2017;390(10101):1550–62. https://doi.org/10.1016/S0140-6736(17)30703-1.
3. Alexander EK, Pearce EN, Brent GA, Brown RS, Chen H, Dosiou C, Grobman WA, Laurberg P, Lazarus JH, Mandel SJ, Peeters RP, Sullivan S. 2017 guidelines of the American Thyroid Association for the diagnosis and management of thyroid disease during pregnancy and the postpartum. Thyroid. 2017;27(3):315–89. https://doi.org/10.1089/thy.2016.0457.

4. Stagnaro-Green A, Abalovich M, Alexander E, Azizi F, Mestman J, Negro R, Nixon A, Pearce EN, Soldin OP, Sullivan S, Wiersinga W, American Thyroid Association Taskforce on Thyroid Disease During Pregnancy and Postpartum. Guidelines of the American Thyroid Association for the diagnosis and management of thyroid disease during pregnancy and postpartum. Thyroid. 2011;21(10):1081–125. https://doi.org/10.1089/thy.2011.0087.
5. Teng W, Shan Z, Patil-Sisodia K, Cooper DS. Hypothyroidism in pregnancy. Lancet Diabetes Endocrinol. 2013;1(3):228–37. https://doi.org/10.1016/S2213-8587(13)70109-8.
6. Dunn D, Turner C. Hypothyroidism in women. Nurs Womens Health. 2016;20(1):93–8. https://doi.org/10.1016/j.nwh.2015.12.002.
7. Li SW, Chan SY. Management of overt hypothyroidism during pregnancy. Best Pract Res Clin Endocrinol Metab. 2020;34(4):101439. https://doi.org/10.1016/j.beem.2020.101439.
8. Dong AC, Stagnaro-Green A. Differences in diagnostic criteria mask the true prevalence of thyroid disease in pregnancy: a systematic review and meta-analysis. Thyroid. 2019;29(2):278–89. https://doi.org/10.1089/thy.2018.0475.
9. Visser WE, Peeters RP. Interpretation of thyroid function tests during pregnancy. Best Pract Res Clin Endocrinol Metab. 2020;34(4):101431. https://doi.org/10.1016/j.beem.2020.101431.
10. Blatt AJ, Nakamoto JM, Kaufman HW. National status of testing for hypothyroidism during pregnancy and postpartum. J Clin Endocrinol Metab. 2012;97(3):777–84. https://doi.org/10.1210/jc.2011-2038.
11. Stricker R, Echenard M, Eberhart R, Chevailler MC, Perez V, Quinn FA, Stricker R. Evaluation of maternal thyroid function during pregnancy: the importance of using gestational age-specific reference intervals. Eur J Endocrinol. 2007;157(4):509–14. https://doi.org/10.1530/EJE-07-0249.
12. Jouyandeh Z, Hasani-Ranjbar S, Qorbani M, Larijani B. Universal screening versus selective case-based screening for thyroid disorders in pregnancy. Endocrine. 2015;48(1):116–23. https://doi.org/10.1007/s12020-014-0385-9.
13. Pearce EN, Lazarus JH, Moreno-Reyes R, Zimmermann MB. Consequences of iodine deficiency and excess in pregnant women: an overview of current knowns and unknowns. Am J Clin Nutr. 2016;104 Suppl 3(Suppl 3):918S–23S. https://doi.org/10.3945/ajcn.115.110429.
14. Zimmermann MB, Boelaert K. Iodine deficiency and thyroid disorders. Lancet Diabetes Endocrinol. 2015;3(4):286–95. https://doi.org/10.1016/S2213-8587(14)70225-6.
15. Asvold BO, Bjøro T, Nilsen TI, Vatten LJ. Tobacco smoking and thyroid function: a population-based study. Arch Intern Med. 2007;167(13):1428–32. https://doi.org/10.1001/archinte.167.13.1428.
16. Derakhshan A, Shu H, Broeren MAC, de Poortere RA, Wikström S, Peeters RP, Demeneix B, Bornehag CG, Korevaar TIM. Reference ranges and determinants of thyroid function during early pregnancy: the SELMA study. J Clin Endocrinol Metab. 2018;103(9):3548–56. https://doi.org/10.1210/jc.2018-00890.
17. Effraimidis G, Tijssen JG, Wiersinga WM. Discontinuation of smoking increases the risk for developing thyroid peroxidase antibodies and/or thyroglobulin antibodies: a prospective study. J Clin Endocrinol Metab. 2009;94(4):1324–8. https://doi.org/10.1210/jc.2008-1548.
18. Andersen SL, Olsen J, Wu CS, Laurberg P. Smoking reduces the risk of hypothyroidism and increases the risk of hyperthyroidism: evidence from 450,842 mothers giving birth in Denmark. Clin Endocrinol. 2014;80(2):307–14. https://doi.org/10.1111/cen.12279.
19. Bryant SN, Nelson DB, McIntire DD, Casey BM, Cunningham FG. An analysis of population-based prenatal screening for overt hypothyroidism. Am J Obstet Gynecol. 2015;213(4):565.e1–6. https://doi.org/10.1016/j.ajog.2015.06.061.
20. Horacek J, Spitalnikova S, Dlabalova B, Malirova E, Vizda J, Svilias I, Cepkova J, McGrath C, Maly J. Universal screening detects two-times more thyroid disorders in early pregnancy than targeted high-risk case finding. Eur J Endocrinol. 2010;163(4):645–50. https://doi.org/10.1530/EJE-10-0516.
21. Taylor PN, Albrecht D, Scholz A, Gutierrez-Buey G, Lazarus JH, Dayan CM, Okosieme OE. Global epidemiology of hyperthyroidism and hypothyroidism. Nat Rev Endocrinol. 2018;14(5):301–16. https://doi.org/10.1038/nrendo.2018.18.

22. Nygaard B. Hypothyroidism (primary). BMJ Clin Evid. 2014;2014:0605.
23. Effraimidis G, Strieder TG, Tijssen JG, Wiersinga WM. Natural history of the transition from euthyroidism to overt autoimmune hypo- or hyperthyroidism: a prospective study. Eur J Endocrinol. 2011;164(1):107–13. https://doi.org/10.1530/EJE-10-0785.
24. Huber G, Staub JJ, Meier C, Mitrache C, Guglielmetti M, Huber P, Braverman LE. Prospective study of the spontaneous course of subclinical hypothyroidism: prognostic value of thyrotropin, thyroid reserve, and thyroid antibodies. J Clin Endocrinol Metab. 2002;87(7):3221–6. https://doi.org/10.1210/jcem.87.7.8678.
25. Strieder TG, Tijssen JG, Wenzel BE, Endert E, Wiersinga WM. Prediction of progression to overt hypothyroidism or hyperthyroidism in female relatives of patients with autoimmune thyroid disease using the thyroid events Amsterdam (THEA) score. Arch Intern Med. 2008;168(15):1657–63. https://doi.org/10.1001/archinte.168.15.1657.
26. Vanderpump MP, Tunbridge WM, French JM, Appleton D, Bates D, Clark F, Grimley Evans J, Hasan DM, Rodgers H, Tunbridge F, et al. The incidence of thyroid disorders in the community: a twenty-year follow-up of the Whickham survey. Clin Endocrinol. 1995;43(1):55–68. https://doi.org/10.1111/j.1365-2265.1995.tb01894.x.
27. Persani L, Brabant G, Dattani M, Bonomi M, Feldt-Rasmussen U, Fliers E, Gruters A, Maiter D, Schoenmakers N, van Trotsenburg ASP. 2018 European Thyroid Association (ETA) guidelines on the diagnosis and management of central hypothyroidism. Eur Thyroid J. 2018;7(5):225–37. https://doi.org/10.1159/000491388.
28. Luongo C, Trivisano L, Alfano F, Salvatore D. Type 3 deiodinase and consumptive hypothyroidism: a common mechanism for a rare disease. Front Endocrinol (Lausanne). 2013;4:115. https://doi.org/10.3389/fendo.2013.00115.
29. Dumitrescu AM, Refetoff S. The syndromes of reduced sensitivity to thyroid hormone. Biochim Biophys Acta. 2013;1830(7):3987–4003. https://doi.org/10.1016/j.bbagen.2012.08.005.
30. López-Muñoz E, Mateos-Sánchez L, Mejía-Terrazas GE, Bedwell-Cordero SE Hypothyroidism and isolated hypothyroxinemia in pregnancy, from physiology to the clinic. Taiwan J Obstet Gynecol. 2019;58(6):757–63. https://doi.org/10.1016/j.tjog.2019.09.005.
31. Carlé A, Pedersen IB, Knudsen N, et al. Gender differences in symptoms of hypothyroidism: a population-based DanThyr study. Clin Endocrinol. 2015;83:717–25.
32. Carlé A, Pedersen IB, Knudsen N, Perrild H, Ovesen L, Laurberg P. Hypothyroid symptoms and the likelihood of overt thyroid failure: a population-based case-control study. Eur J Endocrinol. 2014;171(5):593–602. https://doi.org/10.1530/EJE-14-0481.
33. Pop VJ, Broeren MA, Wiersinga WM, Stagnaro-Green A. Thyroid disease symptoms during early pregnancy do not identify women with thyroid hypofunction that should be treated. Clin Endocrinol. 2017;87(6):838–43. https://doi.org/10.1111/cen.13433.
34. Nazarpour S, Ramezani Tehrani F, Rahmati M, Minooee S, Simbar M, Noroozzadeh M, Azizi F. Validation of Billewicz scoring system for detection of overt hypothyroidism during pregnancy. Int J Endocrinol Metab. 2018;16(3):e64249. https://doi.org/10.5812/ijem.64249. eCollection 2018 Jul.
35. American College of Obstetricians and Gynecologists' Committee on practice bulletins—obstetrics. Thyroid disease in pregnancy: ACOG practice bulletin, number 223. Obstet Gynecol. 2020;135(6):e261–74. https://doi.org/10.1097/AOG.0000000000003893.
36. Vaidya B, Anthony S, Bilous M, Shields B, Drury J, Hutchison S, Bilous R. Detection of thyroid dysfunction in early pregnancy: universal screening or targeted high-risk case finding? J Clin Endocrinol Metab. 2007;92(1):203–7. https://doi.org/10.1210/jc.2006-1748.
37. Taylor PN, Lazarus JH. Hypothyroidism in pregnancy. Endocrinol Metab Clin N Am. 2019;48(3):547–56. https://doi.org/10.1016/j.ecl.2019.05.010.
38. Korevaar TI, Medici M, de Rijke YB, Visser W, de Muinck Keizer-Schrama SM, Jaddoe VW, Hofman A, Ross HA, Visser WE, Hooijkaas H, Steegers EA, Tiemeier H, Bongers-Schokking JJ, Visser TJ, Peeters RP. Ethnic differences in maternal thyroid parameters during pregnancy: the Generation R Study. J Clin Endocrinol Metab. 2013;98(9):3678–86. https://doi.org/10.1210/jc.2013-2005.

39. Velasco I, Soldevila B, Martínez-Mondejar R, Muñoz C, Ferrer L, et al. Thyroid function variability in a cohort of healthy pregnant women: effect of BMI, smoking and iodized salt consumption. LOJ Pharm Clin Res. 2020;2(2):LOJPCR.MS.ID.000134. https://doi.org/10.32474/LOJPCR.2020.02.000134.
40. Korevaar TI, de Rijke YB, Chaker L, Medici M, Jaddoe VW, Steegers EA, Visser TJ, Peeters RP. Stimulation of thyroid function by human chorionic gonadotropin during pregnancy: a risk factor for thyroid disease and a mechanism for known risk factors. Thyroid. 2017;27(3):440–50. https://doi.org/10.1089/thy.2016.0527.
41. Velasco I, Taylor P. Identifying and treating subclinical thyroid dysfunction in pregnancy: emerging controversies. Eur J Endocrinol. 2018;178(1):D1–D12. https://doi.org/10.1530/EJE-17-0598.
42. Krassas GE, Markou KB. The impact of thyroid diseases starting from birth on reproductive function. Hormones (Athens). 2019;18(4):365–81. https://doi.org/10.1007/s42000-019-00156-y.
43. Koyyada A, Orsu P. Role of hypothyroidism and associated pathways in pregnancy and infertility: clinical insights. Tzu Chi Med J. 2020;32(4):312–7. https://doi.org/10.4103/tcmj.tcmj_255_19. eCollection 2020 Oct-Dec.
44. Davis LE, Leveno KJ, Cunningham FG. Hypothyroidism complicating pregnancy. Obstet Gynecol. 1988;72(1):108–12.
45. Leung AS, Millar LK, Koonings PP, Montoro M, Mestman JH. Perinatal outcome in hypothyroid pregnancies. Obstet Gynecol. 1993;81(3):349–53.
46. Unuane D, Velkeniers B. Impact of thyroid disease on fertility and assisted conception. Best Pract Res Clin Endocrinol Metab. 2020;34(4):101378. https://doi.org/10.1016/j.beem.2020.101378.
47. Nazarpour S, Ramezani Tehrani F, Simbar M, Azizi F. Thyroid dysfunction and pregnancy outcomes. Iran J Reprod Med. 2015;13(7):387–96.
48. Shinohara DR, Santos TDS, de Carvalho HC, Lopes LCB, Günther LSA, Aristides SMA, Teixeira JJV, Demarchi IG. Pregnancy complications associated with maternal hypothyroidism: a systematic review. Obstet Gynecol Surv. 2018;73(4):219–30. https://doi.org/10.1097/OGX.0000000000000547.
49. Morreale de Escobar G, Obregon MJ, Escobar del Rey F. Role of thyroid hormone during early brain development. Eur J Endocrinol. 2004;151(Suppl 3):U25–37. https://doi.org/10.1530/eje.0.151u025.
50. Abalovich M, Gutierrez S, Alcaraz G, Maccallini G, Garcia A, Levalle O. Overt and subclinical hypothyroidism complicating pregnancy. Thyroid. 2002;12(1):63–8. https://doi.org/10.1089/105072502753451986.
51. Hirsch D, Levy S, Nadler V, Kopel V, Shainberg B, Toledano Y. Pregnancy outcomes in women with severe hypothyroidism. Eur J Endocrinol. 2013;169(3):313–20. https://doi.org/10.1530/EJE-13-0228.
52. Yang Y, Hou Y, Wang H, Gao X, Wang X, Li J, Teng W, Shan Z. Maternal thyroid dysfunction and gestational anemia risk: meta-analysis and new data. Front Endocrinol (Lausanne). 2020;11:201. https://doi.org/10.3389/fendo.2020.00201. eCollection 2020.
53. Männistö T, Mendola P, Grewal J, Xie Y, Chen Z, Laughon SK. Thyroid diseases and adverse pregnancy outcomes in a contemporary US cohort. J Clin Endocrinol Metab. 2013;98(7):2725–33. https://doi.org/10.1210/jc.2012-4233.
54. Wolfberg AJ, Lee-Parritz A, Peller AJ, Lieberman ES. Obstetric and neonatal outcomes associated with maternal hypothyroid disease. J Matern Fetal Neonatal Med. 2005;17(1):35–8. https://doi.org/10.1080/14767050400028642.
55. Ajmani SN, Aggarwal D, Bhatia P, Sharma M, Sarabhai V, Paul M. Prevalence of overt and subclinical thyroid dysfunction among pregnant women and its effect on maternal and fetal outcome. J Obstet Gynaecol India. 2014;64(2):105–10. https://doi.org/10.1007/s13224-013-0487-y.

56. Cleary-Goldman J, Malone FD, Lambert-Messerlian G, Sullivan L, Canick J, Porter TF, Luthy D, Gross S, Bianchi DW, D'Alton ME. Maternal thyroid hypofunction and pregnancy outcome. Obstet Gynecol. 2008;112(1):85–92. https://doi.org/10.1097/AOG.0b013e3181788dd7.
57. Idris I, Srinivasan R, Simm A, Page RC. Maternal hypothyroidism in early and late gestation: effects on neonatal and obstetric outcome. Clin Endocrinol. 2005;63(5):560–5. https://doi.org/10.1111/j.1365-2265.2005.02382.x.
58. Sahu MT, Das V, Mittal S, Agarwal A, Sahu M. Overt and subclinical thyroid dysfunction among Indian pregnant women and its effect on maternal and fetal outcome. Arch Gynecol Obstet. 2010;281(2):215–20. https://doi.org/10.1007/s00404-009-1105-1.
59. Turunen S, Vääräsmäki M, Männistö T, Hartikainen AL, Lahesmaa-Korpinen AM, Gissler M, Suvanto E. Pregnancy and perinatal outcome among hypothyroid mothers: a population-based cohort study. Thyroid. 2019;29(1):135–41. https://doi.org/10.1089/thy.2018.0311.
60. Wasserstrum N, Anania CA. Perinatal consequences of maternal hypothyroidism in early pregnancy and inadequate replacement. Clin Endocrinol. 1995;42(4):353–8. https://doi.org/10.1111/j.1365-2265.1995.tb02642.x.
61. Ashoor G, Maiz N, Rotas M, Jawdat F, Nicolaides KH. Maternal thyroid function at 11 to 13 weeks of gestation and subsequent fetal death. Thyroid. 2010;20(9):989–93. https://doi.org/10.1089/thy.2010.0058.
62. Su PY, Huang K, Hao JH, Xu YQ, Yan SQ, Li T, Xu YH, Tao FB. Maternal thyroid function in the first twenty weeks of pregnancy and subsequent fetal and infant development: a prospective population-based cohort study in China. J Clin Endocrinol Metab. 2011;96(10):3234–41. https://doi.org/10.1210/jc.2011-0274.
63. Klein RZ, Sargent JD, Larsen PR, Waisbren SE, Haddow JE, Mitchell ML. Relation of severity of maternal hypothyroidism to cognitive development of offspring. J Med Screen. 2001;8:18–20.
64. Wang P, Gao J, Zhao S, Guo Y, Wang Z, Qi F. Maternal thyroxine levels during pregnancy and outcomes of cognitive development in children. Mol Neurobiol. 2016;53(4):2241–8. https://doi.org/10.1007/s12035-015-9189-z.
65. Allan WC, Haddow JE, Palomaki GE, Williams JR, Mitchell ML, Hermos RJ, Faix JD, Klein RZ. Maternal thyroid deficiency and pregnancy complications: implications for population screening. J Med Screen. 2000;7(3):127–30. https://doi.org/10.1136/jms.7.3.127.
66. Wikner BN, Sparre LS, Stiller CO, Källén B, Asker C. Maternal use of thyroid hormones in pregnancy and neonatal outcome. Acta Obstet Gynecol Scand. 2008;87(6):617–27. https://doi.org/10.1080/00016340802075103.
67. Männistö T, Vääräsmäki M, Pouta A, Hartikainen AL, Ruokonen A, Surcel HM, Bloigu A, Järvelin MR, Suvanto-Luukkonen E. Perinatal outcome of children born to mothers with thyroid dysfunction or antibodies: a prospective population-based cohort study. J Clin Endocrinol Metab. 2009;94(3):772–9. https://doi.org/10.1210/jc.2008-1520.
68. Männistö T, Mendola P, Reddy U, Laughon SK. Neonatal outcomes and birth weight in pregnancies complicated by maternal thyroid disease. Am J Epidemiol. 2013;178(5):731–40. https://doi.org/10.1093/aje/kwt031.
69. Andersen SL, Olsen J, Wu CS, Laurberg P. Low birth weight in children born to mothers with hyperthyroidism and high birth weight in hypothyroidism, whereas preterm birth is common in both conditions: a Danish National Hospital Register Study. Eur Thyroid J. 2013;2(2):135–44. https://doi.org/10.1159/000350513.
70. Lee SY, Cabral HJ, Aschengrau A, Pearce EN. Associations between maternal thyroid function in pregnancy and obstetric and perinatal outcomes. J Clin Endocrinol Metab. 2020;105(5):e2015–23. https://doi.org/10.1210/clinem/dgz275.
71. Lai H, Zhan ZY, Liu H. Association between thyroid hormone parameters during early pregnancy and gestational hypertension: a prospective cohort study. J Int Med Res. 2020;48(2):300060520904814. https://doi.org/10.1177/0300060520904814.
72. Sheehan PM, Nankervis A, Araujo Júnior E, Da Silva Costa F. Maternal thyroid disease and preterm birth: systematic review and meta-analysis. J Clin Endocrinol Metab. 2015;100(11):4325–31. https://doi.org/10.1210/jc.2015-3074.

73. Wang S, Li M, Chu D, Liang L, Zhao X, Zhang J. Clinical or subclinical hypothyroidism and thyroid autoantibody before 20 weeks pregnancy and risk of preterm birth: a systematic review. Zhonghua Fu Chan Ke Za Zhi. 2014;49(11):816–22.
74. Batistuzzo A, Ribeiro MO. Clinical and subclinical maternal hypothyroidism and their effects on neurodevelopment, behavior and cognition. Arch Endocrinol Metab. 2020;64(1):89–95. https://doi.org/10.20945/2359-3997000000201.
75. Haddow JE, Palomaki GE, Allan WC, Williams JR, Knight GJ, Gagnon J, O'Heir CE, Mitchell ML, Hermos RJ, Waisbren SE, Faix JD, Klein RZ. Maternal thyroid deficiency during pregnancy and subsequent neuropsychological development of the child. N Engl J Med. 1999;341(8):549–55. https://doi.org/10.1056/NEJM199908193410801.
76. Korevaar TIM, Tiemeier H, Peeters RP. Clinical associations of maternal thyroid function with foetal brain development: epidemiological interpretation and overview of available evidence. Clin Endocrinol. 2018;89(2):129–38. https://doi.org/10.1111/cen.13724.
77. Fetene DM, Betts KS, Alati R. Mechanisms in endocrinology: maternal thyroid dysfunction during pregnancy and behavioural and psychiatric disorders of children: a systematic review. Eur J Endocrinol. 2017;177(5):R261–73. https://doi.org/10.1530/EJE-16-0860.
78. Ge GM, Leung MTY, Man KKC, Leung WC, Ip P, Li GHY, Wong ICK, Kung AWC, Cheung CL. Maternal thyroid dysfunction during pregnancy and the risk of adverse outcomes in the offspring: a systematic review and meta-analysis. J Clin Endocrinol Metab. 2020;105(12):dgaa555. https://doi.org/10.1210/clinem/dgaa555.
79. Jansen TA, Korevaar TIM, Mulder TA, White T, Muetzel RL, Peeters RP, Tiemeier H. Maternal thyroid function during pregnancy and child brain morphology: a time window-specific analysis of a prospective cohort. Lancet Diabetes Endocrinol. 2019;7(8):629–37. https://doi.org/10.1016/S2213-8587(19)30153-6.
80. Korevaar TI, Muetzel R, Medici M, Chaker L, Jaddoe VW, de Rijke YB, Steegers EA, Visser TJ, White T, Tiemeier H, Peeters RP. Association of maternal thyroid function during early pregnancy with offspring IQ and brain morphology in childhood: a population-based prospective cohort study. Lancet Diabetes Endocrinol. 2016;4(1):35–43. https://doi.org/10.1016/S2213-8587(15)00327-7.
81. Päkkilä F, Männistö T, Surcel HM, Ruokonen A, Bloigu A, Pouta A, Hartikainen AL, Vääräsmäki M, Järvelin MR, Suvanto E. Maternal thyroid dysfunction during pregnancy and thyroid function of her child in adolescence. J Clin Endocrinol Metab. 2013;98(3):965–72.
82. Vissenberg R, van den Boogaard E, van Wely M, van der Post JA, Fliers E, Bisschop PH, Goddijn M. Treatment of thyroid disorders before conception and in early pregnancy: a systematic review. Hum Reprod Update. 2012;18(4):360–73. https://doi.org/10.1093/humupd/dms007.
83. Zhou M, Wang M, Li J, Luo X, Lei M. Effects of thyroid diseases on pregnancy outcomes. Exp Ther Med. 2019;18(3):1807–15. https://doi.org/10.3892/etm.2019.7739.
84. Krassas GE, Poppe K, Glinoer D. Thyroid function and human reproductive health. Endocr Rev. 2010;31(5):702–55. https://doi.org/10.1210/er.2009-0041.
85. Abalovich M, Vázquez A, Alcaraz G, Kitaigrodsky A, Szuman G, Calabrese C, Astarita G, Frydman M, Gutiérrez S. Adequate levothyroxine doses for the treatment of hypothyroidism newly discovered during pregnancy. Thyroid. 2013;23(11):1479–83. https://doi.org/10.1089/thy.2013.0024.
86. Okosieme OE, Khan I, Taylor PN. Preconception management of thyroid dysfunction. Clin Endocrinol. 2018;89(3):269–79. https://doi.org/10.1111/cen.13731.
87. Okosieme O, Gilbert J, Abraham P, Boelaert K, Dayan C, Gurnell M, Leese G, McCabe C, Perros P, Smith V, Williams G, Vanderpump M. Management of primary hypothyroidism: statement by the British Thyroid Association Executive Committee. Clin Endocrinol. 2016;84(6):799–808. https://doi.org/10.1111/cen.12824.
88. Khandelwal D, Tandon N. Overt and subclinical hypothyroidism: who to treat and how. Drugs. 2012;72(1):17–33. https://doi.org/10.2165/11598070-000000000-00000.

89. Pop V, Broeren M, Wiersinga W. The attitude toward hypothyroidism during early gestation: time for a change of mind? Thyroid. 2014;24(10):1541–6. https://doi.org/10.1089/thy.2014.0007.
90. Stagnaro-Green A, Dong A, Stephenson MD. Universal screening for thyroid disease during pregnancy should be performed. Best Pract Res Clin Endocrinol Metab. 2020;34(4):101320. https://doi.org/10.1016/j.beem.2019.101320.
91. Lazarus JH, Bestwick JP, Channon S, Paradice R, Maina A, Rees R, Chiusano E, John R, Guaraldo V, George LM, Perona M, Dall'Amico D, Parkes AB, Joomun M, Wald NJ. Antenatal thyroid screening and childhood cognitive function. N Engl J Med. 2012;366(6):493–501. https://doi.org/10.1056/NEJMoa1106104.
92. Maraka S, Singh Ospina NM, O'Keeffe DT, Rodriguez-Gutierrez R, Espinosa De Ycaza AE, Wi CI, Juhn YJ, Coddington CC 3rd, Montori VM. Effects of increasing levothyroxine on pregnancy outcomes in women with uncontrolled hypothyroidism. Clin Endocrinol. 2017;86(1):150–5. https://doi.org/10.1111/cen.13168.
93. Korevaar TIM, Medici M, Visser TJ, Peeters RP. Thyroid disease in pregnancy: new insights in diagnosis and clinical management. Nat Rev Endocrinol. 2017;13(10):610–22. https://doi.org/10.1038/nrendo.2017.93.
94. Shan Z, Teng W. Thyroid hormone therapy of hypothyroidism in pregnancy. Endocrine. 2019;66(1):35–42. https://doi.org/10.1007/s12020-019-02044-2.
95. Taylor PN, Minassian C, Rehman A, Iqbal A, Draman MS, Hamilton W, Dunlop D, Robinson A, Vaidya B, Lazarus JH, Thomas S, Dayan CM, Okosieme OE. TSH levels and risk of miscarriage in women on long-term levothyroxine: a community-based study. J Clin Endocrinol Metab. 2014;99(10):3895–902. https://doi.org/10.1210/jc.2014-1954.
96. Alexander EK, Marqusee E, Lawrence J, Jarolim P, Fischer GA, Larsen PR. Timing and magnitude of increases in levothyroxine requirements during pregnancy in women with hypothyroidism. N Engl J Med. 2004;351(3):241–9. https://doi.org/10.1056/NEJMoa040079.
97. Verga U, Bergamaschi S, Cortelazzi D, Ronzoni S, Marconi AM, Beck-Peccoz P. Adjustment of L-T4 substitutive therapy in pregnant women with subclinical, overt or post-ablative hypothyroidism. Clin Endocrinol. 2009;70(5):798–802. https://doi.org/10.1111/j.1365-2265.2008.03398.x.
98. Loh JA, Wartofsky L, Jonklaas J, Burman KD. The magnitude of increased levothyroxine requirements in hypothyroid pregnant women depends upon the etiology of the hypothyroidism. Thyroid. 2009;19(3):269–75. https://doi.org/10.1089/thy.2008.0413.
99. Yassa L, Marqusee E, Fawcett R, Alexander EK. Thyroid hormone early adjustment in pregnancy (the THERAPY) trial. J Clin Endocrinol Metab. 2010;95(7):3234–41. https://doi.org/10.1210/jc.2010-0013.
100. Hales C, Taylor PN, Channon S, McEwan K, Thapar A, Langley K, Muller I, Draman MS, Dayan C, Gregory JW, Okosieme O, Lazarus JH, Rees DA, Ludgate M. Controlled antenatal thyroid screening II: effect of treating maternal suboptimal thyroid function on child behavior. J Clin Endocrinol Metab. 2020;105(3):dgz098. https://doi.org/10.1210/clinem/dgz098.
101. Stagnaro-Green A. Postpartum management of women begun on levothyroxine during pregnancy. Front Endocrinol (Lausanne). 2015;6:183. https://doi.org/10.3389/fendo.2015.00183. eCollection 2015.
102. Abalovich M, Alcaraz G, Kleiman-Rubinsztein J, Pavlove MM, Cornelio C, Levalle O, Gutierrez S. The relationship of preconception thyrotropin levels to requirements for increasing the levothyroxine dose during pregnancy in women with primary hypothyroidism. Thyroid. 2010;20(10):1175–8. https://doi.org/10.1089/thy.2009.0457.

Gestational Subclinical Hypothyroidism

Creswell J. Eastman and Norman J. Blumenthal

Introduction

Commencing early in the first trimester, pregnancy has a profound effect on the human thyroid gland, characterised by a 25–50% increase in thyroid hormone production with a comparable increase in iodine requirements [1]. Increased thyroid hormone production and secretion is driven by placental human chorionic gonadotrophin (hCG) stimulating the thyroid to increase thyroxine (T4) production resulting in a downward shift of the normal adult reference range for serum thyrotropin (TSH) in the first half of pregnancy [1]. The foetal thyroid does not develop until early in the second trimester and it remains uncertain when the balance of thyroid hormone utilisation in the foetus switches from maternal to foetal thyroid gland production, but it is likely that maternal transfer of T4 contributes to the foetal thyroid hormone requirements up until the time of birth [1].

Impaired maternal thyroid function is a common occurrence during pregnancy and there is strong clinical belief that it should be detected and treated early to prevent adverse obstetrical and foetal outcomes [2]. While the negative impact of overt maternal hypothyroidism (OH) on both the pregnancy and subsequent neurodevelopment of the child is not disputed, the frequency and nature of adverse effects of maternal subclinical hypothyroidism (SCH) on both the pregnancy and the foetus remain controversial. The prevalence, clinical features, and possible adverse outcomes of maternal SCH have attracted a large amount of attention, with numerous

C. J. Eastman (✉)
Faculty of Medicine and Health Sydney Medical School, The University of Sydney NSW Australia and Consultant Emeritus Westmead Hospital, Westmead, NSW, Australia
e-mail: creswell.eastman@sydney.edu.au

N. J. Blumenthal
Consultant Obstetrician and Gynaecologist Blacktown Hospital and Notre Dame University, Sydney, NSW, Australia

F. Azizi, F. Ramezani Tehrani (eds.), *Thyroid Diseases in Pregnancy*,
https://doi.org/10.1007/978-3-030-98777-0_7

publications in recent years, but instead of clarity these efforts have generated more controversy than certainty [3–5].

Several recent systematic reviews and meta-analyses of SCH in pregnancy have concluded that pregnant women with SCH were at higher risk for multiple adverse maternal and neonatal outcomes, including pregnancy loss, placental abruption, premature labour, intrauterine growth retardation and low birth weight infants [3–5]. Despite a large list of obstetric and foetal complications derived from observational studies, these reviews concluded that evidence was lacking for a beneficial effect of LT4 therapy administered to pregnant women with SCH, but they emphasised the inconsistency of definitions used in studies included in the reviews, the paucity of robust therapeutic clinical trials of LT4 replacement and the lack of consensus on these issues among clinicians and researchers [3–5].

Definition of SCH

Confirmation of hypothyroidism, be it overt or subclinical, can only be achieved by measurement of the serum thyroid stimulating hormone (TSH) level as early as possible in gestation. Measurement of serum TSH is generally recommended by most authorities as the appropriate screening test or first-line laboratory investigation for detection of thyroid dysfunction in pregnancy. OH is defined as a serum TSH > 10 mIU/L, usually with a subnormal free thyroxine FT4 level, while SCH is defined as a serum TSH increased above the upper limit of the normal reference range for pregnancy, and characterised by a normal serum FT4 level [2, 6–8]. In the absence of a locally derived and validated pregnancy reference range the American Endocrine Society guidelines recommend a TSH level above 2.5 mIU/L and the ATA recommends a level of 4.0 mIU/L in the first trimester above which LT4 treatment should be instituted or considered [2, 8].

Reference Ranges for Serum TSH for Diagnosis of SCH

The euthyroid reference range for serum TSH undergoes a downward shift early in the first trimester of pregnancy due to the stimulatory effect of hCG on the thyroid gland, via stimulation of the TSH receptor, increasing thyroid hormone secretion and thereby partly suppressing pituitary TSH production. With the decline in hCG stimulation during the second and third trimesters, the serum TSH gradually returns to within the pre-pregnancy range by the time of delivery. Herein lies the first diagnostic challenge for the clinician in decision-making. What reference range for serum TSH should the clinician use? There is consensus that the TSH reference range should be pregnancy and trimester specific and developed from a local population that is iodine sufficient and free from any underlying thyroid disorder [8]. Unfortunately, there is lack of consensus among expert authorities on the upper limit of the normal serum TSH level, or cut-off value, for the diagnosis of SCH, but expert guidelines usually recommend that each laboratory establishes a valid reference range for each trimester of pregnancy derived from its local population [8]. Where locally derived reference ranges have not been developed, default reference TSH ranges have been provided in guideline publications. The American Endocrine Society recommended a serum TSH concentration of 2.5 mIU/L as the upper limit of normal in the first trimester of pregnancy and 3.0 mIU/L in the second trimester [2] and this figure was also the recommended upper limit of normal in the 2011 ATA guidelines [6] and the European Thyroid Association (ETA) guidelines in 2014 [7]. The most recent ATA guidelines, published in 2017, recommends using population-based, trimester-specific TSH reference ranges or, if these trimester and assay-specific ranges are not available, using an upper reference limit of 4.0 mIU/L [8]. The ATA guidelines state that serum TSH reference range determinations should consider iodine intake, TPO (thyroid peroxidase) positivity, and according to other studies, body mass index [8]. Variations in TSH reference ranges with ethnicity are now recognised as being considerable from one population to the next, as judged by the numerous reports of reference ranges from many different countries around the globe. Ethnicity as a determinant is well illustrated in the Generation R Study in the Netherlands, where ethnic differences in pregnant women living in the Netherlands caused significant diagnostic discrepancies depending on whether population or ethnicity-specific reference ranges were used to diagnose thyroid disorders [9].

Another influence on the TSH reference range that has not been well explored is the effect and potential bias of the analytical platform on which the TSH level is measured. Several recent reports of comparisons between some of the results from the more popular commercial platforms have shown consistent differences or bias in measured TSH concentrations, particularly around the upper limit of the normal TSH reference range used for confirming or excluding gestational SCH [10–13]. This issue has not received the attention it deserves in systematic reviews and meta-analyses of gestational SCH, where data from different centres and analytical platforms are aggregated without specific reference to the method and cut-off TSH level used to make the diagnosis of SCH.

In practice, it is our experience that most laboratories either use reference ranges for TSH and FT4 provided by the manufacturer for the analytical platform and their reagents or alternatively they revert to one of the default ranges provided by published guidelines most commonly being the 2017 ATA guidelines [8]. Until recently, reference ranges for pregnancy used by commercial laboratories were essentially the same as reference ranges for the general population. A good example of this variation in pregnancy reference ranges among platforms and analytical methods is shown in Table 1. In the city of Sydney, NSW, Australia, with a population of approximately five million people, there are multiple independent hospital and commercial laboratories with their own TSH and FT4 pregnancy reference ranges, which have traditionally been provided by the manufacturer of the analytical platform on which the assays are performed. Reference ranges for four of the largest reputable commercial laboratories in Sydney are shown in Table 1 and demonstrate how reference ranges and cut-off points for diagnosis of SCH can vary from one laboratory to another. Free T4 reference ranges also differ significantly from one provider to the next as shown in Table 1.

Table 1 Thyroid function reference ranges for pregnancy in Sydney commercial pathology laboratories 2018

Laboratory[a]	TSH reference range (mIU/L)	Free T4 reference range (pmol/L)	Analytical platform
1. Laverty (Trimesters)	0.03–2.5 0.05–3.0 0.3–3.5	10–21 11–18 9.2–17	Bayer Advia Centaur
2. Medlab (Trimesters)	0.1–2.5 0.2–3.0 0.3–3.0	10.0–24	Abbott Architect
3. Aust Clinical Labs	0.1–3.7 0.4–3.8 0.3–3.4	9.0–25	Siemens
4. Douglass Hanly Moir	0.3–2.8 0.1–2.5 0.3–2.9	11.0–19.0	Abbott Architect

[a]Laboratories 1 and 2 provide a cut-off value of >2.5 mIU/L for diagnosis of SCH consistent with the American Endocrine Society Guidelines (Reference 2). Laboratory 3 approximates the ATA Guidelines cut-off value of >4.0 mIU/L for SCH (Reference 8) and Laboratory 4 which has derived its own reference range sits in between

Several studies have shown that serum TSH values vary with different analytical platforms, such that the diagnosis of thyroid dysfunction, particularly SCH, is not consistent or interchangeable between different assays [10–13]. For example, in a comparison of results obtained between the Roche-Cobas and Abbott systems, two of the commonest analytical methods, the determinations on the Cobas system were consistently higher than the Abbott system results [10]. Similarly, in a comparative study of four different platforms (Roche, Abbott, Beckman, and Siemens), the authors again found that TSH levels on the Roche platform measured higher than the Abbott platform in all trimesters of pregnancy, with results from Beckman and Siemens systems sitting in between the Roche and Abbott systems and not being significantly different from one another [12]. It is not clear if assay results from the Roche system may lead to overdiagnosis and likely unnecessary treatment of SCH or if Abbott assays may lead to underdiagnosis and undertreatment of SCH.

The results of a recent online survey of Endocrinologists in the USA provided surprising information from responders, with a majority (52%) stating they used the Endocrine Society TSH cut-off level of 2.5 mIU/L for diagnosis of SCH, 25% used the ATA recommendation of 4.0 mIU/L and a smaller percentage used local population-based levels [13]. The American College of Obstetricians and Gynecologists (ACOG) states that universal screening for thyroid disease in pregnancy is not recommended because identification and treatment of maternal SCH has not been shown to result in improved pregnancy outcomes and/or neurocognitive function in offspring [14]. Other specialist Colleges of Obstetrics and Gynaecology, such as the Royal Australian and New Zealand College of Obstetricians and Gynaecologists (RANZCOG), takes a similar position stating "screening for subclinical hypothyroidism or TPO antibodies and subsequent treatment with thyroxine is not recommended in pregnancy" [15]. In essence, both august bodies are virtually dismissing SCH as a relevant clinical condition in pregnant women, yet paradoxically both recommend maintenance of a serum TSH level below 2.5 mIU/L in patients being treated with LT4 for hypothyroidism [14, 15]. As Maraka and colleagues have stated the real challenge is to establish the TSH level above which women experience adverse pregnancy outcomes and whether the administration of LT4 therapy prevents these adverse outcomes, and this remains an unresolved issue [4].

Measurement of FT4 and Thyroid Autoantibodies in the Diagnosis of SCH

When the TSH concentration is outside the employed pregnancy reference range, measurement of the free T4 level is usually recommended to confirm a diagnosis of OH or SCH. Serum FT4 measurement is not recommended as a frontline or screening test for determining thyroid function during pregnancy because automated immunoassay methods used in clinical diagnostic laboratories are influenced by changes in thyroid hormone binding proteins, such as increases in circulating thyroxine binding globulin (TBG) and decreases in albumin, resulting in potential artefactual errors in FT4 levels [2, 8]. Measurement of free T4 levels by equilibrium dialysis or liquid chromatography/tandem mass spectrometry (LCMS) are more accurate, but these tests are expensive and not readily available in clinical practice [8]. When serum free T4 measurements are performed on pregnant patients, the results should be reported, where possible, according to locally derived, validated, trimester-specific reference ranges. We can only speculate how often this occurs in clinical practice.

Adverse pregnancy outcomes in women with SCH appear to be most influenced by underlying thyroid autoimmunity [8]. In a recent metanalysis of 199 prospective cohort studies comprising 47,045 women, Korevaar and colleagues reported that SCH, isolated hypothyroxinaemia, and thyroid peroxidase antibody (TPOAb) positivity in pregnant women are risk factors for preterm birth [16]. Again, while we express concern about decisions made from aggregated data of patients diagnosed with gestational SCH where different methods have been employed for measurement of TSH, FT4 and TPOAb concentrations, the data derived from the very large number of subjects from the Korevaar study is persuasive. The ATA guidelines state that thyroid autoantibodies have been reported as positive in 2–17% of unselected pregnant women. Prevalence rates vary widely with ethnicity, age, and analytical methods used to detect thyroid antibodies. In our own series of 1025 pregnant patients attending a private obstetrical practice in Sydney, Australia, we found the prevalence to be surprisingly high at 18%, possibly representing some bias because patients were referred for specialist care [17]. Screening pregnant women for thyroid autoantibodies is generally not recommended, but it is clear that antibody testing should be performed if the TSH level is above the upper limit of the reference range [8].

Aetiology of Gestational SCH

It is generally held from observational studies that moderate to severe iodine deficiency is a likely cause of gestational SCH, particularly in women living in areas where the problem is endemic, but there is not a great deal of scientific evidence based upon measurement of maternal thyroid hormone levels during gestation documenting a direct cause-and-effect relationship for minor degrees of gestational iodine deficiency [18]. The accepted definition for population gestational iodine deficiency is a spot median urine iodine concentration (UIC) of <150 ug/L, but the diagnosis in an individual pregnant woman is often uncertain and the evidence for a direct relationship between a UIC and SCH is lacking [18]. Recently, attention has been focussed on the effects of excessive iodine intake on precipitating or causing SCH in regions of China where Universal Salt Iodization has been implemented. Monitoring of the population after the implementation of Universal Salt Iodisation in China has shown a significant increase in SCH consistent with an effect of excessive iodine intake [19, 20]. While all diagnostic and management guidelines for thyroid disorders in pregnancy recommend iodine supplementation for women who are at risk of gestational iodine deficiency and that supplementation should be commenced, where possible, before conception [2, 8]. However, in these guidelines little attention has been paid to warning patients against ingestion of iodine supplements exceeding recommended requirements.

Where thyroid antibody testing has been undertaken in conjunction with TSH testing of pregnant women in the developed world for the diagnosis of SCH, the results show a high prevalence of positive tests consistent with underlying autoimmune thyroid disease, indicating thyroid autoimmunity is the likely cause of SCH in most women with gestational hypothyroidism [8]. Korevaar and colleagues demonstrated that the presence of TPOAb was associated with an impaired thyroidal response to hCG suggesting a mechanism for the development of SCH in pregnant women with thyroid autoimmunity [21]. In our observational study the majority of the women with SCH exhibited positive TPOAb antibodies and all with OH were antibody positive [17]. This strong correlation between the presence of positive TPOAb and impaired thyroid function very likely indicates, but does not prove, a direct cause-and-effect relationship.

The controversial entity of "isolated hypothyroxinaemia" remains an enigma. Much has been written about this biochemical diagnosis, first described by Pop and colleagues where they showed that pregnant women identified with isolated hypothyroxinaemia (serum T4 level below the tenth percentile with a normal serum TSH level in the first trimester) were at risk of giving birth to children suffering from both mental and motor developmental delay [22]. It is difficult to explain why there would not be a reciprocal rise in the TSH level in response to a fall in the circulating T4 level. Some have attempted to explain this by citing preferential T3 secretion over T4, a recognised thyroidal phenomenon to conserve iodine in iodine deficient subjects, with the increased T3 suppressing the compensatory rise in TSH in response to the fall in circulating T4 levels. Experimental evidence to support this phenomenon is lacking. As we have previously commented, isolated hypothyroxinaemia is frequently attributed to iodine deficiency, but there is little evidence to support this [18]. Many authorities take the view that isolated hypothyroxinaemia is not a specific pathological entity, but a methodological artefact arising from changes in thyroid binding proteins in pregnancy invalidating the T4 immunoassay system. It is not recognised as a treatable entity in Endocrine Society and ATA guidelines, so we remain unsure of the pathogenesis and relevance of this entity [2, 8].

Prevalence and Progression of Gestational SCH

Published figures indicate that overt hypothyroidism occurs in less than 0.5% of pregnancies in the developed world [2, 8]. However, prevalence rates in countries in the developing world, where moderate to severe iodine deficiency is endemic, are largely unknown. As we have emphasised, the reported prevalence rates of gestational SCH should be interpreted in the context of, the trimester of pregnancy, ethnicity, body mass index, iodine nutrition, underlying thyroid autoimmunity (TPOAb positivity) and of course what reference range or cut-off level and analytical platform on which the TSH concentration was measured. The Endocrine Society guidelines quote figures of 2–3% for SCH [2], but there are multiple publications reporting much higher prevalence rates. Indeed, many review articles on the subject suggest that SCH is a common diagnosis occurring in 4–8% of women of reproductive age [23]. In our reported data on over 1000 pregnant women the prevalence of SCH was as high as 10% when defined as a TSH >2.5 mIU/L declining to 1.8% when defined as a TSH >4.0 mIU/L as shown in Figs. 1 and 2 [17].

The data concerning progression of severity of gestational SCH is lacking, as is follow-up information on the subsequent development of SCH in future pregnancies and overt hypothyroidism developing in the postpartum period. However, it is self-evident that any pregnant woman known to be TPOAb positive, with or without any discernible rise in serum TSH concentration, should be monitored in the postpartum period and indefinitely if she has any intention of a future pregnancy.

Practical Approach to Management of SCH: Re-analysis of Our Data

In response to these varying laboratory reference ranges, and at times seemingly conflicting expert guidelines recommendations, the clinician managing an individual woman with a marginally elevated serum TSH in the first trimester of pregnancy is frequently confronted with difficult decisions to make [23, 24]. Given this uncertainty, and to illustrate this point in clinical practice, we have reanalysed our published data on a group of 1025 referred pregnant women tested for thyroid function

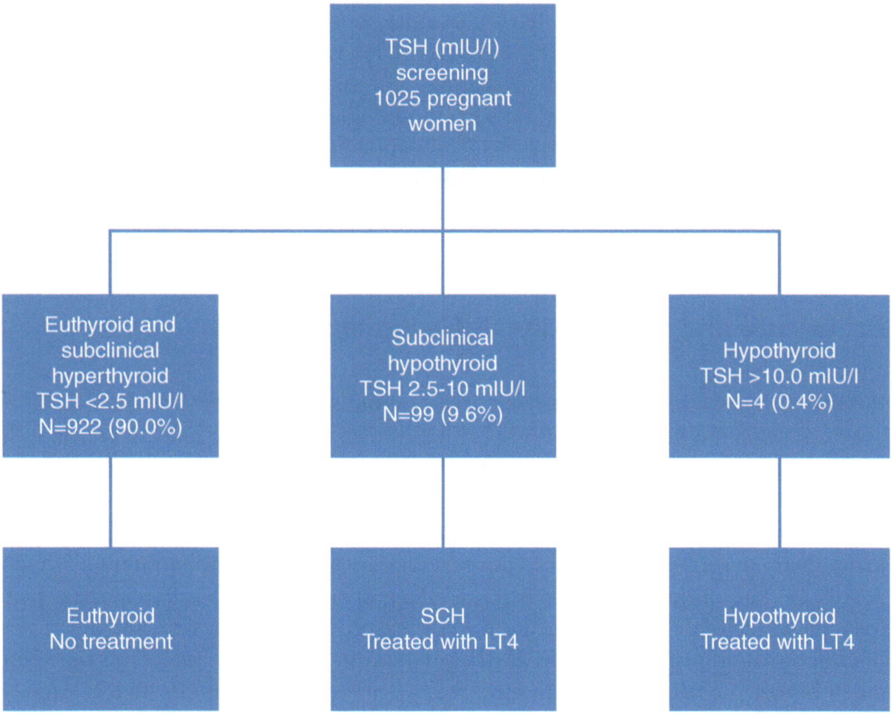

Fig. 1 Results of screening of 1025 consecutive pregnant women by TSH testing during first trimester of pregnancy with application of American Endocrine Society guidelines (2012) for diagnosis and treatment [2, 17]

(TSH and thyroid antibodies) in the first trimester of pregnancy to demonstrate how these different diagnostic reference ranges and recommendations for LT4 therapy, specifically according to the latest ATA Guidelines, would apply to an unselected Australian population of pregnant women living in Western Sydney who were initially diagnosed during the first trimester of pregnancy and treated according to the American Endocrine Society Guidelines published in 2012 [17]. The clinical details, laboratory methods and statistical analyses of the data have previously been described [17]. All the serum TSH concentrations were measured on the Bayer Advia Centaur platform as shown in Table 1, with an upper limit of the reference range for the first trimester being 2.5 mIU/l. We have excluded results of antithyroglobulin antibodies (TgAb) and free T4 levels reported in our original publication, as these parameters are not included in published guidelines.

Of our sample of 1025 pregnant women, 103 patients, or 10.0% of our sample, had a TSH level of ≥2.5 mIU/L. According to the American Endocrine Society Guidelines in place at the time of diagnosis [2], 99 (9.6%) were diagnosed as suffering from SCH and 4 (0.4%) had overt hypothyroidism (OH). Patients diagnosed with OH or SCH were prescribed LT4 therapy to maintain serum TSH levels between 0.5 and 2.5 mIU/L for the remainder of their pregnancies Fig. 1 [17].

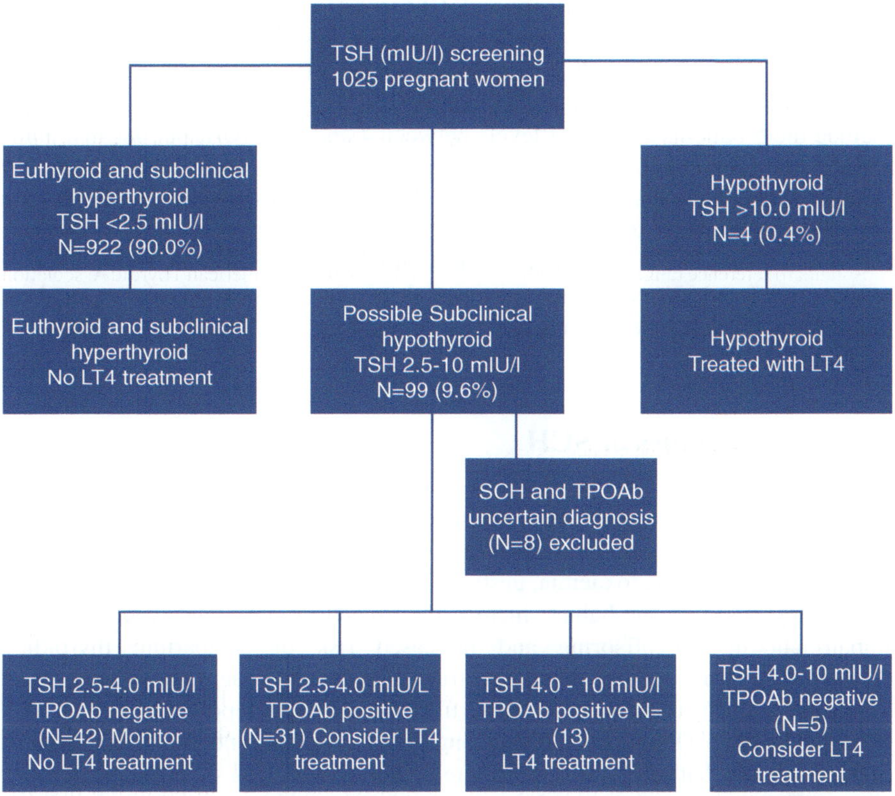

Fig. 2 Retrospective analysis of results of screening of 1025 pregnant women by TSH testing during first trimester of pregnancy, initially diagnosed and treated according to American Endocrine Society guidelines [2, 17], with retrospective application of 2017 American Thyroid Association (ATA) guidelines for diagnosis and treatment of possible hypothyroidism [8]

Subsequently, we have conducted a retrospective analysis of these patients according to ATA guidelines, employing a default TSH cut-off level of 4.0 mIU/L for SCH [8], that has shown most of the patients who had previously been diagnosed with SCH had TSH levels in the range of >2.5–4.0 mIU/L reducing the prevalence of SCH from 9.6 to 1.8% with several patients having insufficient information to classify them (Fig. 2). However, the ATA Guidelines further discriminate for patients with TSH levels between 2.5 and 4.0 mIU/L by the presence or absence of anti-TPOAb and 31 of our 73 patients in this range were anti-TPOAb positive (Fig. 2). According to the ATA Guidelines, it is suggested that these patients should be considered for LT4 replacement therapy. In our series, 18 patients (1.8%) had TSH levels between 4 and 10 mIU/L with 13 of the 18 patients being TPOAb positive. Thus, of the 103 patients originally diagnosed with hypothyroidism and thereby warranting LT4 replacement therapy at the time (99 with SCH and 4 with OH) according to the American Endocrine Society Guidelines, application of the ATA

Guidelines—and offering treatment with LT4 to patients where the ATA guidelines suggest "consider treatment"—would have reduced this number to 48 (44 with SCH and 4 with OH) (Fig. 2) and 8 patients remain unclassified because of uncertain TPOAb data. The number of patients requiring LT4 treatment increases to 53 if we include the 5 patients with TSH levels between 4 and 10 mIU/L but negative anti-TPOAb representing 5.4% of the patients studied, as Nazarpour and colleagues have recently shown that LT4 treatment of thyroid antibody negative SCH patients with TSH >4.0 mIU/L was beneficial in reducing preterm delivery [25]. This exercise demonstrates the large variation that occurs in prevalence of SCH and number of women offered LT4 replacement therapy depending on what criteria are used for diagnosis and replacement therapy.

Adverse Outcomes of SCH

There are numerous reports documenting diverse, but often contested, adverse obstetrical and foetal outcomes resulting from maternal SCH. These include miscarriage, pre-eclampsia toxaemia, gestational glucose intolerance, preterm delivery, small for gestational age babies, increased perinatal mortality and neurocognitive impairment in the offspring and increased risk of postpartum thyroiditis [2, 4, 16, 23]. More recently autism spectrum disorder and epilepsy have been added to this list [26]. An association with infertility has also been reported in women with SCH and positive TPOAb [27]. If this long list of adverse events is a direct result of SCH, it follows that early and appropriate treatment with LT4 should prevent most, if not all, of these disorders. On the contrary, two large randomised controlled therapeutic intervention trials have so far not shown any beneficial effects on the pregnancy or for the offspring [28, 29]. While it is irrational to dismiss the multiple reports of recorded adverse events associated with gestational SCH in observational studies, it has not been possible to reconcile these findings with the results obtained from therapeutic trials.

It was not until 1969 that a clear cause-and-effect relationship was established between maternal hypothyroidism and neurocognitive impairment in the offspring that was not due to iodine deficiency and neurological or myxedematous cretinism [30]. Later a landmark study by Haddow and colleagues confirmed that even mild degrees of undetected, or inadequately treated, maternal thyroid deficiency during pregnancy is associated with lower IQ scores in their offspring in the absence of neonatal hypothyroidism [31]. Most of the hypothyroid women they studied appeared to have suffered from underlying autoimmune thyroiditis. From their study they concluded that "In the absence of objective data, the most prudent policy would be to identify and treat maternal hypothyroidism as early in pregnancy as possible, keeping in mind that the need for thyroxine increases during pregnancy—and that systematic screening for hypothyroidism early in pregnancy may be worthwhile" [31]. Two decades on, what seemed convincing recommendations in 1999 remain controversial to this day. The underlying reason for this controversy is the lack of convincing evidence from randomised controlled trials (RCT) of a beneficial effect of LT4 replacement therapy administered to pregnant women with SCH [28, 29]. Lazarus and colleagues conducted a large multicentre trial of LT4 therapy given to women with SCH, at a median gestational age of just over 12 weeks, that showed no benefit as measured by IQ in the offspring at 3 years of age [28]. The other well-conducted RCT of SCH by Casey and colleagues (defined as a serum TSH >4.0 mIU/L), commencing LT4 treatment between 8- and 20-weeks' gestation, showed LT4 replacement did not result in significantly better cognitive outcomes in children through 5 years of age and no benefit was found in reducing obstetric complications [29]. In short, professional bodies such as ACOG and RANZCOG have recommended against LT4 replacement therapy for SCH on the basis these two RCTs of LT4 replacement therapy did not demonstrate any clinical benefit in gestational SCH [14, 15]. However, there are contrary arguments put forward by those who consider these RCT trials had several potential flaws, most importantly that LT4 treatment may have been commenced too late in gestation. The problem that must now be resolved is how to reconcile the lack of demonstrated clinical benefit from randomised trials of LT4 replacement therapy in gestational SCH with the large body of observational studies showing an association of gestational SCH with multiple adverse maternal and neonatal outcomes. Maraka and colleagues have concluded from a systematic review that the literature supports an association of gestational SCH with adverse maternal and neonatal outcomes, but this association may not be causal, and its magnitude may be overestimated by several factors such as publication bias, to which we would add imprecise definitions and diagnoses of SCH [4].

Treatment Monitoring and Screening

An analysis of treatment practices for gestational SCH in the USA over the period 2010 to 2014 found an increased likelihood of these women being prescribed LT4 replacement therapy, but there were wide variations in treatment practices associated with factors such as ethnicity, place of residence and type of medical specialist group caring for the pregnant patients [23]. Compared with Obstetricians, Endocrinologists appeared more likely to treat patients with SCH and to commence treatment at a lower TSH threshold (TSH levels above 2.5 mIU/L) than other specialities. It is likely these practices reflect an adherence to specialist guidelines both within and between specialties. While there is no disagreement between Endocrinologists and Obstetricians on prescribing LT4 replacement therapy for pregnant women with confirmed OH and the need to ensure appropriate increases in medication during pregnancy to maintain a serum TSH level at <2.5 mIU/L, views continue to diverge when it comes to managing patients with gestational SCH.

The most recent guidelines and recommendations for instituting LT4 replacement therapy for gestational SCH have been provided by the ATA [8]. When a valid local reference range for serum TSH is lacking, the ATA recommends treatment if

Table 2 American Thyroid Association (ATA) recommendations for the diagnosis and management of subclinical hypothyroidism and hypothyroxinaemia in pregnancy[a]

Laboratory data	L-T4 therapy recommended	Recommendation strength	Evidence quality
Anti-TPO positive and TSH level >pregnancy-specific reference range	Yes (>4.0 mIU/L)	Strong	Moderate
Anti-TPO negative and TSH >10 mIU/L	Yes (>10 mIU/L)	Strong	Low
Anti-TPO positive and TSH >2.5 but < upper limit of reference range	Consider (2.5–4.0 mIU/L)	Weak	Moderate
Anti-TPO negative and TSH >upper limit of reference range and <10 mIU/L	Consider (4.0–10 mIU/L)	Weak	Low

[a]Adapted from ATA Guidelines by Cooper and Pearce 2017 [32]

the TSH is >4.0 mIU/L. In addition, measurement of antithyroid peroxidase antibodies (TPOAb) is recommended to be undertaken for those above this cut-off level to assist in decision-making, as illustrated in Fig. 2. The ATA guidelines have been further refined, since the first iteration in 2011, for consideration of L-T4 replacement therapy according to the presence or absence of antithyroid antibodies (TPOAb), as discussed by Cooper and Pearce and shown in Table 2 [32]. These recommendations are based on results of cohort studies showing that TPOAb positivity amplifies the obstetrical risk associated with an elevated maternal serum TSH level [32, 33].

The re-analysis of our data showed that the application of the 2017 ATA guidelines reduced the number of women recommended for LT4 replacement by approximately 50% compared with American Endocrine Society Guidelines. There is much to learn from this exercise. Did the diagnostic criteria we applied lead to unnecessary treatment and increased health care costs for many women? Alternatively, if we had used ATA guidelines would this have resulted in many pregnant women being denied safe interventional care. From our small study we concluded that LT4 replacement therapy in appropriate dosage for women with SCH does prevent certain obstetric and foetal complications and shows no harmful effects [17], a view previously presented by Negro and Stagnaro-Green [33]. To date, most reports of SCH patients treated with low dose LT4 have shown that such treatment when monitored individually appears safe and in most countries this medication is relatively inexpensive.

Screening for Hypothyroidism in Pregnancy

Women with a suspected or known history of a thyroid disorder should be managed by a preconception strategy designed to ensure normal thyroid function before conception followed by careful monitoring throughout the pregnancy [34]. Currently, none of the expert medical bodies providing guidelines for diagnosis and management of gestational hypothyroidism have recommended routine laboratory screening for serum TSH, though opinion was equally divided regarding testing for serum TSH level among the authors of the expert group that wrote the American Endocrine Society guidelines [2]. Case detection, with a long list of risk factors, has been recommended [8] but, in our view adherence to this long list of risk factors in clinical practice is highly unlikely and is probably disregarded or implemented too late in gestation. Most studies have failed to confirm this form of case detection to be a very effective strategy [35]. Our finding of an incidence of 4 per thousand (0.4%) for overt hypothyroidism in our cohort, if confirmed in larger studies across the whole population, would justify universal screening for this disorder alone. It is interesting to compare this figure with rates for neonatal screening for congenital hypothyroidism where screening is universally accepted and promoted.

In a critical appraisal of the literature weighing up the "pros and cons" of universal screening Taylor and colleagues presented several compelling arguments in favour of universal screening, while simultaneously raising uncertainties and practical caveats [36]. Of course, any recommendation for universal screening needs to be considered in the context of the health care system in which this would take place, particularly the availability and cost of TSH testing supported by treatment and monitoring of LT4 replacement during pregnancy. We conclude in the context of current knowledge and until there is more robust evidence to the contrary that systematic screening for hypothyroidism by TSH testing early in pregnancy is likely to be worthwhile, even when the degree of deficiency is mild and does not cause immediate clinical manifestations. If routine TSH screening were to be introduced, the most conservative policy would be to perform testing at the first prenatal visit, preferably in the first trimester as soon as pregnancy has been confirmed. Follow-up of women with positive screening results would need to be prompt by confirming an elevated TSH, testing for free T4 and testing for TPOAb, so that treatment could begin without delay as early as possible in the pregnancy.

Summary

Clinicians left to interpret and apply frequently conflicting recommendations, where consensus is lacking between expert committees and professional bodies, need to proceed prudently with a patient-centred approach, considering any personal or family history of autoimmune thyroid disease and paying particular attention to any previous abnormal reproductive or obstetric history in the individual patient. Arguments for overdiagnosis and overtreatment certainly have merit, but these opinions are more than balanced by those concerned about underdiagnosis and undertreatment. Before commencing LT4 therapy, or deciding against treatment, the patient should be given a summary of current evidence and opinion in a form that is understandable and should take part in the decision to treat or not to treat with LT4 and be supported with that decision until we have better scientific evidence from large, well-conducted diagnostic and therapeutic trials. In the interim, application of the ATA guidelines for diagnosis and management of gestational SCH, while recognising some recommendations are based on low to moderate quality evidence, will assist the clinician in obtaining the best outcome for the individual patient.

References

1. Moleti M, Trimarchi F, Vermiglio F. Thyroid physiology in pregnancy. Endocr Pract. 2014;20:589–59.
2. DeGroot L, Abalovich M, Alexander EK, et al. Management of thyroid dysfunction during pregnancy and the postpartum: Endocrine Society clinical practice guideline. J Clin Endocrinol Metab. 2012;97:2543–65.
3. Van den Boogard E, Vissenberg R, Land JA, Van Wely M, van der Post JAM, Goodijn M, Bisschop PH. Hum Reprod Update. 2011;17(5):605–19.
4. Maraka S, Ospina NM, O'Keeffe DT, et al. Subclinical hypothyroidism in pregnancy: a systematic review and meta-analysis. Thyroid. 2016;26:580–90.
5. Shinohara D, Rosani M, Santos T, de Carvalho HC, Lopes LC, et al. Pregnancy complications associated with maternal hypothyroidism: a systematic review. Obstet Gynaecol Surv. 2018;73:219–30.
6. Stagnaro-Green A, Abalovich M, Alexander E, Azizi F, Mestman J, Negro R, Nixon A, Pearce EN, Soldin OP, Sullivan S, Wiersinga W. American Thyroid Association taskforce on thyroid disease during pregnancy and postpartum 2011 guidelines of the American Thyroid Association for the diagnosis and management of thyroid disease during pregnancy and postpartum. Thyroid. 2011;21:1081–125.
7. Lazarus J, Brown RS, Daumerie C, Hubalewska-Dydejczyk A, Negro R, Vaidya B. 2014 European Thyroid Association guidelines for the management of subclinical hypothyroidism in pregnancy. Eur Thyroid J. 2014;3:76–94.
8. Alexander EK, Pearce EN, Brent GA, Brown RS, Chen H, Dosiou C, Grobman WA, Laurberg P, Lazarus JH, Mandel SJ, Peeters RP, Sullivan S. 2017 guidelines of the American Thyroid Association for the diagnosis and management of thyroid disease during pregnancy and the postpartum. Thyroid. 2017;27:315–89.
9. Korevaar TI, Medici M, de Rijke YB, Visser W, de Munck Keizer-Schrama SMPF, Jaddoe VWV, Hofman A, Ross HA, Visser E, Hooijkaas H, Steegers EAP, Tiemer H, Bongers-Schokking JJ, Visser TJ, Peeters RP. Ethnic differences in maternal thyroid parameters during pregnancy: the Generation R Study. J Clin Endocrinol Metab. 2013;98:3678–86.
10. da Silva VA, de Almeida RJ, Cavalcanta MP, Pereira LA Jr, Reis FM, Pereira MF, Kasamatsu TS, Camacho CP. Two thyroid stimulating hormone assays correlated in clinical practice show disagreement in subclinical hypothyroidism patients. Clin Biochem. 2018;53:13–8.
11. Andersen SL, Christensen PA, Knosgaard L, Andersen S, Handberg A, Hansen AB, Vestergaard P. Classification of thyroid dysfunction in pregnant women differs by analytical method and type of thyroid function test. J Clin Endocrinol Metab. 2020;105:e4012–22.
12. Yuen LY, Chan MHM, Sahota DS, Lit LCW, Ho CS, Ma RCW, Tam WH. Development of gestational age-specific thyroid function test reference intervals in four analytic platforms through multilevel modelling. Thyroid. 2020;30(4):598–608. https://doi.org/10.1089/thy.2019.0323.
13. Toloza F, Ospina NS, Rodriguez-Gutierrez R, O'Keeffe D, Brito J, Montori V, Maraka S. MON-586 practice variation in the management of subclinical hypothyroidism during pregnancy: results from a National Survey of Endocrinologists in the USA. J Endocrine Society. 2019;3(Suppl_1):MON-586.
14. American College of Obstetricians and Gynecologists. Thyroid disease in pregnancy: ACOG practice bulletin; number 223. Obstet Gynecol. 2020;135:e261–74.

15. Royal Australian and New Zealand College of Obstetricians and Gynaecologists (RANZCOG). Subclinical hypothyroidism and hypothyroidism in pregnancy; 2012: Subclinical-hypothyroidism-and-hypothyroidism-in-pregnancy-(C-Obs-46)-Mar18.pdf (ranzcog.edu.au).
16. Korevaar TIM, Derakshan A, Taylor PN, Meima M, Chen L, Bliddal S, McCarty D, et al. Association of thyroid function test abnormalities and thyroid autoimmunity with preterm birth: a systematic review and meta-analysis. JAMA. 2019;322:632–41.
17. Blumenthal N, Eastman CJ. Beneficial effects on pregnancy outcomes of thyroid hormone replacement therapy for subclinical hypothyroidism. J Thyroid Res. 2017;2017:4601365.
18. Eastman CJ, Ma G, Li M. Optimal assessment and quantification of iodine nutrition in pregnancy and lactation: laboratory and clinical methods, controversies, and future directions. Nutrients. 2019;11:2378. https://doi.org/10.3390/nu11102378.
19. Shi X, Han C, Li C, Mao J, Wang W, Xie X, et al. Optimal and safe upper limits of iodine intake for early pregnancy in iodine-sufficient regions: a cross-sectional study of 7190 pregnant women in China. J Clin Endocrinol Metab. 2015;100:1630–8.
20. Sang ZN, Wei W, Zhang GQ, Wen C, Hua L, Jun S, Liu JY, Zhang WQ. Thyroid dysfunction during late gestation is associated with excessive iodine intake in pregnant women. J Clin Endocrinol Metab. 2012;97:E1363–9.
21. Korevaar TIM, Steegers EAP, Pop VJ, Broeren MA, Chaker L, de Rijke YB, Jaddoe WV, Medici M, Vissre TJ, Tiemeier H, Peeters RP. Thyroid autoimmunity impairs the thyroidal response to hCG: two population based prospective cohort studies. J Clin Endocrinol Metab. 2017;102(1):69–77.
22. Pop VJ, Kuijpens JL, van Baar AL, Verkerk G, van Son MM, de Vijlder JJ, et al. Low maternal free thyroxine concentrations during early pregnancy are associated with impaired psychomotor development in infancy. Clin Endocrinol. 1999;50:149–55.
23. Maraka S, Mwangi R, et al. Variations in treatment practices for women with subclinical hypothyroidism in pregnancy: US national assessment. J Clin Endocrinol Metab. 2019;104:3893–901.
24. Maraka S, Singh Ospina NM, Mastorakos G, O'Keeffe DT. Subclinical hypothyroidism in women planning conception and during pregnancy: who should be treated and how? J Endocrine Soc. 2018;2:533–46.
25. Nazarpour S, Tehrani FR, Simbar M, Tohidi M, Minooee S, Rahmati M, Azizi F. Effect of levothyroxine on pregnant women with subclinical hypothyroidism negative for thyroid peroxidase antibodies. J Clin Endocrinol Metab. 2018;103:926–35.
26. Ge GM, Leung MTY, Man KKC, Leung WC, Ip P, Li GHI, Wong ICK, Kung AWC, Cheung CL. Maternal thyroid dysfunction during pregnancy and the risk of adverse outcome in the offspring: a systematic review and meta-analysis. J Clin Endocrinol Metab. 2020; 105:1–21.
27. Dhillon-Smith RK, Tobias A, Smith PP, Middleton LJ, Sunner KK, Baker K, Farrell-Carver S, Bender-Atik R, Agrawal R, Bhatia K, Chu JJ, Edi-Osgaie E, Ewles A, Ghobara T, Gupta P, Jukovic D, Khalaf Y, et al. The prevalence of thyroid dysfunction and autoimmunity in women with history of miscarriage or subfertility. J Clin Endocrinol Metab. 2020;105(8):dgaa302.
28. Lazarus JH, Bestwick JP, Channon S, Paradice R, Maina A, Rees R, Chiusano E, John R, Guaraldo V, George LM, et al. Antenatal thyroid screening and childhood cognitive function. N Engl J Med. 2012;366:493–501.
29. Casey BM, Thom EA, Peaceman AM, VarnerMW SY, Hirtz DG, Reddy UM, Wapner RJ, Thorp JM, Saade G, Tita ATN, Rouse DJ, Sibai B, Lams JD, Mercer BM, Tolosa J, Caritis SN, Van Dorsten JP. Treatment of subclinical hypothyroidism or hypothyroxinemia in pregnancy. N Engl J Med. 2017;376:815–24.
30. Man E, Jones WS. Thyroid function in human pregnancy: incidence of maternal low butanol extractable iodine and of normal TBG and TBPA capacities: retardation of 8-month-old infants. Am J Obstet Gynecol. 1969;104:898–908.

31. Haddow JE, Palomaki GE, Allan WC, Williams JR, Knight GJ, Gagnon J, O'Heir CE, Mitchell M, Hermos RJ, Waisbren SE, Faix JD, Klein RZ. Maternal thyroid deficiency during pregnancy and subsequent neuropsychological development of the child. N Engl J Med. 1999;341:549–55.
32. Cooper DS, Pearce EN. Subclinical hypothyroidism and hypothyroxinemia in pregnancy—still no answers. N Eng J Med. 2017;376:876–7.
33. Negro R, Stagnaro GA. Diagnosis and management of subclinical hypothyroidism in pregnancy. BMJ. 2014;349:g4929.
34. Okosieme OE, Khan I, Taylor PN. Preconception management of thyroid dysfunction. Clin Endocrinol. 2018;89:269–79.
35. Negro R, Schwartz A, Gisomondi R, Tinelli A, Mangieri T, Stagnaro GA. Universal screening versus case finding for detection and treatment for thyroid dysfunction during pregnancy. J Clin Endocrinol Metab. 2010;95:1699–707.
36. Taylor PN, Zouras S, Min T, Nagarahaj K, Lazarus JH, Okosieme O. Thyroid screening in early pregnancy: pros and cons. Front Endocrinol (Lausanne). 2018;9:626. Published 2018 Oct 25. https://doi.org/10.3389/fendo.2018.00626.

Isolated Hypothyroxinemia During Pregnancy

Eunice López-Muñoz

Definition

The criteria for defining isolated maternal hypothyroxinemia (IMH) are heterogeneous and a precise definition is still lacking [1]. IMH has been defined by the American Thyroid Association (ATA) [2] as a free thyroxine (FT4) concentration in the lower 2.5–5th percentile (p) and by the European Thyroid Association (ETA) [3] in the lower than 2.5 p of a given population, despite a normal maternal serum thyroid stimulating hormone (TSH) concentration. Unfortunately, in the studies carried out to date on IMH there are important differences regarding its definition, which considerably modifies the interpretation of the data.

Prevalence

The frequency of IMH varies worldwide, does not follow the frequencies of nonpregnant populations, and has been reported in approximately 2–3% of pregnant women [4, 5]; however, it can be as low as 1.27% and as high as 49.33% [6]. These differences appear to be related to maternal iodine intake, reference ranges for TSH and FT4, gestational age or trimester of pregnancy, and the FT4 measurement method [4–44]. In general, the reported prevalence of IMH is higher in countries with more severe iodine deficiency, in studies that do not use

E. López-Muñoz (✉)
Medical Research Unit in Reproductive Medicine, Unidad Médica de Alta Especialidad Hospital de Gineco Obstetricia No. 4 "Luis Castelazo Ayala", Instituto Mexicano del Seguro Social, Río Magdalena 289, Colonia Tizapan San Angel, Alcaldía Álvaro Obregón, Mexico City, Mexico

F. Azizi, F. Ramezani Tehrani (eds.), *Thyroid Diseases in Pregnancy*,
https://doi.org/10.1007/978-3-030-98777-0_8

pregnancy-specific reference ranges for TSH and FT4 [45], and in which more advanced gestation is evaluated [13, 46]. In addition to iodine status, autoimmune status and ethnic variation in the population significantly affect the prevalence of IMH [47]. The estimated prevalence of IMH in iodine-sufficient areas such as the United States of America and the Netherlands has been estimated at 1.3–9.4% [9, 16], while in mildly or moderately iodine-deficient regions such as China, Iran, and Spain, it has been reported at 4.18–30.4% [5, 14, 41, 48]. Table 1 shows examples of the IMH prevalence reported in large population studies, as well as the status of iodine sufficiency (evaluated or probable), gestational age, and reference values of TSH and FT4 to establish the diagnosis [12, 18, 28, 32, 33, 42].

Table 1 Prevalence of isolated maternal hypothyroxinemia in different populations

N/Country/iodine status	GA	Diagnostic criteria	Reported rate	Ref.
10,990/FASTER Trial, USA/NA probably iodine sufficient	≥10.3 w	TSH (2.5–97.5th p) First *T* 0.036–4.28 mU/L; second *T* 0.213–3.93 mU/L FT4 (<2.5th p) First and second *T* < 0.71 ng/dL	2.1% in first *T* 2.3% in second *T*	[12]
16,346/United Kingdom and 5500/Italy/NA Probably iodine sufficient	<15.6 w	United Kingdom TSH (2.5–97.5th p) 0.15–3.65 mU/L FT4 (<2.5th p) < 0.66 ng/dL Italy TSH (2.5–97.5th p) 0.11–3.5 mU/L FT4 (<2.5th p) < 0.71 ng/dL	1.67%	[18]
6303/Liaoning, China/ Iodine sufficient	4–8 w	TSH 0.29–5.22 mU/L FT4 < 0.95 ng/dL	2.4%	[28]
5435/Generation R Study, the Netherlands/ Iodine sufficient	9.6–17.6 w	TSH (2.5–97.5th p) 0.04–4.55 mU/L FT4 (<2.5th p) < 0.80 ng/dL	2.6%	[32]
97,228/USA/Iodine sufficient	<20 w	TSH (2.5–97.5th p) 0.08–3.99 mU/L FT4 (<2.5th p) < 0.86 ng/dL	3%	[33]
1208 twin pregnancy and 46,834 single pregnancy/Shanghai, China/NA probably iodine sufficient	>8 w	TSH (2.5–97.5th p) first *T* 0.03–3.60 mU/L; third *T* 0.39–3.69 mU/L FT4 (<2.5th p) first *T* < 0.90 ng/dL; third *T* < 0.70 ng/dL	Twin pregnancy 4.7% in first *T* and 3.3% in third *T* Single pregnancy 2.2% in first *T* and 2.0% in third *T*	[42]

GA gestational age, *FASTER* first and second trimester evaluation of risk, *USA* United States of America, *NA* Not assessed, *w* weeks, *TSH* thyroid stimulating hormone, *p* percentile, *FT4* free thyroxine, *T* trimester, *ATA* American Thyroid Association

Etiology

During pregnancy, thyroid hormone requirements and production increase. Physiological adaptation during pregnancy is produced by the increase in the concentration of thyroid binding globulin (TBG), the stimulatory effect of human chorionic gonadotropin (hCG) on thyrocytes and the extrathyroidal thyroxine (T4) distribution space, as well as by the reduction in TSH levels during the first trimester of pregnancy. To maintain the balance in the concentration of T4, the thyroid must produce more hormone, which depends directly on the availability of iodine in the diet and proper functioning of the thyroid gland. Since the increased renal iodine clearance, secondary to a higher glomerular filtration rate, causes a decrease in circulating iodine concentration during pregnancy, adequate supplementation is necessary [49]. Although a single cause of IMH has not been identified, one of the risk factors is iodine deficiency. IMH seems to be pregnancy-specific disease with multifactorial pathophysiology [47].

In addition to iodine deficiency, various risk factors have been reported, such as iron deficiency, placental angiogenic factors, high body mass index (BMI), hCG concentrations, autoimmunity, older age, multiparity, hypertension, lower level of education, smoking, environmental pollutants, anxiety, and twin pregnancy [42, 45, 50].

Iodine Deficiency

Iodine is an element that is needed for the production of thyroid hormone. During normal pregnancy, changes in thyroid function require a balance between hormonal requirements and the availability of iodine [3, 51, 52]. Since iodine levels tend to decrease towards the third trimester of pregnancy, this can result in moderate iodine deficiency and contribute to an increase in the frequency of IMH. In fact, a higher prevalence of IMH has been reported in moderately and severely iodine-deficient regions [5].

Some studies have provided evidence of the importance of iodine supplementation during pregnancy. For example, the risk of developing thyroid disorders during pregnancy, including hypothyroxinemia, was significantly increased with the consumption of non-iodized salt (odds ratio [OR] 14.47; 95% confidence interval [CI] 3.66–57.16) and not consuming iodine supplements during gestation (OR 11.01; 95% CI 1.69–71.79) [44]. A higher prevalence of hypothyroxinemia has been reported in iodine-deficient countries, with a more severe and more frequent tendency to IMH at the end of gestation [5, 13, 52]. This could be due to the tendency of iodine to decrease as pregnancy progresses, particularly in the third trimester [5].

Adequate iodine supplementation is important, even before pregnancy. A study carried out in 100 pregnant women who were classified according to their habits of consumption of iodized salt showed a higher prevalence of maternal thyroid failure

(88.9% of the women with maternal thyroid failure corresponded to IMH, 5.5% to subclinical hypothyroidism, and 5.5% to over hypothyroidism) in the group of women who started iodine supplementation at the diagnosis of pregnancy compared to those who started it up to 24 months before pregnancy (36.8 vs 6.4%, $X^2 = 14.7$, $p = 0.0005$; relative risk [RR] 5.7 CI 95% 2.03–16.08, $z = 3.29$, $p < 0.001$). It appears the time of introduction of iodine supplementation is an important factor in the prevention of maternal thyroid failure, including hypothyroxinemia, during pregnancy [13, 14, 53].

Iron Deficiency

Iron metabolism is related to the metabolism of thyroid hormones. Iron is a component of many enzymes, including thyroid peroxidase (TPO), which is involved in the initial steps of thyroid hormone biosynthesis [54]. Iron deficiency reduces the response to thyrotropin releasing hormone (TRH), lowering serum levels of triiodothyronine (T3) and T4. One proposed mechanism is the impairment of the heme-dependent TPO enzyme, which limits thyroid hormone synthesis, reducing circulating total T3 (TT3) and total T4 (TT4) [27]. Iron deficiency has even been found to reduce effectiveness of iodine prophylaxis, and iron replacement improves it [10]. Low maternal iron levels have been shown to be associated with low TT4 and high TSH concentrations in pregnancy in borderline areas of iodine deficiency [10, 55]. Iron deficiency is considered an independent risk factor for mild (OR = 2.44, CI 95% 1.32–4.49) and severe IMH (OR = 3.72, CI 95% 1.44–7.44) [27].

A study conducted in Brazil with different FT4 (<5th p [<0.86 ng/dL] and < 10th p [<0.92 ng/dL]) and TT4 reference points (<7.8 μg/dL) to establish the diagnosis of IMH showed a higher prevalence in iron-deficient women compared to those without deficiency (20.7 vs 8.4%; 14.8 vs 3.9%; and 17.2 vs 6.5%, respectively) [56].

On the other hand, a study showed an increase in the prevalence of thyroid autoimmunity in pregnant women with iron deficiency [55]. However, another study carried out in women with sufficient iodine and negative TPO antibodies (TPOAb) showed a higher prevalence of hypothyroxinemia in the women with iron deficiency than in those without (18.60% vs 7.96%, $X^2 = 12.56$, $p = 0.001$; OR = 2.64, CI 95% 1.51–4.61), and a higher prevalence of iron deficiency in the women with mild and severe hypothyroxinemia than in those without (5.82% vs 2.30%, $X^2 = 12.20$, $p = 0.007$; OR = 2.62, CI 95% 1.49–4.60) [27].

Placental Angiogenic Factors

During pregnancy, there is an increase in angiogenic factors produced by the placenta, such as placental growth factor (PIGF) (although it can also exert antiangiogenic effects), and antiangiogenic factors, such as the soluble FMS-like tyrosine kinase-1 (sFlt1) [57]. It has been proposed that sFlt1 protects the mother from excessive neovascularization induced by PIGF and vascular endothelial growth factor (VEGF) [58], and in animal models it has been shown that these factors can also influence the thyroid gland, reducing its vascular density and causing an increase in TSH or a decrease in the FT4 [59]. In humans, it has been shown that in newborn umbilical cord blood, a higher level of sFlt1 is associated with an increase in TSH and a decrease in FT4, while a higher level of PIGF is associated with an increase in FT4 [60]. Furthermore, high maternal levels of sFlt1 have been associated with decreased FT4 and TT4 ($p < 0.001$) and an increased risk of IMH (OR 3.05; 95% CI 1.42–6.55; $p = 0.004$), while high maternal levels of PIGF have been associated with decreased TSH and FT4 levels ($p < 0.001$) and an increased risk of IMH (OR 1.77; 95% CI 1.02–3.06; $p = 0.04$) [57].

High BMI

Since high hCG concentration amplifies the association between higher BMI with high TSH and lower FT4 concentrations during pregnancy, it has been proposed that high BMI may be associated with a low thyroid response to hCG stimulation [32], or even a higher concentration in TBG [61]. The increase in TBG may explain the increase that has been observed in TSH and T3 concentrations, as well as the decrease in FT4 between the first and third trimesters in women with a higher BMI [61]. Also, obesity has been proposed to increase peripheral deiodinase activity as an adaptative process to increase metabolic output, resulting in increased conversion of FT4 to free T3 (FT3) [31]. On the other hand, it has been reported that in patients with obesity, the production of cytokines, inflammatory factors, and leptin is increased in adipose tissue. Leptin is a potential regulator of TRH and TSH, as well as of the immune system with an increase in the production of TPOAb, factors that could contribute to the higher prevalence of hypothyroxinemia on women with a high BMI [28].

A higher average weight (178 ± 42 vs 171 ± 33 lbs.; $p = 0.006$) and a higher BMI have been reported in women with hypothyroxinemia than euthyroid women in different populations, for example, United States of America (33 ± 6 vs 32 ± 6 kg/m^2; $p = 0.02$) [9], Ireland (25 ± 3.2 vs 24 ± 4; $p = 0.001$) [23], the Netherlands (23.8–24.2 ± 4.3 vs 22.7 ± 3.6 kg/m^2; $p < 0.001$) [22, 62], and China (21.6 ± 3.0 vs 20.2 ± 2.5 kg/m^2; $p < 0.01$) [39, 41, 63].

In China, even in ethnic minority populations, such as Zhuang, BMI has been positively correlated with IMH (OR 1.08; 95% CI 1.00–1.16; $p < 0.05$) [64]. In Asian populations, a BMI greater than 23 kg/m^2 has been correlated with a low FT4 [65] and a BMI greater than 24 kg/m^2 has been considered as an independent risk factor for mild (OR 2.42, CI 95% 1.84–3.18) and severe IMH (OR 2.88 CI95% 1.87–44.43) [27, 28], similar to that reported in Belgium [31], and the Netherlands, with an increase in the risk of lower FT4 when comparing a BMI of 25 kg/m^2 with one of 20 kg/m^2 (OR 2.20; 95% CI 1.89–2.58), although the risk increases when the BMI is 30 kg/m^2 (OR4.21; 95% CI 3.17–5.59) [66].

hCG Levels

hCG is a specific pregnancy hormone that exerts thyrotropic activity due to its affinity for the TSH receptor. Normally, elevated hCG levels during early pregnancy increase FT4 levels and lower TSH levels. Thyrotropic activity of hCG facilitates increased energy expenditure and metabolic demand, while also protecting the sufficient availability of T4 for the developing fetus. A study carried out in a sufficient population in iodine showed that low hCG concentrations constitute a risk factor for IMH in early pregnancy, even when the thyroid functional capacity to respond to hCG is preserved [32].

Older Age

With aging there may be a gradual decrease in iodine reserves, a situation that could explain the higher prevalence of hypothyroxinemia in older women [5]. Women with IMH have been reported to have an older average age older than euthyroid women in different populations, for example, in United States of America (27.5 ± 6 vs 25.5 ± 6 years, $p < 0.001$) and China (32 vs 30 years; $p < 0.001$) [39, 63], being more frequent an age greater than or equal to 35 years in women with hypothyroxinemia (14 vs 7%; $p < 0.001$) [9]. Older age has even been associated with a higher risk of low FT4, with an increase in risk for each year after age 30 in the Netherlands (OR 1.08; 95% CI 1.03–1.13) [66] and Iran (OR 1.6; 95% CI 1.0–2.5); $p = 0.05$) [5]. However, a study conducted in Spain did not show an association of maternal age ≥ 30 years with a high risk of thyroid alteration (OR 0.85; CI 95% 0.67–1.08; $p = 0.16$) or hypothyroxinemia during pregnancy (OR 0.91; CI 95% 0.68–1.24; $p = 0.54$) [30].

Multiparity

The relationship between parity and increased risk of thyroid disorders during pregnancy, including hypothyroxinemia, may be due to the fact that each pregnancy produces a non-reversible cumulative goitrogenic effect, which requires a greater increase in iodine supplementation in subsequent pregnancies [44]. In fact, an association of multiparity with increased thyroid volume has been reported in different iodine-deficient populations [24, 65, 67].

Multiparity (≥3) has been reported more frequently in women with hypothyroxinemia than euthyroid women in different populations, for example, in United States of America (70 vs 64%; $p = 0.03$) [9] and China (33.1 vs 18.3%; $p < 0.001$) [41, 63]. Multiparity (>1) has even associated with a higher risk for low FT4 (OR 4.92; 95% CI 3.15–7.70) [66] and IMH (OR 1.72; 95% CI 1.04–2.85; $p = 0.03$) [5].

Lower Level of Education

A low educational level can be associated not only with a lower awareness of nutrition during pregnancy, but also with a lower income [5] leading to inadequate dietary intake, as well as iodine and iron deficiency [5, 44]. Differences in years (9.3 ± 3.5 vs 10.2 ± 3.5 years; $p = 0.001$) [62] and level of education (primary 5.8–22.9 vs 2.3–19.1; $p < 0.05$) [22, 63] have been reported among women with hypothyroxinemia compared to euthyroid women, with an increase in the risk of hypothyroxinemia when only primary level is available (OR 6.41; 95% CI 1.04–36.09) [44].

Thyroid Peroxidase Antibodies and Autoimmunity

Thyroid autoimmunity is a risk factor for thyroid dysfunction during pregnancy because of the thyroid inability to meet the increased demands for T4 [45, 53]. Thyroid antibody-positive women have been reported to be more likely to develop hypothyroxinemia [46], with positive TPOAb being the most frequently reported in women with IMH compared to euthyroid women from different populations, for example, in the Netherlands (20 vs 5.3%; $p < 0.001$) [62] and China (12 vs 9.7%; $p = 0.02$) [63]. However, other studies have not reported a higher prevalence of thyroid autoimmunity in women with IMH compared to euthyroid women [48, 68].

Exposure to Environmental Contaminants

Environmental contaminants, such as dioxins (polychlorinated dibenzo-p-dioxins, dibenzofurans) and polychlorinated biophenyls, may affect thyroid function in pregnancy [53, 69]. Organochlorine pesticides activate hepatic uridine diphosphate glucuronyltransferase, which causes an increase in glucuronidation and a decrease in FT4 levels, while polychlorinated biphenyls antagonize the binding of thyroid hormones at the thyroid receptor level [45]. Also, exposure during the first trimester of pregnancy to nitrogen oxide and particulate matter (PM) with an aerodynamic diameter of 2.5 μm or less ($PM_{2.5}$) has been associated with an increased risk of hypothyroxinemia during pregnancy (OR per 5-μg/m^3 change 1.21; 95% CI 1.00–1.47) [70].

Hypertension

A higher frequency of pre-existing hypertension has been reported in women with hypothyroxinemia compared to euthyroid women (7.0–7.4 vs 2.7%; $p < 0.05$) [22, 62].

Smoking

The thiocyanate found in cigarette smoke is a competitive sodium iodine symporter inhibitor, which could explain the lower levels of the FT4 index (FT4I) observed in smokers compared to nonsmokers [71]. Smoking of at least one cigarette per day has been reported more frequently in women with hypothyroxinemia than in euthyroid women (11.5 vs 4.5%; $p < 0.001$) [62]. Smoking discontinued during pregnancy has not been associated with hypothyroxinemia; however, continuing to smoke during pregnancy increases the risk of reduced FT4 levels (OR1.72; 95% CI 1.21–2.45) [66].

Anxiety

It has been reported that in animal models, the metabolism of thyroid hormones is modified by social stress, with the deterioration of the serotoninergic system being the one that could participate in the key events that ultimately lead to hypothyroxinemia [72]. Even in humans, maternal anxiety during pregnancy measured by using the State Trait Anxiety (STA) has been reported more frequently in women with hypothyroxinemia than in euthyroid women (25.4 vs 19.0%; $p = 0.03$) [62].

Twin Pregnancy

Since hCG concentrations are higher in twin pregnancies compared to singleton pregnancies, other mechanisms, such as placental or fetal T4 consumption that could explain the risk of IMH, should be investigated [42]. Compared with single pregnancy, a twin pregnancy has been associated with a higher risk of IMH during early pregnancy (2.2 vs 4.7%, respectively; OR 1.89; 95% CI 1.43–2.49, $p < 0.001$) and during late pregnancy (2.0 vs 3.0%, respectively; OR 1.48; 95% CI 1.04–2.10, $p = 0.028$) [42].

Finally, a study that included women with a pregnancy less than or equal to 18 weeks, from the cohorts of the Generation R study (Rotterdam) ($n = 5985$) and the Amsterdam Born Children and their Development (ABCD) study ($n = 3782$), reported a clinical prediction model that includes risk factors for low FT4 levels. Higher gestational age (per week OR 1.37; 95% CI 1.28–1.46), maternal age $\geq$ 30 years (per year OR 1.06; 95% CI 1.01–1.10), BMI 25 vs 20 kg/m^2 (OR 2.05; 95% CI 1.73–2.42), BMI 30 vs 20 kg/m^2 (OR 3.67; 95% CI 2.70–4.99), parity $\geq$3 (OR 2.21; 95% CI 1.34–3.63), and smoking (OR 1.60; 95% 1.12–2.29) were associated with an increased risk of low FT4 levels. By combining these factors, it was possible to make an adequate discrimination of women at risk of IMH (range c-statistic 0.72–0.76) [66].

Clinical Features

IMH is often asymptomatic and is only identified by laboratory studies [50].

Diagnosis

The diagnosis of IMH during pregnancy is based upon finding a normal maternal TSH concentration and a serum T4 (either TT4 or FT4) concentration in the lower 2.5th–5th p of a given population [2, 3].

The reference range of TSH and T4 can vary significantly in different populations [2] and between trimesters in the same patient [3, 61], as well as show variations depending on the analysis method.

TSH reference range must be defined by each institution or laboratory and must represent the healthy population of pregnant women in each trimester, with negative TPOAb, optimal iodine intake, and without thyroid disease, in whom these ranges will be applied [2, 73–76]. In case of not having specific population ranges, it is suggested to use those of a similar population evaluated with similar TSH assays. If not available, in the first trimester (7–12 weeks) the lower reference range of TSH can be reduced by approximately 0.4 mU/L, while the upper reference range is reduced by 0.5 mU/L, that is, an approximate value of 4.0 mU/L [2, 77]. Later, in the second and third trimesters, the reference ranges should be considered similar to those of nonpregnant women.

Regarding FT4, during the first trimester of gestation, the lower limit (2.5th p) of the reference range reported by immunoassay is around 0.80 ng/dl (10.3 pmol/L) [3]. Given FT4 measurement by automated immunoassay can be complicated during pregnancy due to the decrease in albumin and the increase in circulating TBG, the use of other methods with less influence by serum protein levels, such as equilibrium dialysis, ultrafiltration, or liquid chromatography/tandem mass spectrometry (LC/MS/MS), have been recommended. The reference range reported by direct equilibrium dialysis and LC/MS/MS is approximately 1.08 ng/dL in week 14–0.86 in week 20 [78]. In general, most studies, although showing variability in FT4 concentration with different methods, show lower levels of FT4 in pregnancy compared to nonpregnant women [51]. An FT4 value below the lower reference limit for each measurement method during pregnancy is considered hypothyroxinemia. Because some measurement methods are laborious, expensive, time consuming, and not widely available [2, 3, 76], the clinical practice guidelines for hypothyroidism in adults and the ATA guidelines have also suggested TT4 and FT4I as alternative methods [2, 79, 80].

It has been suggested that TT4 assays are less susceptible to being modified by typical pregnancy binding proteins changes. TT4 levels are more stable throughout pregnancy and may have a better log-linear association with TSH levels than FT4 [81]. It has been shown that the physiological rise in TT4 occurs before 16 weeks of gestation [82]; therefore, the reference range should take into account a 50% increase above the nonpregnant value in TT4 concentration between 7 and 16 weeks of gestation [1–3, 73]. TT4 reference range after 16 weeks of gestation is determined by multiplying the nonpregnant TT4 range (5–12 μg/dL) by 1.5 (7.5–18 μg/dL), while between 7 and 16 weeks it is recommended to increase the reference range by 5% for each week after 7 weeks of gestation [2, 3, 73]. An TT4 value less than 5 μg/dL after 16 weeks or less than the value calculated by increasing 5% in the lower limit for each week after 7 weeks of gestation is considered hypothyroxinemia. Other studies have reported an increase of less than 50% (23–35.5%) in TT4 levels, when comparing those of nonpregnant women or during the first trimester with those of the second or third trimester of gestation [81, 83]. Therefore, the need to establish specific reference ranges for each population and gestation trimester is reinforced, since hypothyroxinemia could be overdiagnosed [83]. Furthermore, Korevaar et al. [81] reported a loss of association of low TT4 levels with preeclampsia, premature delivery (PD), birth weight, and offspring intelligence quotient (IQ), while women with low FT4 had a 2.5- and 3.9-fold higher risk of PD and very PD (VPD), respectively, as well as offspring with lower IQ. Therefore, they considered that TT4 is inferior to FT4 in the evaluation of maternal thyroid function.

FT4I correction for TBG effects is calculated by dividing TT4 values by the T4 binding index (TBR or T-uptake ratio) [84]. The reference range reported in nonpregnant women for FT4I is 4.5–12-5. An increase in the value of the index is normally observed during the first trimester of pregnancy, returning to nonpregnant levels in the second and third trimesters. An FT4 value less than 4.5 is considered hypothyroxinemia [85]. In pregnant women in an area of iodine sufficiency in Iran, specific FT4I reference ranges have also been reported for each trimester of gestation (8.5–12.4 in the first trimester, 9.7–21 in the second trimester, and 8.7–12.9 in the third trimester) [80]. However, one of the impediments to the use of FT4I in clinical practice is that it requires two different tests, which increases the cost [1].

Adverse Outcomes

Some studies have failed to demonstrate a significant association between IMH and adverse perinatal outcomes, while other studies have shown greater frequency and increased risk of complications when IMH is diagnosed in the first 20 weeks of gestation [75, 86, 87]. However, it should not be forgotten that some risk factors for IMH are also associated by themselves with adverse perinatal results. It is also possible that IMH interacts with genetic factors, other endogenous factors, or environmental insults to increase the risk of adverse outcomes, so this situation must be taken into account when evaluating the risks [53, 88–90].

Table 2 shows some of the studies carried out to evaluate the association of IMH with the risk of maternal or fetal complications [6, 9, 12, 15, 17, 22, 23, 29, 31, 39–41, 43, 62, 63, 91–95].

Table 2 Adverse maternal and fetal outcomes associated with isolated maternal hypothyroxinemia

Cases/ Controls or N	GA	Diagnostic criteria	Perinatal and maternal outcomes reported	Ref.
233/16,011	6–20 w	TSH (2.5–97.5th p); FT4 (<2.5th p) < 0.86 ng/dL	IMH was not associated with adverse pregnancy outcomes (hypertensive disorders, GDM, placental abruption, PD or cesarean delivery)	[9]
232/10,990 in first T; 247/10,990 in second T	≥10.3 w	TSH (2.5–97.5th p); FT4 (<2.5th p) first and second T < 0.71 ng/dL	IMH in the first T increases the risk of PD and in the second T increases the risk of GDM	[12]
89/756	15–16 w	TSH 0.15–4.0 mU/L; FT4 (<10th p) < 0.66 ng/dL	IMH was not associated with any adverse effect on fetal growth or pregnancy outcome	[15]
102 PD/4318 ND	11–13.6 w	TPOAb or TgAb positive >60 U/mL	Spontaneous PD was not associated with TPOAb or TgAb positivity, or thyroid dysfunction at 11–13.6 w	[95]
43/845	<20 w	TSH (5–95th p); FT4 (<5th p) 5–8 w < 0.80 ng/dL; 9–12 w < 0.75 ng/dL; 13–16 w < 0.74 ng/dL; 17–20 w < 0.66 ng/dL	IMH increases the risk of fetal distress, SGA and musculoskeletal malformations	[17]
175/1584	IR 83–100 d	TSH (<90th p); FT4 (<10th p)	IMH increases the frequency of gestational hypertension	[22]
18/870	11.3–17 w	TSH (2–98th p); FT4 (<second p) < 0.83 ng/dL	IMH increases the frequency of placental abruption and GDM	[23]
145/5826	9.6–17.6 w	TSH (2.5–97.5th p); FT4 (<2.5th p) first T < 0.84 ng/dL; second T < 0.79 ng/dL; TPOAb positive >60 U/mL	IMH in first or second T increases the risk of spontaneous PD, VPD and PRM in spontaneous delivery	[91]
Meta-analysis 458/19,405	<24 w	Study-specific	IMH does not increase the risk of PD	[93]
50 GDM/60 non-GDM	12–24 w; 24–48 w	SRR: TSH 0.4–4.2 mU/L; FT4 < 0.95 ng/dL RRT: TSH second T 0.2–3.0 mU/L; third T 0.3–3.0 mU/L; FT4 second T < 0.75 ng/dL; third T < 0.65 ng/dL	GDM increases the frequency of IMH using SRR in second T and third T, as well as using RRT in second T and third T. GDM increases the frequency of TPOAb positivity	[94]
82/741	28 w	TSH 0.35–3.00 mU/L; FT4 (<10th p) < 0.80 ng/dL	IMH increases the frequency of adverse metabolic phenotype (BMI, sum of skinfolds, fasting plasma glucose, triglycerides and HOMA-IR)	[29]
55/165	11.9 w	TSH 0.2–2.5 mU/L; FT4 < 1.00 ng/dL	IMH increases the frequency and risk of fetal breech presentation and the frequency of cesarean delivery	[31]

(continued)

Table 2 (continued)

Cases/ Controls or *N*	GA	Diagnostic criteria	Perinatal and maternal outcomes reported	Ref.
220/1800	IR 11.9–14.1 w	FT4 (<5th p) < 0.60 ng/dL; FT4 (< 10th p) < 0.63 ng/dL	Hypothyroxinemia increases the frequency of gestational hypertension.	[62]
228 low first *T*/low third *T*; 608 low first *T*/normal third *T*; 523 normal first *T*/low third *T*; 4672 normal first *T*/ normal third *T*	1st *T* 9–12 w; third *T* 32–36 w	FT4 (< 10th p) first *T* < 1.04 ng/dL; third *T* < 0.80 ng/dL	Low/normal FT4 increases the risk of GDM, and low/low FT4 and normal/low FT4 increases the risk of preeclampsia	[92]
379/513	1st *T* < 12 w; second *T* 13–27 w; third *T* > 28 w	TSH 2011 ATA; FT4 < 0.93 ng/dL	IMH reduces the frequency of miscarriage, and increases the frequency of gestational hypertension and PD	[6]
36/1389	1st *T*	TSH (2.5–97.5th p); FT4 (<2.5th p) < 0.71 ng/dL	IMH increases the frequency of GDM. TSH and FT4 do not increase the risk of GDM	[39]
101/2107 in first *T*; 241/5724 in second *T*	13–20 w	TSH first *T* 0.06–3.83 mU/L; second *T* 0.07–4.08 mU/L; FT4 first *T* < 1.01 ng/dL; second *T* < 0.95 ng/dL	IMH in second *T* increases the risk of hypertensive disorders of pregnancy and placental abruption	[41]
904/37,202	7.0–39.7 w	TSH (2.5–97.5th p); FT4 (<2.5th p)	IMH in second *T* increases the risk of PD and VPD	[40]
67/784 in first *T*; 70/1943 in second *T*	6–13 w; 14–27 w	TSH (2.5–97.5th p); FT4 (<10th p) first *T* < 0.68 ng/dL; second *T* < 0.49 ng/dL	IMH was not associated with adverse pregnancy outcomes (hypertensive disorders, GDM, placenta previa, placental abruption, fetal grow restriction, fetal distress, intrauterine fetal death and PRM)	[43]
936 with FT4 < 2.5th p/40,948; 1987 with FT4 < fifth p/39,924	9–13 w	TSH (2.5–97.5th p); FT4 (<2.5th p) < 0.90 ng/dL; FT4 (<5th p)	IMH increases the frequency of GDM and IMH, and the risk of spontaneous PD with intact membranes. The effects were modified by fetal sex, remaining significant only when fetal sex was female	[63]

Cases pregnant women with isolated maternal hypothyroxinemia (unless otherwise indicated), *Controls* pregnant women with euthyroxinemia (unless otherwise indicated), *GA* gestational age, *w* weeks, *TSH* thyroid stimulating hormone, *FT4* free thyroxine, *p* percentile, *GMD* gestational diabetes mellitus, *PD* premature delivery, *VPD* very premature delivery, *SGA* small for gestational age, *PRM* premature rupture of membranes, *T* trimester, *IMH* isolated maternal hypothyroxinemia, *ND* normal delivery, *IR* interquartile range, *d* day, *TPOAb* thyroid peroxidase antibodies, *TgAb* thyroglobulin antibodies, *BMI* body mass index, *HOMA-IR* homeostatic model assessment for insulin resistance, *HbA1c* glycated hemoglobin, *FT3* free triiodothyronine, *HDL* high density lipoprotein, *SRR* standard reference range, *RRT* reference range per trimester, *ATA* American Thyroid Association

Table 3 shows some studies carried out to evaluate the association of IMH with the risk of postnatal complications [4, 6, 9, 12, 14, 16, 19, 22, 23, 31, 35–37, 41, 43, 62, 89, 90, 96–106].

Some of the adverse effects that have been most frequently associated with IMH are increased risk of PD, higher birth weight, and alterations in the behavioral, mental, language, motor, psychomotor, and cognitive development of the offspring [47, 88].

Table 3 Adverse postnatal outcomes associated with isolated maternal hypothyroxinemia

Cases/controls or *N*	GA	Diagnostic criteria	Offspring outcomes reported	Ref.
57/58	12, 24 and 32 w	TSH 0.15–2.0 mU/L; FT4 (<10th p) < 0.96 ng/dL	IMH at 12 w was associated with a reduction in mental and motor scores at 1 y and 2 y of age in the offspring	[96]
16 from a moderately iodine-deficient area (A)/11 from a marginally iodine-sufficient area (B)	5–10, 11–14 and 18–20 w	TSH 0.4–4.0 mU/L; FT4 (mean ± 2SD) 8 w < 1.02 ng/dL; 13 w < 0.98 ng/dL; 20 w < 0.85 ng/dL	ADHD was more frequent in area A than in area B at 18–36 m and 8–10 y. Mean IQ was lower in children in area A than in children in Area B. FT4 decreased by 20% with gestational age in area A with ADHD and area A without ADHD, but only 8% in area B, always being lower in group B at any time. ADHD would be the ultimate consequence of IMH due to iodine deficiency	[89]
233/16,011	6–20 w	TSH (2.5–97.5th p); FT4 (<2.5th p) < 0.86 ng/dL	IMH was not associated with neonatal complications	[9]
232/10,990 in first *T*; 247/10,990 in second *T*	≥ 10.3 w	TSH (2.5–97.5th p); FT4 (<2.5th p) < 0.71 ng/dL	IMH in the first T increases the frequency of birth weight > 4000 g	[12]
12 with IMH at 12–14 w; 19 with IMH postdelivery; 13 euthyroid at 4–6 w.	≥ 4 w	TSH 0.38–4.80 mU/L; FT4 (<10th p) < 0.82 ng/dL	IMH at 12–14 w and postdelivery was associated with a reduction in the mean developmental quotient at 18 m in the offspring. The later iodine is administered during pregnancy, the greater the risk of delayed neurocognitive development in the offspring	[14]
19/38	16–20 w	TSH (2.5–97.5th p); FT4 (2.5th–97.5th p) 0.92–1.91 ng/dL. TPOAb <50 U/mL; TT4 (<2.5th p) < 7.90 μg/dL	IMH was associated with a reduction in the mean motor and intelligence score in the offspring	[100]

(continued)

Table 3 (continued)

Cases/controls or *N*	GA	Diagnostic criteria	Offspring outcomes reported	Ref.
500	1st *T*	TSH 0.35–2.5 mU/L; TT4 4.5–10.9 µg/L	Maternal TSH and FT4 were not associated with TT4 level or cognitive test score in the offspring	[105]
2736	11.6–15.0 w	TSH 0.03–2.5 mU/L; FT4 (mild IMH < 10th p) < 0.91 ng/dL; (severe IMH < 5th p) < 0.85 ng/dL	IMH was associated with reduced FT4 levels in newborns. Mild IMH increases the risk of expressive language delay across 18 to 30 m. Severe IMH increases the risk of expressive language delay at 18 m, across ages and at 30 m, and of nonverbal cognitive delay at 30 m	[16]
3736	<18 w	TSH 0.03–2.5 mU/L; FT4 (<10th p) < 0.91 ng/dL	IMH was not associated with internalizing or externalizing scores at 1.5 and 3 y	[106]
99/99	2nd *T*	TSH 0.1–3.5 mU/L; FT4 (<3rd p) < 0.92 ng/dL	IMH during second T was not associated with significant changes in BSID at 2 y of age in the offspring	[19]
45/3189	<20 w	TSH first T 0.07–3.1 mU/L; second T 0.10–3.5 mU/L; FT4 first *T* < 0.88 ng/dL; second *T* < 0.86 ng/dL	IMH increases the median TPOAb concentrations in offspring between 7 and 16 y of age. Median TPOAb concentrations were higher in boys than in girls	[4]
175/1584	IR 83–100 d	TSH (<90th p); FT4 (<10th p)	FT4 less than the 10th p at the end of the first T was associated with a slower mean reaction time and a greater reaction time in the offspring, with a greater effect when the TSH level was higher	[22]
18/870	11.3–17.2 w	TSH (2–98th p); FT4 (<2nd p) < 0.83 ng/dL	IMH increases the frequency of birth weight > 4000 g	[23]
4464	11.3–15.0 w	TSH (2.5–97.5th p); FT4 (2.5–97.5th p) 0.80–1.70 ng/dL Cord serum: TSH 3.41–33.8 mU/L; FT4 1.18–2.18 ng/dL	FT4 increases the risk of SGA and lower birth weight	[102]
1643	8–20 w	TSH (2.5–97.5th p); FT4 (<5th p) < 0.65 ng/dL	Low maternal FT4 was associated with a lower mental score in the offspring. TSH levels were not associated with mental or psychomotor scores	[103]

Table 3 (continued)

Cases/controls or *N*	GA	Diagnostic criteria	Offspring outcomes reported	Ref.
4039	5.0–17.9 w	TSH 0.03–2.5 mU/L; FT4 (Mild IMH < 10th p) < 0.91 ng/dL; (Severe IMH < 5th p) < 0.85 ng/dL	Severe IMH increases the risk of children with autism, borderline PDP, and clinical PDP	[104]
455	1st and second *T*	TSH 0.01–5 mU/L; FT4 (<10th p) first *T* < 1.06 ng/dL; second *T* < 0.89 ng/dL	FT4 at the end of the first or second *T* was not associated with intellectual scores at 1 y or 6–8 y of age in the offspring	[99]
3576	6.6–17.9 w	TSH 0.1–2.5 mU/L; FT4 < 0.85 ng/dL	IMH increases ADHD scores at 8 y of age in the offspring	[108]
1010 with schizophrenia/1010 without schizophrenia	1st *T*	TSH (5–95th p); FT4 (<10th p) < 1.09 ng/dL	IMH increases the risk of schizophrenia	[90]
3839	<18 w	TSH (2.5–97.5th p); FT4 (2.5–97.5th p)	FT4 showed an inverted U-shaped association with child IQ, child gray matter volume, and cortex volume	[101]
55/165	11.9 w	TSH 0.2–2.5 mU/L; FT4 < 1.00 ng/dL	IMH increases the frequency and risk of macrosomia	[31]
220/1800	IR 11.9–14.1 w	FT4 (<5th p) < 0.60 ng/dL; FT4 (<10th p) < 0.63 ng/dL	Hypothyroxinemia (FT4 < 5th p) increases the risk of teacher-reported hyperactivity-inattention	[62]
Meta-analysis 168/6442; 32/1159 INMA[a]; 86/3224 generation R[b]; 50/2059 ALSPAC[c]	12.2–14.4[a], 11.4–15.4[b] and 8.1–14.5 w[c]	TSH (2.5–97.5th p); FT4 (<2.5th p) < 0.65 ng/dL[a]; <0.80 ng/dL[b]; <0.97 ng/dLc and TSH (5–95th p); FT4 (<5th p)[a, b, c]	IMH reduces nonverbal IQ and verbal IQ. IMH (TSH 5–95th p; FT4 < 5th p) increases the risk of autistic traits	[97]
93/4169	IR 8–12 w	TSH (2.5–97.5th p); FT4 (<2.5th p)	IMH in early pregnancy was not associated with impaired scholastic performance or educational attainment in the offspring	[35]
78/3002 in first T; 74/2925 in second T	1st and second *T*	TSH (2.5–97.5th p); FT4 (<2.5th p); first *T* < 1.02 ng/dL; second *T* < 0.71 ng/dL	IMH in second *T* increases the risk of large for gestational age	[36]
46/882	1st, second and third *T*	TSH (5–95th p); FT4 (<5th p)	IMH reduces Apgar scores and increases the risk of birth weight > 4000 g	[37]
379/513	1st, second and third *T*	TSH 2011 ATA; FT4 < 0.93 ng/dL	IMH increases the frequency of very low birth weight	[6]

(continued)

Table 3 (continued)

Cases/controls or *N*	GA	Diagnostic criteria	Offspring outcomes reported	Ref.
101/2107 in first *T*; 241/5724 in second *T*	13–20 w	TSH first T 0.06–3.83 mU/L; second T 0.07–4.08 mU/L; FT4 first *T* < 1.01 ng/dL; second *T* < 0.95 ng/dL	IMH increases the risk of birth weight > 4000 g	[41]
67/784 in first *T*; 70/1943 in second *T*	6–13 and 14–27 w	TSH (2.5–97.5th p); FT4 (<10th p) first *T* < 0.68 ng/dL; second *T* < 0.49 ng/dL	IMH does not modify the frequency of low birth weight (<2500 g) and fetal malformations	[43]
Meta-analysis based on 20 international cohorts 929/38,248	7.0–39.7 w	TSH (2.5–97.5th p); FT4 (<2.5th p)	IMH reduces the frequency and risk of SGA and increases mean birth weight. For each SD increase in FT4 concentration, the risk of SGA increases and the mean birth weight decreases	[98]

Cases pregnant women with isolated maternal hypothyroxinemia (unless otherwise indicated), *Controls* pregnant women with euthyroxinemia (unless otherwise indicated), *GA* gestational age, *USA* United States of America, *BSID* Bayley Scale of Infant Development, *y* years, *w* weeks, *TSH* thyroid stimulating hormone, *FT4* free thyroxine, *TT4* total thyroxine, *p* percentile, *IMH* isolated maternal hypothyroxinemia, *ADHD* attention deficit and hyperactivity disorder, *T* trimester, *SGA* small for gestational age, *m* months, *IR* interquartile range, *d* day, *PDP* Pervasive Developmental Problems, *MRI* magnetic resonance imaging, *IQ* intelligence quotient, *TPOAb* thyroid peroxidase antibodies, *INMA* Infancia y Medio Ambiente, *ALSPAC* Avon Longitudinal Study of Parents and Children, *ATA* American Thyroid Association, *SD* standard deviation

Regarding prematurity, various mechanisms have been proposed in hypothyroidism that could be involved in hypothyroxinemia. For example, oxytocin and vasopressin are involved in the onset of labor, and increased vasopressin levels have been observed in animal models and hypothyroid women. Furthermore, in animal models of hypothyroidism, a high amount of surfactant protein A has been observed, which modulates the inflammatory response associated with spontaneous preterm labor [91]. Another factor that can be associated with the occurrence of preterm labor is the increase in oxidative stress, which can also be increased in hypothyroidism [63].

It has been reported that there is an association between low maternal FT4 concentrations in women with IMH during gestation and a higher birth weight, unlike that reported in subclinical hypothyroidism where it is associated with small for gestational age (SGA). The effect observed in IMH is independent of the TSH level, TPOAb status, or hCG effect, so it could not represent a thyroid alteration as such, but rather a possible dysfunction of the utero placental unit [98]. On the other hand, low FT4 levels during pregnancy have been reported to be associated with a higher rate of insulin resistance and gestational diabetes [94], which could favor placental transfer of glucose to the fetal circulation. Excess glucose in the fetus would be stored as body fat, being the potential cause of macrosomia [31].

Finally, in the early stages of fetal life, fundamental process occurs in the central nervous system, including cell migration, differentiation, and the induction of neural tissue in the neocortex, where thyroid hormones are crucial. Before the onset of thyroid hormone production by the fetus in mid-pregnancy, fetal brain development depends on maternal thyroid hormones, so low FT4 levels, mainly in early pregnancy, could be the factor leading to neurodevelopmental disorders [16, 47, 86, 104, 107–111]. In fact, studies in animal models have shown that maternal hypothyroxinemia is responsible for the disruption in cytoarchitecture of the cerebral cortex due to impaired migration and neuronal heterotopy in the progeny [112–115]. By the other hand, low FT4 levels may also indicate suboptimal placental function, so cognitive delay in children of mothers with hypothyroxinemia may also be a consequence of early placental insufficiency [16].

Treatment

Because one of the risk factors for IMH, as well as for alterations in offspring neurodevelopment, is iodine deficiency, many countries have universally adopted salt iodization to ensure sufficient iodine intake in the general population, although it does not imply that it is sufficient during pregnancy [20, 89, 116]. Furthermore, there are still countries with insufficient iodine supplementation during pregnancy, for which the importance of ensuring iodine intake before conception and early pregnancy has been emphasized [20, 74, 110]. An increase of 150–250 μg per day in iodine intake has been recommended by the World Health Organization [117]. A study showed that in addition to the consumption of iodized salt, the use of iodine supplements in conjunction with the daily consumption of eggs and fish reduces the frequency of thyroid dysfunction, including IMH, during pregnancy [44].

It has been suggested that all women should start the intake of iodine supplementation at the first prenatal visit, continue it during pregnancy and lactation, either in the form of potassium iodide (KI) or potassium iodate (KIO_3) tablets or vitamin-mineral mixtures [8, 107]. However, emphasis has been placed on establishing the upper limits of iodine intake. A study reported an increase in the prevalence of subclinical hypothyroidism and TPOAb positivity in pregnant women with more than adequate iodine status (urinary iodine concentrations [UIC] 250–499 μg/L). Although also a higher prevalence of TPOAb positivity was observed in women with insufficient iodin status (UIC $<$ 100 μg/L). In addition, a higher prevalence of IMH was observed in women with excessive iodine status (UCI $\geq$ 500 μg/L). The authors suggest that both iodine deficiency and more than adequate iodine can result in thyroid autoimmunity and subclinical hypothyroidism, and that excess of iodine can trigger the Wolff-Chaikoff effect, with reduced formation and release of thyroid hormone that has been observed in IMH [118].

A study showed lower scores in the evaluation of the mental and motor development of the children of women with hypothyroxinemia in the first 12 weeks and who also showed greater decrease in FT4 during the rest of the gestation, while the children of women with hypothyroxinemia early but whose FT4 levels increased during the rest of the gestation did not show development delay. Therefore, the authors discussed the need to evaluate whether treatment with iodine or thyroxine could be of greater benefit in cases of hypothyroxinemia diagnosed in the first trimester of pregnancy [96].

It has been suggested, if despite iodine supplementation, FT4 persists below the 10th p for gestational age, additional treatment with levothyroxine may be considered to ensure that FT4 levels are within the reference levels of iodine-sufficient euthyroid women in the same gestational age [107]. However, levothyroxine treatment (150 μg daily for a TSH goal of 1.0 mU/L) in women with elevated TSH (but less than 4.68 mU/L), low FT4 (less than 1.03), or both has been reported not to improve their children's cognitive function as assessed at 3 years of age, compared to women not receiving levothyroxine [18].

A randomized controlled clinical trial in 526 pregnant women with hypothyroxinemia diagnosed in the first 20 weeks of gestation evaluated the effect of thyroid hormone replacement at 17.8 weeks of gestation on average (50 μg of levothyroxine with a maximum dose of 200 μg daily, until reaching a FT4 goal of 0.86–1.90 ng/dL) in 265 women vs 261 who received placebo. No differences were found in the frequency of perinatal results (preterm delivery, pregnancy complications, fetal death, neonatal morbidity or mortality), nor in cognitive function or neurodevelopmental indices during the first 5 years of their children [33].

An inverse association has been reported between FT4 concentration and birth weight, which occurs more frequently in the second and third trimesters of gestation and which could be related to a greater metabolic effect of thyroid hormone on fetal growth [98]. It has also been reported that both low and high maternal FT4 during pregnancy are associated with lower child IQ evaluated on average at 6 years of age and lower gray matter and cortex volume evaluated by magnetic resonance imaging (MRI) on average at 8 years of age [101]. These situations must be evaluated and taken into account and avoid overtreatment with levothyroxine.

On the other hand, a study reported a significant reduction in the risk of PD (OR 0.020; 95% CI 0.005–0.085), as well as low birth weight and very low birth weight in newborns (OR 0.019; 95% CI 0.003–0.15) of mothers with hypothyroxinemia, when they received levothyroxine treatment (1.5–2.5 μg/kg per day to ensure serum TSH levels <3 mU/L) during the second and third trimester of gestation, compared to those who did not receive it [6].

So far, in addition to iodine supplementation, there is insufficient evidence to recommend the use of levothyroxine for the treatment of IMH [75]. The clinical guidelines propose different recommendations, the ETA indicates that treatment with levothyroxine can be considered when hypothyroxinemia is detected in the first trimester and the ATA does not recommend any special treatment [2, 3].

Lastly, thyroid hormones are essential in regulating metabolic processes and energy to maintain homeostasis, so small changes in thyroid hormone levels have been associated with adverse metabolic consequences in pregnancy. Changes in thyroid hormone levels in pregnancy have been suggested to be a consequence rather than a cause of changes in body weight, so weight loss and lifestyle-modifying interventions may be associated with desirable changes in thyroid hormone levels [29].

Monitoring

Severe endemic iodine deficiency has been reported to lead to over hypothyroidism, while mild to moderate deficiency is more frequently associated with IMH. Therefore, depending on the country of residence, specific measures must be taken to carry out iodine supplementation in the general population and in pregnant women, making sure to maintain an adequate level of iodine [20]. Although mean urine iodine concentrations can be used to determine the iodine status of populations, there are no biomarkers to diagnose iodine deficiency individually [119]. It may be appropriate to assess the level of thyroid function, including FT4 levels in women during the early pregnancy [16], particularly in the presence of risk factors for hypothyroxinemia [120].

One study reported that IMH before 12 weeks of gestation was not associated with an increased risk of adverse perinatal outcomes, regardless of whether they received 50 μg of levothyroxine daily (oral dose was adjusted during follow-up, to a maximum of 100 μg daily) or not, while hypothyroxinemia in the second trimester was associated with an increased risk of macrosomia (OR 1.94, 95% CI 1.07–3.50; $p = 0.027$) and gestational hypertension (OR 4.20, 95% CI 1.61–10.96; $p < 0.01$), when BMI in the early pregnancy was <25 kg/m^2, for which the authors propose monitoring thyroid function during the second trimester even when thyroid function is reported as normal in the first trimester [111, 121].

On the other hand, TPOAb measurement should always be performed in women with IMH, since TPOAb positivity is an independent risk factor for adverse perinatal outcomes. There is no indication to start treatment with levothyroxine in women with positive TPOAb and TSH within normality, although treatment may be considered during the first trimester of pregnancy in women with a history of pregnancy loss [46, 88].

Summary

IMH has been defined by the American Thyroid Association (ATA) as a free thyroxine (FT4) concentration in the lower 2.5-5th percentile (p) and by the European Thyroid Association (ETA) in the lower than 2.5 p of a given population, despite a normal maternal serum thyroid stimulating hormone (TSH) concentration. The frequency of IMH has been reported in approximately 2–4% of pregnant women; however, it can be as high as 49.33%. Apparently, these differences are related to maternal iodine intake, reference ranges for TSH and FT4, gestational age or trimester of pregnancy and the measurement method of FT4. A single cause of IMH has not been identified, however, various risk factors have been reported such as iodine deficiency, iron deficiency, placental angiogenic factors, high body mass index (BMI), human chorionic gonadotropin (hCG) concentrations, autoimmunity, older age, multiparity, hypertension, lower level of education, smoking, environmental pollutants, anxiety, and twin pregnancy. The diagnosis of IMH during pregnancy is based upon finding a normal maternal TSH concentration and a serum thyroxine (T4) [either total (TT4) or FT4] concentration in the lower 2.5th–5th p of a given population. However, the reference range of TSH and T4 can vary significantly in different populations and between trimesters in the same patient as well as show variations depending on the analysis method. Some studies have failed to demonstrate a significant association between IMH and adverse perinatal outcomes, while other studies have shown greater frequency and increased risk of complications when IMH is diagnosed in the first 20 weeks of gestation. Some of the adverse effects that have been most frequently associated with IMH are increased risk of PD, higher birth weight, and alterations in the behavioral, mental, language, motor, psychomotor, and cognitive development of the offspring. Nevertheless, until now, in addition to iodine supplementation, there is insufficient evidence to recommend the use of levothyroxine for the treatment of IMH.

References

1. Furnica RM, Lazarus JH, Gruson D, Daumerie C. Update on a new controversy in endocrinology: isolated maternal hypothyroxinemia. J Endocrinol Investig. 2015;38(2):117–23.
2. Alexander EK, Pearce EN, Brent GA, Brown RS, Chen H, Dosiou C, et al. 2017 Guidelines of the American Thyroid Association for the diagnosis and management of thyroid disease during pregnancy and the postpartum. Thyroid. 2017;27(3):315–89.
3. Lazarus J, Brown RS, Daumerie C, Hubalewska-Dydejczyk A, Negro R, Vaidya B. 2014 European thyroid association guidelines for the management of subclinical hypothyroidism in pregnancy and in children. Eur Thyroid J. 2014;3(2):76–94.
4. Pakkila F, Mannisto T, Surcel HM, Ruokonen A, Bloigu A, Pouta A, et al. Maternal thyroid dysfunction during pregnancy and thyroid function of her child in adolescence. J Clin Endocrinol Metab. 2013;98(3):965–72.
5. Etemadi A, Amouzegar A, Mehran L, Tohidi M, Azizi F, Moradi K, et al. Isolated hypothyroxinemia in iranian pregnant women, the role of iodine deficiency: a population-based cross-sectional study. Thyroid. 2020;30(2):262–9.
6. Zhou M, Wang M, Li J, Luo X, Lei M. Effects of thyroid diseases on pregnancy outcomes. Exp Ther Med. 2019;18(3):1807–15.
7. Teng W, Shan Z, Patil-Sisodia K, Cooper DS. Hypothyroidism in pregnancy. Lancet Diabetes Endocrinol. 2013;1(3):228–37.
8. Negro R, Mestman JH. Thyroid disease in pregnancy. Best Pract Res Clin Endocrinol Metab. 2011;25(6):927–43.
9. Casey BM, Dashe JS, Spong CY, McIntire DD, Leveno KJ, Cunningham GF. Perinatal significance of isolated maternal hypothyroxinemia identified in the first half of pregnancy. Obstet Gynecol. 2007;109(5):1129–35.
10. Zimmermann MB, Burgi H, Hurrell RF. Iron deficiency predicts poor maternal thyroid status during pregnancy. J Clin Endocrinol Metab. 2007;92(9):3436–40.
11. Vaidya B, Anthony S, Bilous M, Shields B, Drury J, Hutchison S, et al. Detection of thyroid dysfunction in early pregnancy: universal screening or targeted high-risk case finding? J Clin Endocrinol Metab. 2007;92(1):203–7.

12. Cleary-Goldman J, Malone FD, Lambert-Messerlian G, Sullivan L, Canick J, Porter TF, et al. Maternal thyroid hypofunction and pregnancy outcome. Obstet Gynecol. 2008;112(1):85–92.
13. Moleti M, Lo Presti VP, Campolo MC, Mattina F, Galletti M, Mandolfino M, et al. Iodine prophylaxis using iodized salt and risk of maternal thyroid failure in conditions of mild iodine deficiency. J Clin Endocrinol Metab. 2008;93(7):2616–21.
14. Berbel P, Mestre JL, Santamaria A, Palazon I, Franco A, Graells M, et al. Delayed neurobehavioral development in children born to pregnant women with mild hypothyroxinemia during the first month of gestation: the importance of early iodine supplementation. Thyroid. 2009;19(5):511–9.
15. Hamm MP, Cherry NM, Martin JW, Bamforth F, Burstyn I. The impact of isolated maternal hypothyroxinemia on perinatal morbidity. J Obstet Gynaecol Can. 2009;31(11):1015–21.
16. Henrichs J, Bongers-Schokking JJ, Schenk JJ, Ghassabian A, Schmidt HG, Visser TJ, et al. Maternal thyroid function during early pregnancy and cognitive functioning in early childhood: the generation R study. J Clin Endocrinol Metab. 2010;95(9):4227–34.
17. Su PY, Huang K, Hao JH, Xu YQ, Yan SQ, Li T, et al. Maternal thyroid function in the first twenty weeks of pregnancy and subsequent fetal and infant development: a prospective population-based cohort study in China. J Clin Endocrinol Metab. 2011;96(10):3234–41.
18. Lazarus JH, Bestwick JP, Channon S, Paradice R, Maina A, Rees R, et al. Antenatal thyroid screening and childhood cognitive function. N Engl J Med. 2012;366(6):493–501.
19. Craig WY, Allan WC, Kloza EM, Pulkkinen AJ, Waisbren S, Spratt DI, et al. Mid-gestational maternal free thyroxine concentration and offspring neurocognitive development at age two years. J Clin Endocrinol Metab. 2012;97(1):E22–8.
20. Oguz Kutlu A, Kara C. Iodine deficiency in pregnant women in the apparently iodine-sufficient capital city of Turkey. Clin Endocrinol. 2012;77(4):615–20.
21. Altomare M, La Vignera S, Asero P, Recupero D, Condorelli RA, Scollo P, et al. High prevalence of thyroid dysfunction in pregnant women. J Endocrinol Investig. 2013;36(6):407–11.
22. Finken MJ, van Eijsden M, Loomans EM, Vrijkotte TG, Rotteveel J. Maternal hypothyroxinemia in early pregnancy predicts reduced performance in reaction time tests in 5- to 6-year-old offspring. J Clin Endocrinol Metab. 2013;98(4):1417–26.
23. Breathnach FM, Donnelly J, Cooley SM, Geary M, Malone FD. Subclinical hypothyroidism as a risk factor for placental abruption: evidence from a low-risk primigravid population. Aust N Z J Obstet Gynaecol. 2013;53(6):553–60.
24. Gowachirapant S, Melse-Boonstra A, Winichagoon P, Zimmermann MB. Overweight increases risk of first trimester hypothyroxinaemia in iodine-deficient pregnant women. Matern Child Nutr. 2014;10(1):61–71.
25. Saki F, Dabbaghmanesh MH, Ghaemi SZ, Forouhari S, Ranjbar Omrani G, Bakhshayeshkaram M. Thyroid function in pregnancy and its influences on maternal and fetal outcomes. Int J Endocrinol Metab. 2014;12(4):e19378.
26. Habimana L, Twite KE, Daumerie C, Wallemacq P, Donnen P, Kalenga MK, et al. High prevalence of thyroid dysfunction among pregnant women in Lubumbashi, Democratic Republic of Congo. Thyroid. 2014;24(3):568–75.
27. Yu X, Shan Z, Li C, Mao J, Wang W, Xie X, et al. Iron deficiency, an independent risk factor for isolated hypothyroxinemia in pregnant and nonpregnant women of childbearing age in China. J Clin Endocrinol Metab. 2015;100(4):1594–601.
28. Han C, Li C, Mao J, Wang W, Xie X, Zhou W, et al. High body mass index is an indicator of maternal hypothyroidism, hypothyroxinemia, and thyroid-peroxidase antibody positivity during early pregnancy. Biomed Res Int. 2015;2015:351831.
29. Knight BA, Shields BM, Hattersley AT, Vaidya B. Maternal hypothyroxinaemia in pregnancy is associated with obesity and adverse maternal metabolic parameters. Eur J Endocrinol. 2016;174(1):51–7.
30. Dieguez M, Herrero A, Avello N, Suarez P, Delgado E, Menendez E. Prevalence of thyroid dysfunction in women in early pregnancy: does it increase with maternal age? Clin Endocrinol. 2016;84(1):121–6.
31. Furnica RM, Gruson D, Lazarus JH, Maiter D, Bernard P, Daumerie C. First trimester isolated maternal hypothyroxinaemia: adverse maternal metabolic profile and impact on the obstetrical outcome. Clin Endocrinol. 2017;86(4):576–83.

32. Korevaar TI, de Rijke YB, Chaker L, Medici M, Jaddoe VW, Steegers EA, et al. Stimulation of thyroid function by human chorionic gonadotropin during pregnancy: a risk factor for thyroid disease and a mechanism for known risk factors. Thyroid. 2017;27(3):440–50.
33. Casey BM, Thom EA, Peaceman AM, Varner MW, Sorokin Y, Hirtz DG, et al. Treatment of subclinical hypothyroidism or hypothyroxinemia in pregnancy. N Engl J Med. 2017;376(9):815–25.
34. Hernandez-Mariano JA, Torres-Sanchez L, Bassol-Mayagoitia S, Escamilla-Nunez MC, Cebrian ME, Villeda-Gutierrez EA, et al. Effect of exposure to p,p -DDE during the first half of pregnancy in the maternal thyroid profile of female residents in a Mexican floriculture area. Environ Res. 2017;156:597–604.
35. Nelson SM, Haig C, McConnachie A, Sattar N, Ring SM, Smith GD, et al. Maternal thyroid function and child educational attainment: prospective cohort study. BMJ. 2018;360:k452.
36. Zhu YD, Han Y, Huang K, Zhu BB, Yan SQ, Ge X, et al. The impact of isolated maternal hypothyroxinaemia on the incidence of large-for-gestational-age infants: the Ma'anshan Birth Cohort study. BJOG. 2018;125(9):1118–25.
37. Yang J, Liu Y, Liu H, Zheng H, Li X, Zhu L, et al. Associations of maternal iodine status and thyroid function with adverse pregnancy outcomes in Henan Province of China. J Trace Elem Med Biol. 2018;47:104–10.
38. Dong AC, Stagnaro-Green A. Differences in diagnostic criteria mask the true prevalence of thyroid disease in pregnancy: a systematic review and meta-analysis. Thyroid. 2019;29(2):278–89.
39. Huang K, Xu Y, Yan S, Li T, Xu Y, Zhu P, et al. Isolated effect of maternal thyroid-stimulating hormone, free thyroxine and antithyroid peroxidase antibodies in early pregnancy on gestational diabetes mellitus: a birth cohort study in China. Endocr J. 2019;66(3):223–31.
40. Consortium on T, Pregnancy-Study Group on Preterm B, Korevaar TIM, Derakhshan A, Taylor PN, Meima M, et al. Association of thyroid function test abnormalities and thyroid autoimmunity with preterm birth: a systematic review and meta-analysis. JAMA. 2019;322(7):632–41.
41. Su X, Zhao Y, Cao Z, Yang Y, Duan T, Hua J. Association between isolated hypothyroxinaemia in early pregnancy and perinatal outcomes. Endocr Connect. 2019;8(4):435–41.
42. Chen Z, Yang X, Zhang C, Ding Z, Zhang Y, Korevaar TIM, et al. Thyroid function test abnormalities in twin pregnancies. Thyroid. 2020;
43. Chen L, Yang H, Ye E, Lin Z, Peng M, Lin H, et al. Insignificant effect of isolated hypothyroxinemia on pregnancy outcomes during the first and second trimester of pregnancy. Front Endocrinol (Lausanne). 2020;11:528146.
44. Refaat B, Azzeh F. Factors Associated with Thyroid Disorders and Iodine Adequacy in Pregnant Saudi Women. Biol Trace Elem Res. 2020;
45. Dosiou C, Medici M. Management of endocrine disease: isolated maternal hypothyroxinemia during pregnancy: knowns and unknowns. Eur J Endocrinol. 2017;176(1):R21–38.
46. Poppe K, Glinoer D. Thyroid autoimmunity and hypothyroidism before and during pregnancy. Hum Reprod Update. 2003;9(2):149–61.
47. Ramezani Tehrani F, Nazarpour S, Behboudi-Gandevani S. Isolated maternal hypothyroxinemia and adverse pregnancy outcomes: a systematic review. J Gynecol Obstet Hum Reprod. 2021;50(7):102057.
48. Shan ZY, Chen YY, Teng WP, Yu XH, Li CY, Zhou WW, et al. A study for maternal thyroid hormone deficiency during the first half of pregnancy in China. Eur J Clin Investig. 2009;39(1):37–42.
49. Krassas G, Karras SN, Pontikides N. Thyroid diseases during pregnancy: a number of important issues. Hormones (Athens). 2015;14(1):59–69.
50. Lopez-Munoz E, Mateos-Sanchez L, Mejia-Terrazas GE, Bedwell-Cordero SE. Hypothyroidism and isolated hypothyroxinemia in pregnancy, from physiology to the clinic. Taiwan J Obstet Gynecol. 2019;58(6):757–63.
51. Glinoer D. The regulation of thyroid function in pregnancy: pathways of endocrine adaptation from physiology to pathology. Endocr Rev. 1997;18(3):404–33.

52. Vermiglio F, Lo Presti VP, Castagna MG, Violi MA, Moleti M, Finocchiaro MD, et al. Increased risk of maternal thyroid failure with pregnancy progression in an iodine deficient area with major iodine deficiency disorders. Thyroid. 1999;9(1):19–24.
53. Henrichs J, Ghassabian A, Peeters RP, Tiemeier H. Maternal hypothyroxinemia and effects on cognitive functioning in childhood: how and why? Clin Endocrinol. 2013;79(2):152–62.
54. Dahiya B. ASEAN economic integration and sustainable urbanization. J Urban Cult Res. 2016;3(1):8–15. https://doi.org/10.14456/JUCR.2016.10.
55. Veltri F, Decaillet S, Kleynen P, Grabczan L, Belhomme J, Rozenberg S, et al. Prevalence of thyroid autoimmunity and dysfunction in women with iron deficiency during early pregnancy: is it altered? Eur J Endocrinol. 2016;175(3):191–9.
56. Rosario PW, Oliveira LFF, Calsolari MR. Maternal hypothyroxinemia in the first trimester of gestation and association with obstetric and neonatal outcomes and iron deficiency: a prospective Brazilian study. Arch Endocrinol Metab. 2018;62(3):332–6.
57. Korevaar TI, Steegers EA, de Rijke YB, Visser WE, Jaddoe VW, Visser TJ, et al. Placental angiogenic factors are associated with maternal thyroid function and modify hCG-mediated FT4 stimulation. J Clin Endocrinol Metab. 2015;100(10):E1328–34.
58. Clark DE, Smith SK, He Y, Day KA, Licence DR, Corps AN, et al. A vascular endothelial growth factor antagonist is produced by the human placenta and released into the maternal circulation. Biol Reprod. 1998;59(6):1540–8.
59. Kamba T, Tam BY, Hashizume H, Haskell A, Sennino B, Mancuso MR, et al. VEGF-dependent plasticity of fenestrated capillaries in the normal adult microvasculature. Am J Physiol Heart Circ Physiol. 2006;290(2):H560–76.
60. Korevaar TI, Steegers EA, Schalekamp-Timmermans S, Ligthart S, de Rijke YB, Visser WE, et al. Soluble Flt1 and placental growth factor are novel determinants of newborn thyroid (dys)function: the generation R study. J Clin Endocrinol Metab. 2014;99(9):E1627–34.
61. Fan J, Zhang Y, Zhang C, Barjaktarovic M, Yang X, Peeters RP, et al. Persistency of thyroid dysfunction from early to late pregnancy. Thyroid. 2019;29(10):1475–84.
62. Oostenbroek MHW, Kersten RHJ, Tros B, Kunst AE, Vrijkotte TGM, Finken MJJ. Maternal hypothyroxinaemia in early pregnancy and problem behavior in 5-year-old offspring. Psychoneuroendocrinology. 2017;81:29–35.
63. Yang X, Yu Y, Zhang C, Zhang Y, Chen Z, Dubois L, et al. The association between isolated maternal hypothyroxinemia in early pregnancy and preterm birth. Thyroid. 2020;30(12):1724–31.
64. Sheng Y, Huang D, Liu S, Guo X, Chen J, Shao Y, et al. Reference intervals of thyroid hormones and correlation of BMI with thyroid function in healthy zhuang ethnic pregnant women. Biomed Res Int. 2018;2018:2032413.
65. Knudsen N, Bulow I, Laurberg P, Ovesen L, Perrild H, Jorgensen T. Parity is associated with increased thyroid volume solely among smokers in an area with moderate to mild iodine deficiency. Eur J Endocrinol. 2002;146(1):39–43.
66. Korevaar TI, Nieboer D, Bisschop PH, Goddijn M, Medici M, Chaker L, et al. Risk factors and a clinical prediction model for low maternal thyroid function during early pregnancy: two population-based prospective cohort studies. Clin Endocrinol. 2016;85(6):902–9.
67. Rotondi M, Amato G, Biondi B, Mazziotti G, Del Buono A, Rotonda Nicchio M, et al. Parity as a thyroid size-determining factor in areas with moderate iodine deficiency. J Clin Endocrinol Metab. 2000;85(12):4534–7.
68. Moleti M, Lo Presti VP, Mattina F, Mancuso A, De Vivo A, Giorgianni G, et al. Gestational thyroid function abnormalities in conditions of mild iodine deficiency: early screening versus continuous monitoring of maternal thyroid status. Eur J Endocrinol. 2009;160(4):611–7.
69. Koopman-Esseboom C, Morse DC, Weisglas-Kuperus N, Lutkeschipholt IJ, Van der Paauw CG, Tuinstra LG, et al. Effects of dioxins and polychlorinated biphenyls on thyroid hormone status of pregnant women and their infants. Pediatr Res. 1994;36(4):468–73.
70. Ghassabian A, Pierotti L, Basterrechea M, Chatzi L, Estarlich M, Fernandez-Somoano A, et al. Association of exposure to ambient air pollution with thyroid function during pregnancy. JAMA Netw Open. 2019;2(10):e1912902.

71. Pearce EN, Oken E, Gillman MW, Lee SL, Magnani B, Platek D, et al. Association of first-trimester thyroid function test values with thyroperoxidase antibody status, smoking, and multivitamin use. Endocr Pract. 2008;14(1):33–9.
72. Olivares EL, Silva-Almeida C, Pestana FM, Sonoda-Cortes R, Araujo IG, Rodrigues NC, et al. Social stress-induced hypothyroidism is attenuated by antidepressant treatment in rats. Neuropharmacology. 2012;62(1):446–56.
73. De Groot L, Abalovich M, Alexander EK, Amino N, Barbour L, Cobin RH, et al. Management of thyroid dysfunction during pregnancy and postpartum: an Endocrine Society clinical practice guideline. J Clin Endocrinol Metab. 2012;97(8):2543–65.
74. Krassas GE, Poppe K, Glinoer D. Thyroid function and human reproductive health. Endocr Rev. 2010;31(5):702–55.
75. Dong AC, Stephenson MD, Stagnaro-Green AS. The need for dynamic clinical guidelines: a systematic review of new research published after release of the 2017 ATA guidelines on thyroid disease during pregnancy and the postpartum. Front Endocrinol (Lausanne). 2020;11:193.
76. Stagnaro-Green A, Abalovich M, Alexander E, Azizi F, Mestman J, Negro R, et al. Guidelines of the American Thyroid Association for the diagnosis and management of thyroid disease during pregnancy and postpartum. Thyroid. 2011;21(10):1081–125.
77. Rotondi M, Capelli V, Chiovato L, Nappi RE. 2017 ATA guidelines on the management of thyroid dysfunctions in pregnancy: what do OB/GYNs need to know? Gynecol Endocrinol. 2019;35(4):276–9.
78. Yue B, Rockwood AL, Sandrock T, La'ulu SL, Kushnir MM, Meikle AW. Free thyroid hormones in serum by direct equilibrium dialysis and online solid-phase extraction--liquid chromatography/tandem mass spectrometry. Clin Chem. 2008;54(4):642–51.
79. Garber JR, Cobin RH, Gharib H, Hennessey JV, Klein I, Mechanick JI, et al. Clinical practice guidelines for hypothyroidism in adults: cosponsored by the American Association of Clinical Endocrinologists and the American Thyroid Association. Endocr Pract. 2012;18(6):988–1028.
80. Azizi F, Mehran L, Amouzegar A, Delshad H, Tohidi M, Askari S, et al. Establishment of the trimester-specific reference range for free thyroxine index. Thyroid. 2013;23(3):354–9.
81. Korevaar TI, Chaker L, Medici M, de Rijke YB, Jaddoe VW, Steegers EA, et al. Maternal total T4 during the first half of pregnancy: physiologic aspects and the risk of adverse outcomes in comparison with free T4. Clin Endocrinol. 2016;85(5):757–63.
82. Weeke J, Dybkjaer L, Granlie K, Eskjaer Jensen S, Kjaerulff E, Laurberg P, et al. A longitudinal study of serum TSH, and total and free iodothyronines during normal pregnancy. Acta Endocrinol. 1982;101(4):531–7.
83. Pramanik S, Mukhopadhyay P, Ghosh S. Total T4 rise in pregnancy: a relook? Thyroid Res. 2020;13:14.
84. Pantalone KM, Hatipoglu B, Gupta MK, Kennedy L, Hamrahian AH. Measurement of serum free thyroxine index may provide additional case detection compared to free thyroxine in the diagnosis of central hypothyroidism. Case Rep Endocrinol. 2015;2015:965191.
85. Lee RH, Spencer CA, Mestman JH, Miller EA, Petrovic I, Braverman LE, et al. Free T4 immunoassays are flawed during pregnancy. Am J Obstet Gynecol 2009;200(3):260 e1–6.
86. Zoeller RT, Rovet J. Timing of thyroid hormone action in the developing brain: clinical observations and experimental findings. J Neuroendocrinol. 2004;16(10):809–18.
87. Yazbeck CF, Sullivan SD. Thyroid disorders during pregnancy. Med Clin North Am. 2012;96(2):235–56.
88. Taylor PN, Muller I, Nana M, Velasco I, Lazarus JH. Indications for treatment of subclinical hypothyroidism and isolated hypothyroxinaemia in pregnancy. Best Pract Res Clin Endocrinol Metab. 2020;34(4):101436.
89. Vermiglio F, Lo Presti VP, Moleti M, Sidoti M, Tortorella G, Scaffidi G, et al. Attention deficit and hyperactivity disorders in the offspring of mothers exposed to mild-moderate iodine deficiency: a possible novel iodine deficiency disorder in developed countries. J Clin Endocrinol Metab. 2004;89(12):6054–60.

90. Gyllenberg D, Sourander A, Surcel HM, Hinkka-Yli-Salomaki S, McKeague IW, Brown AS. hypothyroxinemia during gestation and offspring Schizophrenia in a National Birth Cohort. Biol Psychiatry. 2016;79(12):962–70.
91. Korevaar TI, Schalekamp-Timmermans S, de Rijke YB, Visser WE, Visser W, de Muinck Keizer-Schrama SM, et al. Hypothyroxinemia and TPO-antibody positivity are risk factors for premature delivery: the generation R study. J Clin Endocrinol Metab. 2013;98(11):4382–90.
92. Zhang Y, Dai X, Yang S, Zhang C, Han M, Huang HF, et al. Maternal low thyroxin levels are associated with adverse pregnancy outcomes in a Chinese population. PLoS One. 2017;12(5):e0178100.
93. Sheehan PM, Nankervis A, Araujo Junior E, Da Silva CF. Maternal thyroid disease and preterm birth: systematic review and meta-analysis. J Clin Endocrinol Metab. 2015;100(11):4325–31.
94. Oguz A, Tuzun D, Sahin M, Usluogullari AC, Usluogullari B, Celik A, et al. Frequency of isolated maternal hypothyroxinemia in women with gestational diabetes mellitus in a moderately iodine-deficient area. Gynecol Endocrinol. 2015;31(10):792–5.
95. Ashoor G, Maiz N, Rotas M, Jawdat F, Nicolaides KH. Maternal thyroid function at 11–13 weeks of gestation and spontaneous preterm delivery. Obstet Gynecol. 2011;117(2 Pt 1):293–8.
96. Pop VJ, Brouwers EP, Vader HL, Vulsma T, van Baar AL, de Vijlder JJ. Maternal hypothyroxinaemia during early pregnancy and subsequent child development: a 3-year follow-up study. Clin Endocrinol. 2003;59(3):282–8.
97. Levie D, Korevaar TIM, Bath SC, Dalmau-Bueno A, Murcia M, Espada M, et al. Thyroid function in early pregnancy, child IQ, and autistic traits: a meta-analysis of individual participant data. J Clin Endocrinol Metab. 2018;103(8):2967–79.
98. Derakhshan A, Peeters RP, Taylor PN, Bliddal S, Carty DM, Meems M, et al. Association of maternal thyroid function with birthweight: a systematic review and individual-participant data meta-analysis. Lancet Diabetes Endocrinol. 2020;8(6):501–10.
99. Grau G, Aguayo A, Vela A, Aniel-Quiroga A, Espada M, Miranda G, et al. Normal intellectual development in children born from women with hypothyroxinemia during their pregnancy. J Trace Elem Med Biol. 2015;31:18–24.
100. Li Y, Shan Z, Teng W, Yu X, Li Y, Fan C, et al. Abnormalities of maternal thyroid function during pregnancy affect neuropsychological development of their children at 25–30 months. Clin Endocrinol. 2010;72(6):825–9.
101. Korevaar TI, Muetzel R, Medici M, Chaker L, Jaddoe VW, de Rijke YB, et al. Association of maternal thyroid function during early pregnancy with offspring IQ and brain morphology in childhood: a population-based prospective cohort study. Lancet Diabetes Endocrinol. 2016;4(1):35–43.
102. Medici M, Timmermans S, Visser W, de Muinck Keizer-Schrama SM, Jaddoe VW, Hofman A, et al. Maternal thyroid hormone parameters during early pregnancy and birth weight: the Generation R Study. J Clin Endocrinol Metab. 2013;98(1):59–66.
103. Julvez J, Alvarez-Pedrerol M, Rebagliato M, Murcia M, Forns J, Garcia-Esteban R, et al. Thyroxine levels during pregnancy in healthy women and early child neurodevelopment. Epidemiology. 2013;24(1):150–7.
104. Roman GC, Ghassabian A, Bongers-Schokking JJ, Jaddoe VW, Hofman A, de Rijke YB, et al. Association of gestational maternal hypothyroxinemia and increased autism risk. Ann Neurol. 2013;74(5):733–42.
105. Oken E, Braverman LE, Platek D, Mitchell ML, Lee SL, Pearce EN. Neonatal thyroxine, maternal thyroid function, and child cognition. J Clin Endocrinol Metab. 2009;94(2):497–503.
106. Ghassabian A, Bongers-Schokking JJ, Henrichs J, Jaddoe VW, Visser TJ, Visser W, et al. Maternal thyroid function during pregnancy and behavioral problems in the offspring: the generation R study. Pediatr Res. 2011;69(5 Pt 1):454–9.
107. Morreale de Escobar G, Obregon MJ, Escobar del Rey F. Is neuropsychological development related to maternal hypothyroidism or to maternal hypothyroxinemia? J Clin Endocrinol Metab. 2000;85(11):3975–87.

108. Modesto T, Tiemeier H, Peeters RP, Jaddoe VW, Hofman A, Verhulst FC, et al. Maternal mild thyroid hormone insufficiency in early pregnancy and attention-deficit/hyperactivity disorder symptoms in children. JAMA Pediatr. 2015;169(9):838–45.
109. Chang K, Shin JI. Association of gestational maternal hypothyroxinemia and increased autism risk: the role of brain-derived neurotrophic factor. Ann Neurol. 2014;75(6):971.
110. Negro R, Soldin OP, Obregon MJ, Stagnaro-Green A. Hypothyroxinemia and pregnancy. Endocr Pract. 2011;17(3):422–9.
111. Moleti M, Vermiglio F, Trimarchi F. Maternal isolated hypothyroxinemia: to treat or not to treat? J Endocrinol Investig. 2009;32(9):780–2.
112. Auso E, Lavado-Autric R, Cuevas E, Del Rey FE, Morreale De Escobar G, Berbel P. A moderate and transient deficiency of maternal thyroid function at the beginning of fetal neocorticogenesis alters neuronal migration. Endocrinology. 2004;145(9):4037–47.
113. Lavado-Autric R, Auso E, Garcia-Velasco JV, Arufe Mdel C, Escobar del Rey F, Berbel P, et al. Early maternal hypothyroxinemia alters histogenesis and cerebral cortex cytoarchitecture of the progeny. J Clin Invest. 2003;111(7):1073–82.
114. Goodman JH, Gilbert ME. Modest thyroid hormone insufficiency during development induces a cellular malformation in the corpus callosum: a model of cortical dysplasia. Endocrinology. 2007;148(6):2593–7.
115. Lazarus JH, Taylor PN. Hypothyroxinaemia and brain development. Acta Endocrinol (Buchar). 2016;12(1):1–6.
116. Koyuncu K, Turgay B, Soylemez F. Iodine deficiency in pregnant women at first trimester in Ankara. J Turk Ger Gynecol Assoc. 2019;20(1):37–40.
117. Harding KB, Pena-Rosas JP, Webster AC, Yap CM, Payne BA, Ota E, et al. Iodine supplementation for women during the preconception, pregnancy and postpartum period. Cochrane Database Syst Rev 2017;3:CD011761.
118. Shi X, Han C, Li C, Mao J, Wang W, Xie X, et al. Optimal and safe upper limits of iodine intake for early pregnancy in iodine-sufficient regions: a cross-sectional study of 7190 pregnant women in China. J Clin Endocrinol Metab. 2015;100(4):1630–8.
119. Chang DL, Pearce EN. Screening for maternal thyroid dysfunction in pregnancy: a review of the clinical evidence and current guidelines. J Thyroid Res. 2013;2013:851326.
120. Taylor PN, Okosieme OE, Premawardhana L, Lazarus JH. Should all women be screened for thyroid dysfunction in pregnancy? Womens Health (Lond). 2015;11(3):295–307.
121. Gong X, Liu A, Li Y, Sun H, Li Y, Li C, et al. The impact of isolated maternal hypothyroxinemia during the first and second trimester of gestation on pregnancy outcomes: an intervention and prospective cohort study in China. J Endocrinol Investig. 2019;42(5):599–607.

Maternal Hyperthyroidism

K. Gkastaris and G. E. Krassas

Definition

Thyrotoxicosis is the clinical syndrome of hypermetabolism and hyperactivity that occurs when a person is exposed to supraphysiological concentrations of thyroid hormones (TH). *Hyperthyroidism* is the hyperfunction of the thyroid gland leading to sustained increases in TH biosynthesis from the thyroid gland and it represents the commonest cause of thyrotoxicosis. Even though thyrotoxicosis in pregnancy is relatively rare and certainly much less common than hypothyroidism, it can pose a challenge to the clinician given its diagnostic and therapeutic difficulties as well as the possible maternal and foetal complications.

Prevalence and Aetiology

Overt thyrotoxicosis can affect between 0.2 and 0.4% of pregnancies [1–3] although the prevalence of subclinical thyrotoxicosis can be as high as 1% [3, 4]. Gestational thyrotoxicosis can be caused by a number of conditions: autoimmune, non-autoimmune and iatrogenic (Table 1). *Transient gestational thyrotoxicosis* is a condition caused by elevated human chorionic gonadotropin (hCG) levels [5] leading to suppressed serum thyroid stimulating hormone (TSH) and raised free-thyroxine (FT4) levels. It is frequently associated with *hyperemesis gravidarum (HG)*, it does not lead to the clinical syndrome of thyrotoxicosis and is typically limited to the first

K. Gkastaris (✉)
Royal United Hospitals Bath NHS, Bath, UK

G. E. Krassas
IASEIO, Medical Center, Thessaloniki, Greece
e-mail: gkra34@otenet.gr

F. Azizi, F. Ramezani Tehrani (eds.), *Thyroid Diseases in Pregnancy*,
https://doi.org/10.1007/978-3-030-98777-0_9

Table 1 Causes of thyrotoxicosis in pregnancy

Cause	Aetiology
Immune thyroid disease	
Graves' disease	Circulating TSH receptor antibodies
Sporadic silent thyroiditis	Autoimmune destruction of thyroid gland
Non-autoimmune thyroid disease	
Toxic multinodular goitre (MNG)	Autonomous function—Some due to activating mutations in TSH receptor
Toxic solitary adenoma	
Subacute painful thyroiditis	Release of stored TH – aetiology possibly viral
Familial gestational thyrotoxicosis	Mutant TSH receptor hypersensitivity to hCG
Transient thyrotoxicosis associated with hyperemesis gravidarum	Circulating hCG
Hyperplacentosis	Increased placental weight and high circulating hCG levels
Hyperreactio luteinalis	Enlargement of both ovaries due to benign cysts leading to high hCG levels
Trophoblastic tumour	High circulating hCG
Hydatidiform mole	Trophoblastic disease leading to high hCG levels
Choriocarcinoma	High circulating hCG
Struma ovarii (ovarian teratoma)	Thyroid hormone produced outside the thyroid gland
Functional metastases of thyroid cancer	
Resistance to thyroid hormone	Inappropriate TSH secretion
Pituitary tumour producing TSH (TSHoma)	
Iatrogenic	
Excessive levothyroxine intake	Excess exogenous thyroid hormone (iatrogenic/overtreatment or factitious)
Drug-induced thyroiditis	Amiodarone, lithium, interferon α
Jod-Basedow effect	Iodine-induced hyperthyroidism (iodine, iodine-containing drugs, radiographic contrast agents)

half of pregnancy. On the other hand, the commonest cause of clinical hyperthyroidism in pregnancy is *Graves' disease* (GD) (80–90%). Other causes of thyrotoxicosis [6–8] in pregnancy include *toxic multinodular goitre, toxic adenoma and subacute thyroiditis*. Finally, some other conditions which are less common are summarised in Table 1. Another cause of thyrotoxicosis that has to be considered by the clinician is overtreatment with or factitious intake of thyroid hormone.

Foetal-Maternal Relationships

Pregnancy is associated with significant physiologic changes that affect the thyroid function tests. These changes are reversible but in combination with the hypermetabolic state of pregnancy can cause diagnostic difficulties as they mimic the clinical signs and symptoms of thyrotoxicosis. The physiologic changes are summarised in Table 2.

Table 2 Physiologic changes in pregnancy that influence thyroid function tests [9]

Physiologic change	Thyroid function test change
↑ Thyroid-binding globulin (TBG)	↑ Serum total T4 and T3 concentrations
First trimester hCG elevation	↑ Free T4 and ↓TSH
↑ Plasma volume	↑ T4 and T3 pool size
↑ Type III 5-deiodinase (inner ring deiodination) due to increased placental mass	↑ T4 and T3 degradation resulting in requirement for increased hormone production
Thyroid enlargement (in some women)	Serum thyroglobulin
↑ Iodine clearance	↕ Hormone production in iodine-deficient areas

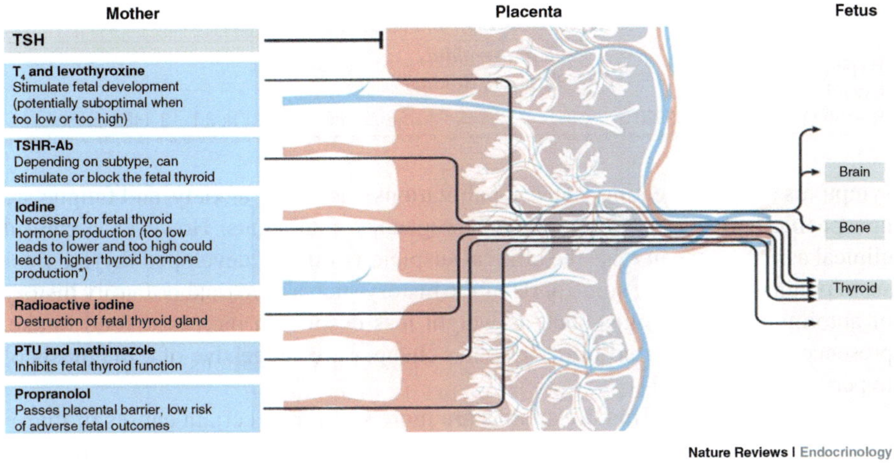

Fig. 1 The role of the placenta in thyroid hormone delivery to the foetus

TH is important to the foetus for the development of many organs, particularly the brain. The foetus does not possess a functioning thyroid in early pregnancy but it is now well documented that maternal T4 crosses the placenta at all stages of pregnancy. This is particularly important during the first trimester of pregnancy since the foetal thyroid begins concentrating iodine at 10–12 weeks of gestation and the foetal pituitary TSH takes over the control of the axis by about week 20 of gestation [9].

The placenta plays a key role not merely as an exchange unit for TH but also in the regulation of transplacental TH transfer [10] through its expression of placental TH transporters, thyroid hormone binding proteins, iodothyronine deiodinases, sulphotransferases, and sulphatases (Fig. 1).

Clinical Presentation

Diagnostically, on some occasions the diagnosis is already known prior to the gestation, for example, established GD or toxic nodule(s). In contrast, the diagnosis of thyrotoxicosis first occurring during pregnancy can pose a challenge, as many of its

Table 3 Common clinical symptoms of thyrotoxicosis and manifestations which are present only in specific causes

General symptoms and signs	Clinical manifestations of specific causes of thyrotoxicosis
Anxiety/nervousness	***Graves autoimmune disease***
Hyperactivity	Diffuse goitre
Fatigue/exhaustion	Ophthalmopathy
Weakness	Thyroid bruit
Tremor	Localised dermopathy
Palpitations	Thyroid acropachy
Heat intolerance	***Thyroid autonomy***
Nausea	Uninodular or multinodular goitre
Increased appetite	***Subacute thyroiditis***
Tachycardia/arrhythmia	Thyroid pain and tenderness
Tremor	***Silent thyroiditis***
Hyperreflexia	Diffuse thyroiditis
Eyelid retraction	
Systolic hypertension	

symptoms such as sweating, nausea, palpitations, insomnia, anxiety, and fatigue are nonspecific and can "mimic" frequent pregnancy complaints. However, a careful clinical assessment can raise the clinical suspicion of newly developed thyrotoxicosis in pregnancy because some parts of the history such as personal or family history of autoimmunity and signs such as weight loss despite an increased food intake, presence of goitre, thyroid bruit or ocular changes are suggestive of a diagnosis of hyperthyroidism [1, 11].

Some of the clinical manifestations are more specific to certain causes of thyrotoxicosis (Table 3): diffuse goitre, thyroid bruit, thyroid ophthalmopathy, acropachy and/or dermopathy are typical of GD. Thyroid ophthalmopathy can present with upper eyelid retraction, oedema, erythema of the periorbital tissues and conjunctivae. Acropachy presents with soft tissue swelling, finger clubbing, and periosteal reaction of the extremities. Thyroid dermopathy refers to localised lesions of the skin resulting from the deposition of hyaluronic acid. Although it is most often confined to the pretibial area, it may occur anywhere on the skin. On the other hand, a sore and painful thyroid typically accompanies subacute thyroiditis [12].

Diagnosis

The diagnosis of hyperthyroidism should always be confirmed by elevated serum thyroid hormone concentrations and suppressed serum TSH levels. A downward shift of the TSH reference range occurs during pregnancy, with a reduction in both the lower (decreased by about 0.1–0.2 mU/L) and the upper limit of maternal TSH (decreased by about 0.5–1.0 mU/L), relative to the typical non-pregnant TSH reference range [1]. The largest decrease in serum TSH is observed during the first trimester because of elevated levels of serum hCG directly stimulating the TSH receptor and thereby increasing thyroid hormone production. Thereafter, serum TSH and its reference range gradually rise in the second and third trimesters, but nonetheless remain lower than in non-pregnant women [1]. There are pregnant women with low (but detectable) TSH who demonstrate no clinical signs of thyrotoxicosis and require no treatment. If the exact diagnosis is uncertain, measurement of TSH receptor antibodies (TRAbs) is indicated, since the presence of these antibodies differentiates GD from other causes of gestational thyrotoxicosis. Furthermore, in cases of GD the measurement of TRAbs has prognostic significance for the development of GD in the foetus [1, 11, 13].

It should be noted that serum T4 levels vary during normal pregnancy [14] with significant geographic and ethnic diversity. As a consequence, there has been a considerable debate and controversies regarding which cut-off levels for TSH in pregnancy should be adopted as normal [1, 11, 13]. When possible, laboratories are strongly encouraged to develop population and trimester-specific normal ranges for TSH as well as triiodothyronine (T3) and T4 (both total and free) [1, 11, 13]. Nonetheless, acknowledging that this is not widely possible, the latest American guidelines recommend suggest that, in the first trimester, the lower reference range of TSH can be reduced by approximately 0.4 mU/L, while the upper reference range is reduced by approximately 0.5 mU/L. For the typical patient in early pregnancy, this corresponds to a TSH upper reference limit of 4.0 mU/L. This reference limit should generally be applied beginning with the late first trimester, weeks 7–12, with a gradual return towards the non-pregnant range in the second and third trimesters [1].

Management

The overall goal of management is to maintain or achieve euthyroidism as early as possible in pregnancy. Antithyroid drugs (ATDs) are the cornerstone of treatment of hyperthyroidism in pregnancy [1, 13]. Thyroidectomy should be preserved as second-line option in selected cases and radioactive iodine (RAI) treatment is contraindicated in pregnancy [1, 13].

(a) *Antithyroid drugs (ATDs)* have been used for the treatment of hyperthyroidism in pregnancy for several decades now even though recent large observational studies have raised concerns about the risk of birth defects. Women should be maintained at a high euthyroid level [1, 11, 13, 15] using the smallest possible dose of ATDs in order to reduce the risk of birth defects and of foetal hypothyroidism. Methimazole (MMI) and propylthiouracil (PTU) cross the placenta equally [16–18] whereas thyroid hormones' crossing is negligible. For this reason, the "block and replace" strategy should be avoided in pregnancy. PTU and MMI are thought to be equally effective in maintaining maternal euthyroidism [19]. The focus of the debate in the recent years has been the side effects and the possible teratogenic potential of these medications. Over the last decade, a number of large observational studies have come to light evaluating the possible link between treatment with ATDs in the first trimester of pregnancy and birth defects. These studies had a number of methodological differences [20] and covered different populations: some of them reported an association between ATDs and birth defects [21–24] whereas some did not [25–28]. The most common birth defects associated with MMI use in the first trimester of pregnancy are aplasia cutis and choanal and oesophageal atresia and developmental delay [1, 19]. Historically, PTU had not been linked to birth defects. Despite the fact that some recent studies [21, 22] reported that PTU was associated with a higher frequency of birth defects compared to non-exposed, a meta-analysis including 12 studies showed no differences between PTU exposure and no ATD exposure [29]. In general, PTU is recommended drug of choice for the first 16 weeks of pregnancy [1, 13, 30].

In terms of side effects of the ATDs, fortunately the vast majority of them are mild and mostly cutaneous [15, 16]. The first exception, luckily rare (<0.5%) is agranulocytosis. The patient should be warned that if she develops fever, mouth ulcers and/or sore throat, she should be tested immediately for a full blood count (FBC). If the FBC results confirm neutropaenia, the ATDs should be discontinued. Additionally, broad spectrum antibiotics and granulocyte colony stimulating factor should be initiated in febrile, septic or high-risk patients [1, 13]. The second severe side effect of the ATDs is hepatotoxicity. It has been traditionally thought that PTU causes hepatocellular pattern of liver injury whereas MMI causes cholestatic pattern. Recent studies have challenged this belief [31, 32]. Nonetheless, a recent larger study from Japan [33] and a meta-analysis of 30 studies [34] have shown significantly higher rates of liver injury associated with PTU rather than MMI. Some deaths have also been reported in adolescents and adults [31, 35, 36]. For these reasons, the European guidelines recommend change of PTU to MMI after 16 weeks of gestation [11, 13]. The American guidelines suggest PTU for the first 16 weeks of gestation but do not specify the recommended ATDs for the rest of the pregnancy [1].

Further study and clinical data on the timing and type of ATDs are required but with the current evidence, the authors' view is to switch from MMI to PTU during the pre-conception period (at the period of pregnancy planning) and at most during the first 5 weeks of gestation, to continue treatment with PTU for the first 16 weeks of gestation and to switch back to MMI for the remainder of the pregnancy. Furthermore, the authors' experience is that the use of MMI is preferable to carbimazole (CBZ) during pregnancy as CBZ is a pro-drug, which converts to MMI after absorption. The usual doses required are summarised in Table 4.

(b) *β-blockers, and in particular propranolol,* can be of help with amelioration of symptoms of hyperthyroidism and its additional effect of blocking the peripheral conversion of inactive T4 to active form T3. In the context of pregnancy, it can be used transiently at a dose of 10–40 mg every 6–8 h in cases of symptomatic thyrotoxicosis and also for preoperative preparation. There are no significant teratogenic effects of propranolol reported in the literature. Long-term use in pregnancy was historically avoided due to a possible association with intrauterine growth restriction but a recent retrospective cohort study from the U.S. showed that the risk of small growth for age (SGA) associated with propranolol exposure was not significantly different from the non-exposed group [37]. It is probably logical to monitor the foetal growth closely in cases of long-term propranolol use until more data become available. The usual doses required are summarised in Table 4.

(c) *Thyroidectomy* during pregnancy should be avoided if possible and reserved only as second-line option in specific circumstances: (1) anaphylactic or severe allergic reaction to ATDs, (2) agranulocytosis or hepatotoxicity with ATDs, (3) failure to control thyrotoxicosis despite high dose of ATDs, (4) rarely compressive symptoms (stridor or dysphagia) from a large goitre (Table 5). The optimal timing for thyroidectomy in pregnancy is the second trimester when the foetus is at smaller risk and the uterus resistant to contraction [1, 13]. If the woman is still thyrotoxic prior to the surgery and/or unable to tolerate ATDs, preparation for surgery includes propranolol and a short (10–14 day) course of potassium iodide solution (50–100 mg/day) [1, 9]. It should be noted that following thyroidectomy a gradual, but not immediate, disappearance of TRAbs is observed; therefore, there is a small risk of transient foetal thyrotoxicosis [38]. The indications for thyroidectomy in pregnancy are summarised in Table 5. However, according to the authors' experience, in the vast majority of cases thyroidectomy in pregnancy is not needed.

Table 4 Pharmacological approach to hyperthyroidism in pregnancy (adjusted from [1, 13])

Medication	Initial dose range	Typical dose range for majority	Notes
Propylthiouracil (PTU)	50–400 mg/day	50–200 mg/day	First 16 weeks of gestation
			Equivalent potency of MMI to PTU is approx 1:10
Methimazole (MMI)	5–30 mg/day	5–20 mg/day	After week 16 of gestation
Carbimazole (CBZ)	5–40 mg/day	10–25 mg/day	10 mg of CBZ are rapidly metabolised to 6 mg of MMI
Propranolol	10–40 mg × 3–4/day		For symptomatic relief or prior to thyroidectomy
Potassium iodide	50–100 mg/day for 10–14 days		Mainly for preparation for thyroidectomy

Table 5 Indications for thyroidectomy in pregnancy

Anaphylactic or severe allergic reactions to ATDs
Agranulocytosis or hepatotoxicity with ATDs
Failure to control thyrotoxicosis despite high dose of ATDs (400 mg/day of PTU and 30–40 mg/day of MMI)
Compressive symptoms (stridor or dysphagia) from a large goitre

(d) *Potassium iodide* has been used in Japan for the treatment of mild thyrotoxicosis [39, 40]. However, there are no data from other parts of the world with lower diet intake and currently the main European and American authorities do not recommend it during pregnancy [1, 13].

Low concentration of selenium has been reported in pregnant women with hyperthyroidism compared with euthyroid ones [41, 42]. However, no clear data on the therapeutic role of selenium administration are available to date.

Radioactive iodine (RAI) is obviously contraindicated in pregnancy as the foetus is exposed to significant radiation from transplacental transfer of 131-I as well as from the isotope form in the maternal excretory system. However the protocols surrounding the administration of RAI vary widely worldwide and cases of GD inadvertently treated with RAI in early gestation have been reported. The maternal thyroid uptake, the gestational age and the ability of the foetal thyroid to concentrate iodine are essential in determining the radioiodine exposure in the utero. Foetal exposure to radioiodine before implantation may increase the risk of miscarriage and death of the embryo in a dose-dependent manner, but surviving embryos will probably escape any major malformations or thyroid problems. Exposure during thyroid development, from 10 weeks of gestation onwards, will result in foetal hypothyroidism and foetal thyroid ablation needing lifelong thyroxine replacement. In these cases the management includes maintain maternal thyroxine levels towards the upper end of normal for the rest of the pregnancy and immediate treatment of the neonate with thyroxine [43]. The neonatal screening programmes for congenital hypothyroidism ensure that mental retardation can be avoided by prompt initiation of levothyroxine (LT4) treatment.

The pharmacological options to hyperthyroidism in pregnancy are summarised in Table 4.

Management Goals and Monitoring

Clinical Scenarios

Autoimmune Disease (Graves' Disease)

The overall target of treatment is to maintain euthyroidism throughout pregnancy. Typically, measurement of thyroid function tests (TFTs) is required every 4–6 weeks. The clinician can encounter different clinical scenarios and different parameters have to be taken into account:

1. *The woman with newly diagnosed GD in pregnancy.* Fortunately, these cases are relatively rare as thyroid immunity is suppressed in pregnancy. However, if a new diagnosis of GD is made in pregnancy, the goal of the management is (a) to achieve maternal euthyroidism as soon as possible using the smallest possible

ATDs dose (PTU for the first trimester and MMI afterwards) and (b) to assess the risk of neonatal thyrotoxicosis with TRAbs measurement (as discussed in detail in another section of this chapter).

2. The *woman with active hyperthyroidism (more commonly GD) diagnosed prior to the onset of pregnancy who currently receives ATDs treatment.* In this case euthyroidism should be achieved before conception and maintained throughout pregnancy. The recommendation is to switch from MMI to PTU during the pre-conception period (at the period of pregnancy planning) and at most during the first 5 weeks of gestation, to continue treatment with PTU for the first 16 weeks of gestation and to switch back to MMI for the remainder of the pregnancy. The recommended approach is the use the smallest possible ATDs dose that will allow for controlling maternal thyrotoxicosis rather than "block and LT4 replacement" approach. This is because the transplacental passage of ATDs is high and can cause ATD-induced foetal hypothyroidism. On the other hand, addition of LT4 will not be protective as its transplacental passage is negligible. Furthermore, it is recommended that the maternal TRAbs status is assessed to ascertain the risk of neonatal thyrotoxicosis (as discussed in detail in another section of this chapter).

   It should be noted that many GD cases tend to get better in pregnancy and subsequently there has been extensive debate about the appropriate approach to the well-controlled mild GD cases. It is recommended that the clinician considers the possibility of withdrawing ATDs prior to conception or in the first weeks of pregnancy if the patient is well controlled on a small dose of ATDs [1]. It is the authors' view that assessment of the TRAbs titre can be very useful in that respect: Women with negative TRAbs status who require small doses of ATDs are more likely to go into remission; therefore, in these women it would be safe to consider withdrawing ATDs. It is also the authors' view that, should the clinician decide to proceed with a trial off ATDs, thyroid function tests should be performed at 2, 4 and 6 weeks after treatment withdrawal in order to detect an early relapse.

3. *The woman with hyperthyroidism in the past who received permanent treatment.* In this case the woman with GD or nodular thyroid disease who received RA or underwent total thyroidectomy is currently on treatment with LT4 for acquired hypothyroidism (although a percentage of women treated with RAI might be euthyroid without replacement therapy). The aim of the management here is to maintain the desired TSH levels with LT4 dose adjustment. Additionally, the potential presence of TRAbs should be considered if the original diagnosis was GD as the neonate can still be at risk of autoimmune thyroid dysfunction.

4. *The woman with previous GD who is currently in remission.* In this case the woman should be monitored throughout pregnancy with TSH and fT4 measurements every 4–6 weeks for any evidence of relapse of GD. Fortunately this risk is relatively small as during pregnancy thyroid autoimmunity is usually suppressed. However, TRAbs should again be measured due to the risk of neonatal thyrotoxicosis.

5. *The woman with a history of a previous birth of a child with neonatal thyroid dysfunction.* In the last 30 years a number of case reports have been published reporting neonates diagnosed with central hypothyroidism, i.e. insufficient production of TSH leading to T4/T3 deficiency [44, 45]. In some of these cases, the mother was not tested for or diagnosed with any thyroid issues during pregnancy [46, 47]. There are two probable mechanisms of the central neonatal hypothyroidism: (a) Suppression of the foetal TSH levels secondary to higher T4/T3 levels during intrauterine life resulting from suboptimally treated or untreated maternal hyperthyroidism and increased transplacental maternal-foetal T4/T3 transport [48]. (b) Possible conversion of the maternal TRAbs from stimulating to inhibitory ones which cause neonatal hypothyroidism rather than hyperthyroidism [49–52]. In these rare cases, it is important that the mother is carefully monitored in subsequent pregnancies for any signs of thyroid dysfunction and, even if she is euthyroid, for evidence of thyroid immunity with measurement of the TRAbs.

Other Non-autoimmune Clinical Scenarios

6. *Transient gestational hyperthyroidism associated with hyperemesis gravidarum (HG)* is typically self-limiting even though around 5% of these women require hospitalisation for rehydration and administration of antiemetic medications due to the risk of ketosis. In a small number of women, ATDs may be given transiently as there is a correlation between FT4/FT3 levels and the severity of the hyperemesis and in extreme cases HG has been associated with cardiovascular complications [53] and even cardiac arrest [54].
7. *Subacute thyroiditis.* The presentation is fairly characteristic with a painful swollen neck, biochemical evidence of inflammation [leucocytosis, elevated C-reactive protein (CRP) and erythrocyte sedimentation rate (ESR)] and hyperthyroidism. Nuclear medicine uptake scan is contraindicated, but ultrasonography may also assist diagnostically. In cases that the diagnosis is still uncertain, fine-needle aspiration (FNA) of the thyroid may be of further help. The treatment consists of analgesia and oral prednisolone. These women should be monitored closely as some will develop hypothyroidism.
8. *Nodular thyroid disease (pre-existing toxic adenoma and toxic multinodular disease)* should be treated with ATDs during pregnancy. Thyroidectomy is not recommended. However, if it is essential, for example, in the presence of compressive symptoms (stridor or dysphagia), it should be performed during the second trimester.
9. *Graves' orbitopathy (GO).* Fortunately, as thyroid autoimmunity is usually suppressed in pregnancy, GO tends to improve during gestation. However some pregnant women, usually nicotine smokers, may develop symptoms or signs of GO: pain, dryness, irritation, chemosis, periorbital oedema, proptosis and in extreme cases ophthalmoplegia and optic neuropathy. The treatment consists of topical eye lubricants, smoking cessation, selenium administration and, in severe

cases, oral or intravenous steroids [13, 55–57]. In cases of sight-threatening orbitopathy, if there is no response after 2 weeks of intravenous glucocorticoids, urgent decompressive surgery is indicated, whereas in stable and inactive cases, rehabilitative surgery may be required but that can usually be postponed until post-partum.

Importance of TRAbs Assessment During Pregnancy

Graves' disease (GD) is an autoimmune condition caused by circulating *TRAbs* that can cross the placenta and have an effect on the foetal thyroid. The activity level of GD fluctuates in pregnancy reflecting fluctuations in TRAbs concentrations. Overall the thyroid immunity tends to decrease in pregnancy with many women GD going into complete remission, especially in late gestation [58, 59]. The spontaneous improvement in the immunity is likely to be multifactorial, but it has been advocated that one of the main mechanisms is the progressive reduction in TRAbs which is observed in pregnancy [13]. The TRAbs can cross the placenta from 18 weeks of gestation and at the 30th week of development, the foetal TRAbs levels are almost equal to that of the mother. In the vast majority of cases these antibodies have a stimulating effect on foetal thyroid causing hyperthyroidism; however in rare cases their action can be inhibitory causing hypothyroidism [49, 50, 52].

It is recommended to measure the TRAbs titres in pregnant women with known or suspected GD [1, 13]. The measurement can serve different purposes depending on the stage of the gestation and whether the cause of the hyperthyroidism is known or not: in the case of a new diagnosis of hyperthyroidism in pregnancy, measurement of TRAbs can be a very useful tool to differentiate between GD and other causes of abnormal TFTs, mainly transient gestational hyperthyroidism. In actual fact, women with de novo GD in pregnancy tend to have higher titres compared with women with pre-existing GD. On the other hand, in known cases of GD, measurement of TRAbs mainly helps clinicians to assess the risk of foetal (FD) and neonatal dysthyroidism (ND), even though it also reflects the immunological activity and the subsequent aggressiveness of the disease for the mother.

One of the main goals of the clinician treating a pregnant woman with GD is the prediction of the risk of developing FD and ND. The TRAb levels in the mother are one of the main predictors because their action can directly activate the foetal or neonatal thyroid gland. However there is an ongoing debate on two questions concerning the measurement of TRAbs: (1) when and in whom to measure TRAbs and (2) what the predictive for development of FD/ND TRAbs cut-offs should be.

1. *When and in whom should TRAbs be measured?*

   The European [11, 13] and American [1] guidelines for the management of hyperthyroidism in pregnancy describe different clinical situations: First, in women with newly diagnosed hyperthyroidism in pregnancy to assist the clinician with his differential diagnosis, principally between GD and transient gestational hyperthyroidism. Second, in pregnant women with known and active GD who receive treatment with ATDs already prior to conception. Third, in pregnant women who are currently euthyroid but have previously received definitive treatment for GD with surgery or RAI. These women may still maintain elevated TRAbs [60, 61]; therefore the risk of FD/ND remains. Fourth, in pregnant women with previous history of delivering an infant with hyperthyroidism. In a fifth and final situation, in pregnant women who were previously treated for GD with ATDs and are currently euthyroid off ATDs, the recommendations suggest that, even though the thyroid function should be measured, TRAbs testing is not necessary as the risk is negligible. Regarding the timing of TRAbs measurement, the recommendation is for measurement of the antibodies in early pregnancy. If maternal TRAbs are undetectable or low in early pregnancy, no further TRAbs testing is needed as the risk is thought to be negligible. If maternal TRAb concentration is elevated in early pregnancy, repeat testing should occur at weeks 18–22. Finally, if elevated TRAbs are detected at weeks 18–22 or the mother is taking ATDs in the third trimester, a TRAbs measurement should again be performed in late pregnancy (weeks 30–34) to evaluate the need for neonatal and postnatal monitoring.

2. *What are the optimal maternal TRAbs concentration cut-offs for prediction of FD/ND?*

   There is an ongoing debate about the levels of TRAbs more accurately predicting the risk for FD and ND. Recently, a large retrospective study of 417 women with GD and positive TRAbs during gestation reported that the risk of FD was best predicted by a maternal TRAbs concentration of ≥2.5 IU/L or ≥2.5 times the upper limit of the reference interval since the second-generation human assay had a reference interval upper limit of 1.0 IU/L [59]. In terms of predicting ND the optimal maternal TRAbs concentration cut-off is less clear. In the same study [59], the authors reported an optimal concentration of ≥5.9 times the upper limit of the reference interval as optimal predictor of ND. However, a systematic review of 20 articles (53 cases) suggested a lower cut-off point at ≥3.7 times the upper limit of the reference interval [62]. The American guidelines advocate a cut-off of three times the upper limit of normal for the assay [1]. Given the seriousness of ND it seems reasonable to adopt the lower cut-off point until more data become available. It is therefore recommended the foetuses of mothers with GD and TRAbs ≥2.5 times the upper limit of the reference interval to be monitored closely for signs of thyrotoxicosis.

The authors' view is that TRAbs should be measured in early pregnancy and, if negative, they don't need to be repeated. If they are positive, they should be repeated at week 18–22 of gestation and, if they remain positive, at week 30–34. Furthermore, it is also the authors' view that, given the seriousness of ND, any TRAbs titre above the laboratory's cut-off should be considered "positive" and the neonatologists should be alerted.

Foetal Ultrasonography

Serial ultrasound testing should be performed in the presence of elevated TRAbs and uncontrolled hyperthyroidism for the assessment of gestational age, foetal viability, amniotic fluid volume, foetal anatomy, and detection of malformations [1]. Alarming signs of potential foetal hyperthyroidism include foetal tachycardia (heart rate >170 bpm), intrauterine growth restriction, presence of foetal goitre, signs of congestive heart failure, and foetal hydrops [63, 64].

Umbilical Cord Sampling

Elevated TRAbs alone is not an indication for umbilical cord sampling (cordocentesis) [65] as it is associated with foetal mortality and morbidity [66, 67] and a relatively high recall rate [68]. It should be used in rare circumstances and performed in an appropriate setting [1]. Possibly its only role lies in women who are TRAbs positive and receive ATDs and the foetal thyroid status is unclear but overall it is not recommended [1, 38, 69, 70].

Maternal and Foetal Aspects, Pregnancy Outcomes

It is well documented that overt hyperthyroidism was directly linked with adverse pregnancy outcomes and that the duration and inadequate control of maternal thyrotoxicosis were clear determinants of maternal and foetal/neonatal complications [28, 58, 71, 72]. Early recognition and appropriate treatment of maternal hyperthyroidism is therefore of paramount importance to prevent these complications [1, 11]. On the other hand, subclinical hyperthyroidism, i.e. suppressed TSH and normal/upper end of normal fT4 levels, does not seem to be associated with adverse pregnancy outcomes [73, 74]. The adverse outcomes of uncontrolled hyperthyroidism are summarised in Table 6.

Maternal Aspects of Uncontrolled Thyrotoxicosis

The two main maternal complications of uncontrolled hyperthyroidism are congestive cardiac failure (CCF) and thyroid storm. Thyroid storm is discussed in detail in chapter "Thyroid Storm and Neonatal Hyperthyroidism" of this book. CCF can complicate up to 5–10% of pregnancies with untreated or uncontrolled hyperthyroidism

Table 6 Maternal, obstetric and neonatal complications of uncontrolled hyperthyroidism

Complications of gestational hyperthyroidism
Maternal
Side effects of antithyroid drugs
Cardiovascular (tachyarrhythmias, left ventricular dysfunction)
Thyroid storm
Obstetric
Miscarriage
Still birth
Preterm labour or delivery
Gestational hypertension
Foetal dysthyroidism
Foetal distress/intrauterine growth restriction
Placental abruption
Haemorrhage
Neonatal
Low birth weight (2.500 g) or macrosomia (>4.500 g)
Respiratory distress syndrome
Admission to neonatal intensive care unit
Neonatal dysthyroidism
Congenital abnormalities/neurobehavioural disorders of the offspring

[75, 76]. This frequency is significantly higher compared to non-pregnant thyrotoxic women, which implies that this is due to the increased cardiac workload secondary to thyrotoxic and pregnancy cardiovascular effects [75]. In many cases an additional precipitant is present, for example, anaemia, sepsis, bleeding or preeclampsia [75]. In the majority of cases of CCF in pregnancy an additional precipitating event is identified, for example, sepsis, trauma, bleeding or labour.

CCF should be managed in an intensive care unit. Almost always supportive treatment is required such as diuretics, vasopressors/inotropes, controlled cooling and aggressive management of any precipitating factors (sepsis, anaemia, trauma, etc.).

Foetal Aspects and Pregnancy Outcomes

Hyperthyroidism also impacts on foetal health. For some time there has been a debate in the literature whether it is hyperthyroidism per se or the underlying autoimmunity accompanying GD that is responsible for the adverse foetal outcomes. On one hand it has been shown that the presence of antibodies is associated with higher frequency of obstetric complications [58, 71]. On the other hand, a previous large prospective (cohort) study [73] and a recent systematic review and meta-analysis has shown that subclinical autoimmune hyperthyroidism is not linked with higher frequency of intrauterine growth restriction [74]. Furthermore elegant studies of women with a diagnosis of resistance to thyroid hormone (RTH) showed that elevated maternal T4 levels can directly adversely affect foetal development (miscarriage rate and birth weight) [7, 8, 77]. It is therefore more likely that adverse pregnancy outcomes are directly related to the duration and inadequate control of maternal thyrotoxicosis rather than the autoimmunity per se.

Several case studies and large retrospective studies have shown that inadequately controlled thyrotoxicosis is associated with a risk of spontaneous abortion, preterm delivery, low birth weight, and stillbirth [28, 72, 78–84].

Conclusions

Over the last two decades there has been an increase in the knowledge and our appreciation of the physiological and immunological aspects of thyroid function in relation to pregnancy. This accumulating knowledge has led to a different approach to gestational thyrotoxicosis with close maternal and foetal surveillance. Uncontrolled thyrotoxicosis can lead to adverse maternal, obstetrical and foetal outcomes; therefore prompt diagnosis and timely initiation of treatment is essential to reduce the risk. On the other hand, the use of ATDs during pregnancy is associated with potential hazard to the foetus so their unnecessary use should be avoided. The complexity of the different clinical scenarios of thyrotoxicosis during gestation makes close follow-up by a specialist crucial. Maternal hyperthyroidism due to GD poses the foetus at an additional risk, that of neonatal dysthyroidism due to maternal thyroid receptor antibodies crossing the placenta and entering the foetus. As a consequence the management of the pregnant woman with GD has two goals: First, the restoration and maintenance of maternal euthyroidism throughout pregnancy using the recommended ATDs according to the stage of gestation. Second, the appropriate risk stratification and close monitoring of the foetus for evidence of hyperthyroidism.

Measurement of TRAbs has become a very useful tool in pregnancy, not only when the diagnosis is unclear, for example, in newly developed thyrotoxicosis in early pregnancy, but also for neonatal thyrotoxicosis risk stratification purposes. The TRAbs titre in pregnancy allows an individualised approach to each mother and foetus. Although rarely, offspring of mothers with GD can develop foetal/neonatal thyrotoxicosis. The complexity of the condition and the emerging evidence require close collaboration between endocrinologists, obstetricians and neonatologists.

Despite the accumulating evidence over the last two decades and the comprehensive available guidelines, there are still questions to be answered and critical issues to be addressed. It needs to be clarified what are the optimal maternal TRAbs concentration cut-offs for prediction of FD/ND. In our opinion, given the seriousness of ND, it seems reasonable to adopt the lower cut-off point until more data become available. Additionally, further studies evaluating the safety of alternative therapies of thyrotoxicosis in pregnancy (e.g. potassium iodide) will be valuable.

Summary

Normal maternal thyroid function is essential not only for maternal health, but also for foetal development. Thyrotoxicosis, which is the clinical syndrome of hypermetabolism and hyperactivity that occurs when a person is exposed to supraphysiological concentrations of thyroid hormones (TH), can present during pregnancy. Albeit less common than hypothyroidism in pregnancy, it can pose a challenge to the clinician given its diagnostic and therapeutic difficulties as well as the possible maternal and foetal complications. One of the main challenges is the prompt differential diagnosis between transient thyrotoxicosis often due to hyperemesis gravidarum and Graves' disease (GD) if the woman is not already known to have thyrotoxicosis prior to the pregnancy. This is crucial in pregnancy as Graves' disease is linked with various maternal and foetal complications, some of which can be serious or life-threatening especially in case of late recognition and poor management. An additional difficulty is that many of the symptoms of thyrotoxicosis such as sweating, nausea, palpitations, insomnia, anxiety, fatigue are nonspecific and can "mimic" frequent pregnancy complaints. However, a careful clinical assessment can raise the clinical suspicion of newly developed thyrotoxicosis in pregnancy. The diagnosis should be confirmed with measurement of the levels of the TSH as well as of the free-T4/free-T3. If the exact diagnosis is uncertain, measurement of TSH receptor antibodies (TRAbs) is indicated, since the presence of these antibodies differentiates GD from other causes of gestational thyrotoxicosis. Furthermore, in cases of GD the measurement of TRAbs has prognostic significance for the development of GD in the foetus. The overall goal of management is to maintain or achieve euthyroidism as early as possible in pregnancy. Anti-thyroid drugs (ATDs) are the cornerstone of treatment of hyperthyroidism in pregnancy. Thyroidectomy should be preserved as second line option in selected cases and radioactive iodine (RAI) treatment is contraindicated in pregnancy.

References

1. Alexander EK, Pearce EN, Brent GA, Brown RS, Chen H, Dosiou C, et al. 2017 guidelines of the American Thyroid Association for the diagnosis and management of thyroid disease during pregnancy and the postpartum. Thyroid. 2017;27:315–89.
2. Cooper DS, Laurberg P. Hyperthyroidism in pregnancy. Lancet Diabetes Endocrinol. 2013;1:238–49.
3. Krassas G, Karras SN, Pontikides N. Thyroid diseases during pregnancy: a number of important issues. Hormones (Athens). 2015;14:59–69. https://doi.org/10.1007/BF03401381.
4. Andersen SL, Olsen J, Carlé A, Laurberg P. Hyperthyroidism incidence fluctuates widely in and around pregnancy and is at variance with some other autoimmune diseases: a Danish population-based study. J Clin Endocrinol Metab. 2015;100:1164–71.
5. Tan JY, Loh KC, Yeo GS, Chee YC. Transient hyperthyroidism of hyperemesis gravidarum. BJOG. 2002;109:683–8.

6. Bolz M, Korber S, Schober HC. TSH secreting adenoma of pituitary gland (TSHom)—rare cause of hyperthyroidism in pregnancy. Dtsch Med Wochenschr. 2013;138:362–6.
7. Pappa T, Anselmo J, Mamanasiri S, Dumitrescu AM, Weiss RE, Refetoff S. Prenatal diagnosis of resistance to thyroid hormone and its clinical implications. J Clin Endocrinol Metab. 2017;102:3775–82.
8. Srichomkwun P, Anselmo J, Liao XH, Hönes GS, Moeller LC, Alonso-Sampedro M, et al. Fetal exposure to high maternal thyroid hormone levels causes central resistance to thyroid hormone in adult humans and mice. J Clin Endocrinol Metab. 2017;102:3234–40.
9. Lazarus JH. Thyroid disease during pregnancy. In: Krassas GE, Rivkees SA, Kiess W, editors. Diseases of the thyroid in childhood and adolescence, pediatric and adolescent medicine, vol. 11. Basel: Karger; 2007. p. 27.
10. Chan SY, Vasilopoulou E, Kilby MD. The role of the placenta in thyroid hormone delivery to the fetus. Nat Clin Pract Endocrinol Metab. 2009;5:45–54.
11. De Groot L, Abalovich M, Alexander EK, Amino N, Barbour L, Cobin RH, et al. Management of thyroid dysfunction during pregnancy and postpartum: an Endocrine Society clinical practice guideline. J Clin Endocrinol Metab. 2012;97:2543–65.
12. Braverman LE, Cooper DS. Introduction to thyrotoxicosis. In: Braverman LE, Cooper DS, editors. Thyroid. A fundamental and clinical text. 10th ed. Alphen aan den Rijn: Wolters Kluwer; 2001. p. 354–5.
13. Kahaly GJ, Bartalena L, Hegedüs L, Leenhardt L, Poppe K, Pearce SH. 2018 European Thyroid Association guideline for the management of graves' hyperthyroidism. Eur Thyroid J. 2018;7:167–86.
14. Krassas GE, Poppe K, Glinoer D. Thyroid function and human reproductive health. Endocr Rev. 2010;31:702–55. https://doi.org/10.1210/er.2009-0041.
15. Francis T, Francis N, Lazarus JH, Okosieme OE. Safety of antithyroid drugs in pregnancy: update and therapy implications. Expert Opin Drug Saf. 2020;19:565–76.
16. Abdi H, Amouzegar A, Azizi F. Antithyroid drugs. Iran J Pharm Res. 2019;18(Suppl 1):1–12.
17. Gardner DF, Cruikshank DP, Hays PM, Cooper DS. Pharmacology of propylthiouracil (PTU) in pregnant hyperthyroid women: correlation of maternal PTU concentrations with cord serum thyroid function tests. J Clin Endocrinol Metab. 1986;62:217–20.
18. Mortimer RH, Cannell GR, Addison RS, Johnson LP, Roberts MS, Bernus I. Methimazole and propylthiouracil equally cross the perfused human term placental lobule. J Clin Endocrinol Metab. 1997;82:3099–102.
19. Wing DA, Millar LK, Koonings PP, Montoro MN, Mestman JH. A comparison of propylthiouracil versus methimazole in the treatment of hyperthyroidism in pregnancy. Am J Obstet Gynecol. 1994;170:90–5.
20. Andersen SL, Andersen S. Antithyroid drugs and birth defects. Thyroid Res. 2020;13:11.
21. Yoshihara A, Noh J, Yamaguchi T, Ohye H, Sato S, Sekiya K, et al. Treatment of graves' disease with antithyroid drugs in the first trimester of pregnancy and the prevalence of congenital malformation. J Clin Endocrinol Metab. 2012;97:2396–403.
22. Andersen SL, Olsen J, Wu CS, Laurberg P. Birth defects after early pregnancy use of antithyroid drugs: a Danish nationwide study. J Clin Endocrinol Metab. 2013;98:4373–81.
23. Seo GH, Kim TH, Chung JH. Antithyroid drugs and congenital malformations: a Nationwide Korean cohort study. Ann Intern Med. 2018;168:405–13.
24. Andersen SL, Knosgaard L, Olsen J, Vestergaard P, Andersen S. Maternal thyroid function, use of antithyroid drugs in early pregnancy and birth defects. J Clin Endocrinol Metab. 2019;104:6040–8.
25. Andersen SL, Lonn S, Vestergaard P, Torring O. Birth defects after use of antithyroid drugs in early pregnancy: a Swedish nationwide study. Eur J Endocrinol. 2017;177:369–78.
26. Gianetti E, Russo L, Orlandi F, Chiovato L, Giusti M, Benvenga S, et al. Pregnancy outcome in women treated with methimazole or propylthiouracil during pregnancy. J Endocrinol Invest. 2015;38:977–85.

27. Korelitz JJ, McNally DL, Masters MN, Li SX, Xu Y, Rivkees SA. Prevalence of thyrotoxicosis, antithyroid medication use, and complications among pregnant women in the United States. Thyroid. 2013;23:758–65.
28. Lo JC, Rivkees SA, Chandra M, Gonzalez JR, Korelitz JJ, Kuzniewicz MW. Gestational thyrotoxicosis, antithyroid drug use and neonatal outcomes within an integrated healthcare delivery system. Thyroid. 2015;25:698–705.
29. Song R, Lin H, Chen Y, Zhang X, Feng W. Effects of methimazole and propylthiouracil exposure during pregnancy on the risk of neonatal congenital malformations: a meta-analysis. PLoS One. 2017;12:e0180108.
30. Kahaly GJ. Management of Graves thyroidal and extrathyroidal disease: an update. J Clin Endocrinol Metab. 2020;105:3704–20.
31. Wang MT, Lee WJ, Huang TY, Chu CL, Hsieh CH. Antithyroid drug-related hepatotoxicity in hyperthyroidism patients: a population-based cohort study. Br J Clin Pharmacol. 2014;78:619–29.
32. Yang J, Li LF, Xu Q, Zhang J, Weng WW, Zhu YJ, et al. Analysis of 90 cases of antithyroid drug-induced severe hepatotoxicity over 13 years in China. Thyroid. 2015;25:278–83.
33. Suzuki N, Noh JY, Hiruma M, Kawaguchi A, Morisaki M, Ohye H, et al. Analysis of antithyroid drug-induced severe liver injury in 18,558 newly diagnosed patients with Graves' disease in Japan. Thyroid. 2019;29:1390–8.
34. Yu W, Wu N, Li L, Wang J, OuYang H, Shen H. Side effects of PTU and MMI in the treatment of hyperthyroidism: a systematic review and meta-analysis. Endocr Pract. 2020;26:207–17. https://doi.org/10.4158/EP-2019-0221.
35. Cooper DS, Rivkees SA. Putting propylthiouracil in perspective. J Clin Endocrinol Metab. 2009;94:1881–2.
36. Perros P, Hegedüs L, Bartalena L, Marcocci C, Kahaly GJ, Baldeschi L, et al. Graves' orbitopathy as a rare disease in Europe: a European Group on Graves' Orbitopathy (EUGOGO) position statement. Orphanet J Rare Dis. 2017;12:72.
37. Duan L, Ng A, Chen W, Spencer HT, Lee MS. Beta-blocker subtypes and risk of low birth weight in newborns. J Clin Hypertens (Greenwich). 2018;20:1603–9. https://doi.org/10.1111/jch.13397.
38. Laurberg P, Bournaud C, Karmisholt J, Orgiazzi J. Management of Graves' hyperthyroidism in pregnancy: focus on both maternal and foetal thyroid function, and caution against surgical thyroidectomy in pregnancy. Eur J Endocrinol. 2009;160:1–8.
39. Yoshihara A, Noh JY, Watanabe N, Mukasa K, Ohye H, Suzuki M, et al. Substituting potassium iodide for methimazole as the treatment for Graves' disease during the first trimester may reduce the incidence of congenital anomalies: a retrospective study at a single medical institution in Japan. Thyroid. 2015;25:1155–61.
40. Yoshihara A, Noh JY, Watanabe N, Kunii Y, Suzuki M, Matsumoto M, et al. Characteristics of patients with Graves' disease whose thyroid hormone levels increase after substituting potassium iodide for methimazole in the first trimester of pregnancy. Thyroid. 2020;30:451–6.
41. Hofstee P, James-McAlpine J, McKeating DR, Vanderlelie JJ, Cuffe JS, Perkins AV. Low serum selenium in pregnancy is associated with reduced T3 and increased risk of GDM. J Endocrinol. 2021;248(1):45–57.
42. Pop V, Krabbe J, Maret W, Rayman M. Plasma mineral (selenium, zinc or copper) concentrations in the general pregnant population, adjusted for supplement intake, in relation to thyroid function. Br J Nutr. 2020;14:1–8.
43. Lazarus JH. Thyroid disease during pregnancy. In: Krassas GE, Rivkees SA, Kiess W, editors. Diseases of the thyroid in childhood and adolescence, pediatric and adolescent medicine, vol. 11. Basel: Karger; 2007. p. 25–40, table 1.
44. Mandel SH, Hanna CE, LaFranchi SH. Diminished thyroid-stimulating hormone secretion associated with neonatal thyrotoxicosis. J Pediatr. 1986;109:662–5.

45. Hashimoto H, Maruyama H, Koshida R, et al. Central hypothyroidism resulting from pituitary suppression and peripheral thyrotoxicosis in a premature infant born to a mother with Graves disease. J Pediatr. 1995;127:809–11.
46. Kempers MJE, van Trotsenburg ASP, van Tijn DA, et al. Disturbance of the fetal thyroid hormone state has long-term consequences for treatment of thyroidal and central congenital hypothyroidism. J Clin Endocrinol Metab. 2005;90:4094–100.
47. Nguyen CT, Mestman JH. Graves' hyperthyroidism in pregnancy. Curr Opin Endocrinol Diabetes Obes. 2019;26:232–40.
48. Matsuura N, Harada S, Ohyama Y, et al. The mechanisms of transient hypothyroxinemia in infants born to mothers with Graves' disease. Pediatr Res. 1997;42:214–8.
49. Van Trotsenburg ASP. Management of neonates born to mothers with thyroid dysfunction, and points for attention during pregnancy. Best Pract Res Clin Endocrinol Metab. 2020;34:101437.
50. Decallonne B, Martens PJ, Van den Bruel A, Vanhole C, Kahaly GJ. Graves disease with thyroid-stimulating hormone receptor-blocking autoantibodies during pregnancy. Ann Intern Med. 2020;172:767–9.
51. Kiefer FW, Klebermass-Schrehof K, Steiner M, Worda C, Kasprian G, Diana T, et al. Fetal/neonatal thyrotoxicosis in a newborn from a hypothyroid woman with Hashimoto thyroiditis. J Clin Endocrinol Metab. 2017;102:6–9.
52. Ohira S, Miyake M, Kobara H, Kikuchi N, Osada R, Ashida T, et al. Fetal goitrous hypothyroidism due to maternal thyroid stimulation-blocking antibody: a case report. Fetal Diagn Ther. 2010;28:220–4.
53. Nannaka VB, Lvovsky D. A rare case of gestational thyrotoxicosis as a cause of acute myocardial infarction. Endocrinol Diabetes Metab Case Rep. 2016;2016:16–0063.
54. Kuryłowicz A, Niewiński G, Kański A, Derlatka P, Czajkowski K, Bednarczuk T, et al. Severe gestational hyperthyroidism complicated by cardiac arrest—a case report. Ginekol Pol. 2017;88:43–4.
55. Marcocci C, Kahaly GJ, Krassas GE, Bartalena L, Prummel M, Stahl M, et al.; European Group on Graves' Orbitopathy. Selenium and the course of mild Graves' orbitopathy. N Engl J Med. 2011;364:1920–31.
56. Bartalena L, Baldeschi L, Dickinson AJ, Eckstein A, Kendall-Taylor P, Marcocci C, et al. Consensus statement of the European group on Graves' orbitopathy (EUGOGO) on management of Graves' orbitopathy. Thyroid. 2008;18:333–46.
57. Perros P, Wiersinga WM. The Amsterdam declaration on Graves' orbitopathy. Thyroid. 2010;20(3):245–6.
58. Moleti M, Di Mauro M, Sturniolo G, Russo M, Vermiglio F. Hyperthyroidism in the pregnant woman: maternal and fetal aspects. J Clin Transl Endocrinol. 2019;16:100190.
59. Banigé M, Estellat C, Biran V, et al. Study of the factors leading to fetal and neonatal dysthyroidism in children of patients with Graves Disease. J Endocr Soc. 2017;1:751–61.
60. Nakada K, Mizukoshi T, Tamura M, Katoh N, Sakurai M. Longitudinal changes in TSH receptor antibodies after radioiodine therapy for Graves' hyperthyroidism: relationship with thyroid weight and therapeutic efficacy. J Nucl Med. 2018;59(Suppl 1):1345.
61. Nakada K, Mizukoshi T, Hattori N, Tamura M, Kato K, Kato N. The effect of changes of serum thyrotropin receptor antibody on the outcome of radioactive iodide therapy for Graves' hyperthyroidism. J Nucl Med. 2020;61(Suppl 1):45.
62. van Dijk MM, Smits IH, Fliers E, Bisschop PH. Maternal thyrotropin receptor antibody concentration and the risk of fetal and neonatal thyrotoxicosis: a systematic review. Thyroid. 2018;28:257–64.
63. Polak M, Le Gac I, Vuillard E, Guibourdenche J, Leger J, Toubert ME, et al. Fetal and neonatal thyroid function in relation to maternal Graves' disease. Best Pract Res Clin Endocrinol Metab. 2004;18:289–302.
64. Illouz F, Luton D, Polak M, Besançon A, Bournaud C. Graves' disease and pregnancy. Ann Endocrinol (Paris). 2018;79:636–46.

65. Kilpatrick S. Umbilical blood sampling in women with thyroid disease in pregnancy: is it necessary? Am J Obstet Gynecol. 2003;189:1–2.
66. Porreco RP, Bloch CA. Fetal blood sampling in the management of intrauterine thyrotoxicosis. Obstet Gynecol. 1990;76(3 Pt 2):509–12.
67. Sasahara J, Ishii K, Fujikawa E, Mitsuda N. Current status of percutaneous umbilical cord blood sampling in Japan. J Obstet Gynaecol Res. 2019;45:1821–7.
68. Abduljabbar M, Al Shahri A, Afifi A. Is umbilical cord blood total thyroxin measurement effective in newborn screening for hypothyroidism? J Med Screen. 2009;16:119–23.
69. Luton D, Le Gac I, Vuillard E, Castanet M, Guibourdenche J, Noel M, et al. Management of Graves' disease during pregnancy: the key role of fetal thyroid gland monitoring. J Clin Endocrinol Metab. 2005;90:6093–8.
70. van der Kaay DC, Wasserman JD, Palmert MR. Management of neonates born to mothers with Graves' disease. Pediatrics. 2016;137:e20151878.
71. Moleti M, Sturniolo G, Di Mauro M, Russo M, Vermiglio F. Autoimmune thyroid diseases and pregnancy. Ann Thyroid. 2018;3:18.
72. Nazarpour S, Ramezani Tehrani F, Simbar M, Azizi F. Thyroid dysfunction and pregnancy outcomes. Iran J Reprod Med. 2015;13:387–96.
73. Casey BM, Dashe JS, Wells CE, McIntire DD, Leveno KJ, Cunningham FG. Subclinical hyperthyroidism and pregnancy outcomes. Obstet Gynecol. 2006;107(2 Pt 1):337–41.
74. Tong Z, Xiaowen Z, Baomin C, Aihua L, Yingying Z, Weiping T, et al. The effect of subclinical maternal thyroid dysfunction and autoimmunity on intrauterine growth restriction: a systematic review and meta-analysis. Medicine (Baltimore). 2016;95:e3677.
75. Sheffield JS, Cunningham FG. Thyrotoxicosis and heart failure that complicate pregnancy. Am J Obstet Gynecol. 2004;190:211–7.
76. Khoo CM, Lee KO. Endocrine emergencies in pregnancy. Best Pract Res Clin Obstet Gynaecol. 2013;27:885–91.
77. Anselmo J, Cao D, Karrison T, Weiss RE, Refetoff S. Fetal loss associated with excess thyroid hormone exposure. JAMA. 2004;292:691–5.
78. Nguyen CT, Mestman JH. A look at Graves' hyperthyroidism in pregnancy. Ann Thyroid. 2018;3:28.
79. Smith C, Thomsett M, Choong C, Rodda C, McIntyre HD, Cotterill AM. Congenital thyrotoxicosis in premature infants. Clin Endocrinol. 2001;54:371–6.
80. Männistö T, Mendola P, Grewal J, Xie Y, Chen Z, Laughon SK. Thyroid diseases and adverse pregnancy outcomes in a contemporary US cohort. J Clin Endocrinol Metab. 2013;98:2725–33.
81. Turunen S, Vääräsmäki M, Lahesmaa-Korpinen AM, Leinonen MK, Gissler M, Männistö T, et al. Maternal hyperthyroidism and pregnancy outcomes: a population-based cohort study. Clin Endocrinol. 2020;93:721–8.
82. Luewan S, Chakkabut P, Tongsong T. Outcomes of pregnancy complicated with hyperthyroidism: a cohort study. Arch Gynecol Obstet. 2011;283:243–7.
83. Andersen SL, Olsen J, Wu CS, Laurberg P. Spontaneous abortion, stillbirth and hyperthyroidism: a Danish population-based study. Eur Thyroid J. 2014;3:164–72.
84. LeBeau SO, Mandel SJ. Thyroid disorders during pregnancy. Endocrinol Metab Clin N Am. 2006;35:117–36, vii.

Gestational Transient Hyperthyroidism

Spyridon N. Karras and Themistoklis Tzotzas

Introduction

Pregnancy is an ongoing dynamic state, where the developing child is under the influence of a continuum of biologic events that enables tissue adaptation. This multifactorial process represents interplay between genetic, environmental, and hormonal influences, which regulate the function of a specific tissue [1]. It has been demonstrated that this critical time frame of intrauterine development comprises a "window of vulnerability": the developing fetus is susceptible to a changing environment, enabling a phenotypic diversity and aiming for a maximum adaptation at future life. At this time of endometrial plasticity, certain mother-related parameters, including disorders of thyroid function, could significantly affect the optimal course of pregnancy and the in utero fetal development [2]. In the case of thyrotoxicosis, an in-depth knowledge of the pathophysiology of the disease, patient's clinical symptoms and signs is required, as well as the inherent ability of the clinician, to integrate available findings, with laboratory results [3].

The most common cause of thyrotoxicosis during pregnancy results from autoimmune hyperthyroidism [Graves' disease (GD)], and rarely from autonomous thyroid nodules or toxic multinodular goiter [3]. In the pregnant state, however, physiological hormonal changes, induced by pregnancy per se, might lead to misleading laboratory findings, including a significant decrease of thyroid stimulating hormone (TSH) as well as an increase in total thyroxine (T4) and free T4 (FT4) concentrations, which in combination with some of the clinical symptoms of early pregnancy could comprise a significant clinical dilemma [4]. These adaptive

S. N. Karras (✉)
National Scholarship Foundation, Thessaloniki, Greece

T. Tzotzas
Department of Endocrinology, Diabetes, and Metabolism, St Luke's General Hospital, Thessaloniki, Greece
e-mail: tzotzas@otenet.gr

F. Azizi, F. Ramezani Tehrani (eds.), *Thyroid Diseases in Pregnancy*,
https://doi.org/10.1007/978-3-030-98777-0_10

responses affect reference range values for TSH in pregnant women, and the use of pregnancy-specific reference ranges is recommended [1, 2].

Apart from the unique laboratory findings, mimicking hyperthyroidism, in some cases, pregnant women with no previous or present history of autoimmune hyperthyroidism, manifest a wide range of clinical signs and symptoms, including morning sickness, different degrees of vomiting, palpitations, and weight loss [5]. These findings, in conjunction with "abnormal" thyroid tests that are often found in early pregnancy, might suggest the diagnosis of hyperthyroidism; however, during pregnancy differential diagnosis is often intriguing, since there are some forms of gestational hyperthyroidism, resulting primarily from the sharp increase and TSH-like activity of human chorionic gonadotropin (hCG) [6]. The latter "physiological" changes manifest a transient course of hyperthyroidism, requiring no antithyroid drug (ATD) treatment or other intervention. This form of gestational transient hyperthyroidism (GTH), as a result of adaptive responses during pregnancy, with no autoimmune background or the presence of autonomous thyroid nodules, will be the objective of this chapter.

Definition

A plethora of previous definitions have been used to describe this clinical entity, with an initial attempt to be incorporated in the syndrome of hyperemesis gravidarum (HG) [7], comprising a severe form of nausea, vomiting, and weight loss, which often requires hospitalization. However, this term might not be representative for the milder forms of gestational hyperthyroidism, as well as for the other causes of gestational transient hyperthyroidism. Kimura et al. [8] proposed the term "gestational thyrotoxicosis," whereas the terms "gestational hyperthyroidism" and "gestational transient thyrotoxicosis" have also been suggested, previously. In our opinion, we consider the term thyrotoxicosis not physiologically entirely sound, whereas the term used by Goldman et al. [9], "transient non-immune hyperthyroidism of early pregnancy," could be considered as the most holistic terminology to describe the key characteristics of this entity. More precisely the term "non-immune" needs to be confirmed by future mechanistic studies. In this chapter, the term "gestational transient hyperthyroidism (GTH)" will be used to describe this entity.

Prevalence

The prevalence of hyperthyroidism resulting from GD is approximately 0.1–0.4% of patients [2], whereas the overall prevalence of all forms of thyrotoxicosis in pregnancy is 3–4% [3]. GTH comprises the most common form of hyperthyroidism in the early stages of pregnancy, with about 70% of cases diagnosed in the time frame of the first 12–16 weeks of pregnancy.

The prevalence of GTH varies among populations worldwide, indicating potential effects of different iodine status, obstetrical routine laboratory evaluation, ethnic or TSH-receptor polymorphism variations and prevalence of thyroid autoimmunity. Glinoer [10] reported a prevalence of 2–3% in Belgian women during 8th to 14th week of pregnancy, whereas the prevalence of gestational thyrotoxicosis in Asian women was found to be 11.0% and was significantly higher in subjects at 8–11 weeks of gestation than at 12–14 weeks [11]. Similarly, non-European populations, including those of Indian ethnic origin (Pakistani, Bangladeshi, and Indian) and Pacific Islanders [12–14], have also been reported to manifest a prevalence of approximately 15% of women at early pregnancy, compared to 4.8% of European women [12], highlighting its high prevalence in pregnant populations worldwide.

Pathophysiology

Pregnancy is characterized by a profound increase in plasma flow and glomerular filtration rate [1, 2]. This phenomenon results in a significant increase of extracellular pool of distribution of total T4 and triiodothyronine (T3), which are required to increase their concentrations to a new steady state, in order to adapt to the new plasma equilibrium [2, 15]. The enhanced biological production of T4 and T3 is facilitated mainly through the estrogen-mediated increased production of thyroxine-binding globulin (TBG) and the hCG stimulation of the thyroid gland [16].These necessary adaptive responses, which result in a positive net-load of thyroid equilibrium, are also required to overcome the increased thyroid turnover observed during pregnancy.

In the case of high maternal-fetal concentration gradient [17], a significant transfer of T4 can occur, since fetal brain has the ability to induce the efficiency of T4-to-T3 conversion. The main adaptive response, which protects the fetus from inappropriate intrauterine exposure of T4, is the upregulation of type iodothyronine deiodinase (D3) expression, in the fetal-placental-uterine unit, which deactivates T3 and T4 [18].

In addition, the increased iodine clearance results in increased iodine requirements during pregnancy [19]. It becomes evident that during early stages of pregnancy, a tightly coordinated biological balance is evident, which on one hand maximizes optimal thyroidal status through maternal stores for the brain development of the fetus, and on the other hand protects the embryo from exposure to high T4 concentrations.

At that basis, hCG plays an integral role in the establishment of this physiological interplay, during early pregnancy [1]. It belongs to the glycoprotein family hormone, sharing similarities with other members of this family.

These hormones are composed of two non-covalently linked subunits, α and β: α subunit is shared by all of them, whereas β subunit is characteristic of each hormone. HCG β subunit is encoded by a cluster of genes located on chromosome 19 [20]. Therefore, hCG is a heterodimeric protein synthesized mainly by the syncytiotrophoblast [21]. It has been reported that hCG mRNA is detected at six- to eight-cell embryo stage, so its production in human embryos begins before implantation [22]. From day 8 after fertilization, hCG is detectable in maternal serum, and its levels peak at tenth week of gestation, decreasing then slowly until the end of pregnancy [21]. Moreover, in first-trimester placental explants, it was reported that the secretion of this glycoprotein is pulsatile [23]. B-hCG subunit detection in serum and urine is commonly used as a pregnancy test [21], being higher in multiple pregnancies [23] in trophoblastic tumors and in HG [1, 2]. HCG binds to G protein-coupled receptor luteinizing hormone–hCG, and mainly activates the enzyme adenylyl cyclase, increasing concomitantly cyclic adenosine monophosphate (cAMP) levels and protein kinase A (PKA) activity. By its activation, hCG plays several pleiotropic roles during gestation, owing to its autocrine and paracrine actions, interfering with several processes that are vital for the pregnancy outcome, including immunotolerance.

It suppresses the maternal immunological system through an increase of T regulatory cell number at the fetal–maternal interface [24, 25]. This effect has been associated with the high remission rates of autoimmune disorders, often observed due to the suppression of the maternal immune system associated with pregnancy [25].

HCG is also a weak agonist of the human thyroid receptor (h TSHR), with less potency compared to TSH (1 U H hCG = 0.7 μU of human TSH), thereby increasing thyroid hormone production in normal pregnancy, which is usually not associated with clinical symptoms [26, 27]. In cases where high concentrations of hCG are evident, this agonist activity is enhanced, resulting in some cases in clinical and laboratory findings of hyperthyroidism, including diffuse goiter, elevated free T4 concentrations, and suppressed TSH [3]. The amount of desialylated hCG produced modulates its thyrotropic actions, since molecules that are less sialylated activate the TSH receptor to a greater extent [27].

Recent results however expand the association of hCG thyrotropic actions during early pregnancy and GTH beyond this hypothesis, implicating genetic and additional hormonal factors involved in this interaction. In detail, growth differentiation factor 15 (GDF15), a divergent member of the transforming growth factor-β (TGF-β) superfamily, which has been reported to exert a significant role in the regulation of energy substrate utilization or energy expenditure [28], has been increased in patients with hyperthyroidism compared with healthy subjects and dramatically declined after thionamide treatment [29], confirming an independent association between serum GDF15 levels and hyperthyroidism.

GDF15 and IGFBP7 are critical factors involved in early placentation, but are also unregulated in early pregnancy and cause loss of appetite in animal models [30–32]. GDF15 receptor GFRAL was recently identified and is localized in the brainstem where feeding behavior, nausea, and vomiting are regulated [33]. They are also upregulated in early pregnancy and cause loss of appetite in animal models [30–32, 34].

In a recent genome-wide association study meta-analysis, these factors have been found to be important pathogenetic contributors for HG [35],which comprises the most severe form of nausea and vomiting of pregnancy (NVP).

Although hCG concentrations are considered the main determinant of HG, this hypothesis is currently challenged by studies that involved additional parameters, including GDF15 and IGFBP7. These factors, due to their thyrotropic activity, are likely to provide an additional link between adaptive hormonal changes in early pregnancy and GTH development.

On the other hand, hCG manifests a central and peripheral regulatory action in appetite control and gastric emptying through cholecystokinin 1 receptors [36], whereas gut-derived regulatory peptides, ghrelin and PPY-3 have been also implicated in the pathogenesis of HG [37]. Thyroid hormones are well-established regulators of these appetite-regulatory hormones [37, 38]. It becomes evident that additional metabolic pathways are likely to mediate the interplay between the development of GTH and hCG, in early pregnancy, that remain to be elucidated.

In addition, familial mutations at the lysine 183 amino acid in the extracellular N-terminal domain of human TSH receptor (h TSHR) have been associated with hypersensitivity to hCG and familial gestational hyperthyroidism [39]. It has also been proposed that hCG may trigger the onset of GD in susceptible individuals [40], as well as the worsening or relapse in women with known GD, who become pregnant [41]. It becomes evident that genetic factors as well as autoimmunity are vital components of this complex association, which lies well beyond a simple concentration-derived effect of hCG, during early pregnancy.

Clinical Features

NVP affects 50–90% of all pregnant women [42] and has been considered as a protective mechanism against the toxicity induced by ingestion of harmful compounds and "palatable" foods for the developing fetus. It has been previously reported that the severity of nausea and vomiting correlates with the degree of hyperthyroidism in early pregnancy [43]. HG, the most severe form of NVP, occurs in 0.3–2% of pregnancies and leads to significant weight loss, dehydration, electrolyte imbalance, and ketonuria [44] and is associated with maternal morbidity such as Wernicke's encephalopathy, renal and liver function abnormalities, esophageal rupture, postpartum posttraumatic stress, and depression. HG is also associated with a four-fold increased risk of adverse fetal outcome including low birth weight, intrauterine growth restriction, preterm delivery, fetal and neonatal death, and a three-fold increased risk of neurodevelopmental delay in children [45, 46]. As mentioned above, hCG plays an integral part in the pathogenesis of GTH [44] and has been also involved in the development of GTH. GTH is diagnosed in 1–3% of pregnancies and is observed more frequently in pregnant women suffering from HG and usually resolves by 18 weeks gestation [9].

The severity of nausea and vomiting often determines the pattern of clinical symptoms, since fatigue, palpitations, and muscle cramps are likely to occur. Clinical signs are also intimately correlated with the degree of dehydration, including hypotension, tachycardia, fine tremor, and myopathy, which improve after fluid and electrolyte replacement. Common signs of thyrotoxicosis, including goiter and exophthalmos, are in the vast majority of cases absent, with the exception of patients with previous autoimmune hyperthyroidism and co-existent GTH. In rare cases of hyperplacentosis or trophoblastic disease due to molar pregnancy or trophoblastic tumors, symptoms and signs also correlate with the degree of hCG concentrations. In this case, the most common manifestation is vaginal bleeding with preexistent amenorrhea, and under these circumstances a careful obstetrical evaluation is required [9].

Clinical, Laboratory, and Imaging Diagnosis

A holistic approach for diagnosing GTH presupposes a detailed report of previous medical history of the future mother, including absence of autoimmune thyroid disease or associated symptoms before pregnancy, history of significant nausea and vomiting in previous pregnancies, family history of HG, Helicobacter pylori infection, and a low body mass index [2, 9]. As noted above, goiter or firm thyroid at palpation and ophthalmopathy are absent, whereas signs of dehydration might be evident. Prominent nausea and vomiting favor a diagnosis of HG, although these symptoms might co-exist in women with pre-existing Graves' disease. In this case, additional signs of thyroid disease would be expected (Table 1).

Laboratory evaluation is crucial for differential diagnosis of GTH and first trimester Graves' disease. Whereas in both situations concentrations of FT4 or FTI are increased and TSH is maximally suppressed or undetectable, in the case of GTH, titers of antithyroid antibodies, thyroid peroxidase (TPO), and TRAbs are low or negative [1, 2, 9]. Measurements of TT3 or FT3 and FT4 are particularly useful, since a higher FT3/FT4 ratio has been reported in active GD compared to GTH, identifying a cut-off ratio of 2.7 [47], with a sensitivity and specificity of 77% and 88%, respectively.

HCG concentrations have been also reported to be significantly higher in GTH, compared [48] with active GD, with values above 400.000 IU/L suppressing TSH

Table 1 Differences between gestational transient hyperthyroidism (GTH) and preexistent Graves' disease (GD)

	GTH	GD
Etiology	HCG's thyrotropic action	Autoimmunity
Prepregnancy symptoms	Absent	Usually present
Nausea/hyperemesis	Present	Rare
Electrolytes/liver abnormalities	Often present	Absent
Goiter/Ophthalmopathy	Absent	Usually present
Anti-TPO/TSHRAbs	Absent	Present
FT3/FT4 ratio	<2.7	>2.7
Antithyroid drug intervention	Not needed	Usually needed
Maternal/fetal complications	Usually absent	Present

concentrations [6]. A hCG cut-off of 70.000 miu/L has been also reported to differentiate GTH and GD, however, with a lower specificity (51%) compared to FT3/FT4 ratio, in ROC curves [48]. Transient electrolytes abnormalities (60%) and liver abnormalities (50%) of patients are also a common manifestation of HG [44], which differentiates GTH from active GD [1, 9].

The course of GTH is also clinically useful, since in the vast majority of situations, vomiting subsides after 14–18 weeks gestation, and serum FT4 returns to normal values by the 15th week gestation, although in some cases, NVP might subside a few weeks later [40, 41]. Thyroid ultrasound in women with active GD might reveal a heterogeneous pattern of the gland as found in autoimmune thyroiditis, as well as an increased vascularity, which is however also found during pregnancy as a result of the increase in the plasma blood flow [49]. Thyroid scintigraphy is not indicated during pregnancy. Abdominal ultrasound could be considered in collaboration with a gynecologist, to rule out multiple pregnancies or the presence of a hydatidiform mole (molar pregnancy).

Management

GTH is a condition that in most cases does not require ATD intervention. Propylthiouracil was used in selected cases, with no improvement in outcomes, whereas larger studies comparing conservative and drug approach are warranted. However, in cases with difficulty to differentiate early GD from GTH, low doses of propylthiouracil (100–200 mg) might be useful for a few weeks. Pregnant women could be re-assured regarding the benign course of this entity, resulting from adaptive changes [9, 40, 41]. Close collaboration with the obstetrician is required. In cases of HG, management includes intravenous hydration, containing vitamin B complex and nausea medications: for women with persistent vomiting, significant weight loss, and presence of ketones in urine, hospitalization is very frequently required [44].

Pregnancy and Neonatal Outcomes

Due to its short and self-limiting course, GTH does not appear to associate with significant adverse pregnancy or neonatal outcomes as is the case in GD [50, 51]. However, few studies have found that the gestation period was shorter in mothers with GTH and that their infants had significant lower birth weight compared to mothers with normal thyroid function [52, 53]. In such cases, a negative correlation was found between the FT4 values in the early pregnancy and the gestational period [52].The lower birth weight in these infants is related to severity of hyperemesis and degree of weight loss but not correlated to GTH per se [53]. Therefore, specific prenatal care is not necessary in infants of mothers with GTH but can be considered in cases of mothers presenting the abovementioned hypercatabolic symptoms.

In the table, differences in the etiology, clinical manifestations, laboratory diagnosis, and management between GTH and GD are presented.

Summary

GTH is a self-limiting condition resulting from adaptive responses during pregnancy, with no autoimmune background or the presence of autonomous thyroid nodules.

It requires an in-depth knowledge of the hCG pleiotropic actions during early pregnancy, as well as the ability of the clinician to differentiate early GD, based on patient's clinical picture and laboratory results. Optimal collaboration, with the obstetrical team and neonatologists, as well as close prospective follow-up is warranted in most cases.

References

1. Barker DJ. The fetal and infant origins of adult disease. BMJ. 1990;301:1111.
2. Glinoer D, De Nayer P, Bourdoux P, Glinoer D, de Nayer P, Bourdoux P, et al. Regulation of maternal thyroid during pregnancy. J Clin Endocrinol Metab. 1990;71:276–87. https://doi.org/10.1210/jcem-71-2-276.
3. Krassas GE, Poppe K, Glinoer D. Thyroid function and human reproductive health. Endocr Rev. 2010;31:702–55. https://doi.org/10.1210/er.2009-0041.
4. Glinoer D, Spencer CA. Serum TSH determinations in pregnancy: how, when and why. Nat Rev Endocrinol. 2010;6:526–9. https://doi.org/10.1038/nrendo.2010.91.
5. Goodwin TM, Montoro M, Mestman JH. Transient hyperthyroidism and hyperemesis gravidarum: clinical aspects. Am J Obstet Gynecol. 1992;167:648–52. https://doi.org/10.1016/S0002-9378(11)91565-8.
6. Lockwood CM, Grenache DG, Gronowski AM. Serum human chorionic gonadotropin concentrations greater than 400,000 IU/L are invariably associated with suppressed serum thyrotropin concentrations. Thyroid. 2009;19:863–8. https://doi.org/10.1089/thy.2009.0079.
7. Goodwin TM, Hershman JM. Hyperthyroidism due to inappropriate production of human chorionic gonadotropin. Clin Obstet Gynecol. 1997;40:32–44. https://doi.org/10.1097/00003081-199703000-00006.
8. Kimura M, Amino N, Tamaki H, Ito E, Mitsuda N, Miyai K, et al. Gestational thyrotoxicosis and hyperemesis gravidarum: possible role of hCG with higher stimulating activity. Clin Endocrinol. 1993;38:345–50. https://doi.org/10.1111/j.1365-2265.1993.tb00512.x.
9. Goldman AM, Mestman JH. Transient non autoimmune hyperthyroidism of early pregnancy. J Thyroid Res. 2011;2011:142413. https://doi.org/10.4061/2011/142413.
10. Glinoer D. The regulation of thyroid function in pregnancy: pathways of endocrine adaptation from physiology to pathology. Endocr Rev. 1997;18:404–33. https://doi.org/10.1210/edrv.18.3.0300.
11. Yeo CP, Khoo DH, Eng PH, Tan HK, Yo SL, Jacob E. Prevalence of gestational thyrotoxicosis in Asian women evaluated in the 8th to 14th weeks of pregnancy: correlations with total and free beta human chorionic gonadotrophin. Clin Endocrinol. 2001;55:391–8. https://doi.org/10.1046/j.1365-2265.2001.01353.x.

12. Price A, Davies R, Heller SR, Milford-Ward A, Weetman AP. Asian women at increased risk of gestational thyrotoxicosis. J Clin Endocrinol Metab. 1996;81:1160–3. https://doi.org/10.1210/jcem.81.3.8772593.
13. Vangen S, Stoltenberg C, Stray-Pedersen B. Complaints and complications in pregnancy: a study of ethnic Norwegian and ethnic Pakistani women in Oslo. Ethn Health. 1999;4:19–28. https://doi.org/10.1080/13557859998155.
14. Jordan V, Grebe SK, Cooke RR, Ford HC, Larsen PD, Stone PR, et al. Acidic isoforms of chorionic gonadotrophin in European and Samoan women are associated with hyperemesis gravidarum and may be thyrotrophic. Clin Endocrinol. 1999;50:619–27. https://doi.org/10.1046/j.1365-2265.1999.00702.x.
15. LeBeau SO, Mandel SJ. Thyroid disorders during pregnancy. Endocrinol Metab Clin North Am. 2006;35:117–36. https://doi.org/10.1016/j.ecl.2005.09.009.
16. Dashe JS, Casey BM, Wells CE, McIntire DD, Byrd EW, Leveno KJ, et al. Thyroid-stimulating hormone in singleton and twin pregnancy: importance of gestational age-specific reference ranges. Obstet Gynecol. 2005;106:753–7. https://doi.org/10.1097/01.AOG.0000175836.41390.73.
17. Stagnaro-Green A. Maternal thyroid disease and preterm delivery. J Clin Endocrinol Metab. 2009;94:21–5. https://doi.org/10.1210/jc.2008-1288.
18. Huang SA, Dorfman DM, Genest DR, Salvatore D, Larsen PR. Type 3 iodothyronine deiodinase is highly expressed in the human uteroplacental unit and in fetal epithelium. J Clin Endocrinol Metab. 2003;88:1384–8. https://doi.org/10.1210/jc.2002-021291.
19. Alexander EK, Marqusee E, Lawrence J, Jarolim P, Fischer GA, Larsen PR. Timing and magnitude of increases in levothyroxine requirements during pregnancy in women with hypothyroidism. N Engl J Med. 2004;351:241–9. https://doi.org/10.1056/nejmoa040079.
20. Policastro PF, Daniels-McQueen S, Carle G, Boime I. A map of the hCG beta-LH beta gene cluster. J Biol Chem. 1986;261:5907–16.
21. Cole LA. Immunoassay of human chorionic gonadotropin, its free subunits, and metabolites. Clin Chem. 1997;43:2233–43.
22. Bonduelle ML, Dodd R, Liebaers I, Van Steirteghem A, Williamson R, Akhurst R. Chorionic gonadotrophin-beta mRNA, a trophoblast marker, is expressed in human 8-cell embryos derived from tripronucleate zygotes. Hum Reprod. 1988;3:909–14. https://doi.org/10.1093/oxfordjournals.humrep.a136808.
23. Barnea ER, Kaplan M. Spontaneous, gonadotropin-releasing hormone-induced, and progesterone-inhibited pulsatile secretion of human chorionic gonadotropin in the first trimester placenta in vitro. J Clin Endocrinol Metab. 1989;69:215–7. https://doi.org/10.1210/jcem-69-1-215.
24. Schumacher A, Brachwitz N, Sohr S, Engeland K, Langwisch S, Dolaptchieva M, et al. Human chorionic gonadotropin attracts regulatory T cells into the fetal maternal interface during early human pregnancy. J Immunol. 2009;182:5488–97. https://doi.org/10.4049/jimmunol.0803177.
25. Weetman A. Autoimmune thyroid disease. Endocrine. 2020;68:258–60. https://doi.org/10.1007/s12020-020-02188-6.
26. Davies TF, Taliadouros GS, Catt KJ, Nisula BC. Assessment of urinary thyrotropin-competing activity in choriocarcinoma and thyroid disease: further evidence for human chorionic gonadotropin interacting at the thyroid cell membrane. J Clin Endocrinol Metab. 1979;49:353–7. https://doi.org/10.1210/jcem-49-3-353.
27. Yoshimura M, Hershman JM. Thyrotropic action of human chorionic gonadotropin. Thyroid. 1995;5:425–34. https://doi.org/10.1089/thy.1995.5.425.
28. Tsai VWW, Husaini Y, Sainsbury A, Brown DA, Breit SN. The MIC-1/GDF15-GFRAL pathway in energy homeostasis: implications for obesity, cachexia, and other associated diseases. Cell Metab. 2018;28:353–68. https://doi.org/10.1016/j.cmet.2018.07.018.
29. Jiejie Z, Min L, Ying C, Zhang S, Ying H, Song Z, et al. Elevated serum growth differentiation factor 15 levels in hyperthyroid patients. Front Endocrinol (Lausanne). 2019;9:793. https://doi.org/10.3389/fendo.2018.00793.

30. Hsu JY, Crawley S, Chen M, Ayupova DA, Lindhout DA, Higbee J, et al. Non-homeostatic body weight regulation through a brainstem-restricted receptor for GDF15. Nature. 2017;550:255–9. https://doi.org/10.1038/nature24042.
31. Marjono AB, Brown DA, Horton KE. Macrophage inhibitory cytokine-1 in gestational tissues and maternal serum in normal and pre-eclamptic pregnancy. Placenta. 2003;24:100–6. https://doi.org/10.1053/plac.2002.0881.
32. Xiong Y, Walker K, Min X. Long-acting MIC-1/GDF15 molecules to treat obesity: evidence from mice to monkeys. Sci Transl Med. 2017;9:eaan8732. https://doi.org/10.1126/scitranslmed.aan8732.
33. Moore AG, Brown DA, Fairlie WD. The transforming growth factor-ss superfamily cytokine macrophage inhibitory cytokine-1 is present in high concentrations in the serum of pregnant women. J Clin Endocrinol Metab. 2000;85:4781–8. https://doi.org/10.1210/jcem.85.12.7007.
34. Liu ZK, Wang RC, Han BC. A novel role of IGFBP7 in mouse uterus: regulating uterine receptivity through Th1/Th2 lymphocyte balance and decidualization. PLoS One. 2012;7:e45224. https://doi.org/10.1371/journal.pone.0045224.
35. Fejzo MS, Sazonova OV, Sathirapongsasuti JF, Hallgrímsdóttir IB, Vacic V, MacGibbon KW, et al. Placenta and appetite genes GDF15 and IGFBP7 are associated with hyperemesis gravidarum. Nat Commun. 2018;9:1178. https://doi.org/10.1038/s41467-018-03258-0.
36. Kok-Min S, Jyun-Lin L, Ming-Luen D, Huang SW, Hwang JL, Huang WJ, et al. Human chorionic gonadotropin regulates gastric emptying in ovariectomized rats. J Endocrinol. 2013;216:307–14. https://doi.org/10.1530/joe-12-0421.
37. Albayrak M, Karatas A, Demiraran Y, Erman H, Topuz S, Bıyık I, et al. Ghrelin, acylated ghrelin, leptin and PYY-3 levels in hyperemesis gravidarum. J Matern Fetal Neonatal Med. 2013;26:866–70. https://doi.org/10.3109/14767058.2013.766699.
38. Mullur R, Liu YY, Brent GA. Thyroid hormone regulation of metabolism. Physiol Rev. 2014;94:355–82. https://doi.org/10.1152/physrev.00030.2013.
39. Caron P, Broussaud S, Galano-Frutos JJ, Sancho J, Savagner F. New variant (Val597Ile) in transmembrane region of the TSH receptor with human chorionic gonadotropin hypersensitivity in familial gestational hyperthyroidism. Clin Endocrinol. 2020;93:339–45. https://doi.org/10.1111/cen.14215.
40. Iijima S. Pitfalls in the assessment of gestational transient thyrotoxicosis. Gynecol Endocrinol. 2020;36:662–7. https://doi.org/10.1080/09513590.2020.1754391.
41. Kobaly K, Mandel SJ. Hyperthyroidism and pregnancy. Endocrinol Metab Clin North Am. 2019;48:533–45. https://doi.org/10.1016/j.ecl.2019.05.002.
42. Clark SM, Costantine MM, Hankins GD. Review of NVP and HG and early pharmacotherapeutic intervention. Obstet Gynecol Int. 2012;2012:252676. https://doi.org/10.1155/2012/252676.
43. Mori M, Amino N, Tamaki H, Miyai K, Tanizawa O. Morning sickness and thyroid function in normal pregnancy. Obstet Gynecol. 1988;72:355–9.
44. Verberg MF, Gillott DJ, Al-Fardan N, Grudzinskas JG. Hyperemesis gravidarum, a literature review. Hum Reprod Update. 2005;11:527–39. https://doi.org/10.1093/humupd/dmi021.
45. Fejzo MS, Magtira A, Schoenberg FP. Antihistamines and other prognostic factors for adverse outcome in hyperemesis gravidarum. Eur J Obstet Gynecol Reprod Biol. 2013;170:71–6. https://doi.org/10.1016/j.ejogrb.2013.04.017.
46. Fejzo MS, Magtira A, Schoenberg FP. Neurodevelopmental delay in children exposed in utero to hyperemesis gravidarum. Eur J Obstet Gynecol Reprod Biol. 2015;189:79–84. https://doi.org/10.1016/j.ejogrb.2015.03.028.
47. Yoshihara A, Noh JY, Mukasa K, Suzuki M, Ohye H, Matsumoto M, et al. Serum human chorionic gonadotropin levels and thyroid hormone levels in gestational transient thyrotoxicosis: is the serum hCG level useful for differentiating between active Graves' disease and GTT? Endocrine J. 2015;62:557–60. https://doi.org/10.1507/endocrj.ej14-0596.
48. Tagami T, Hagiwara H, Kimura T, Usui T, Shimatsu A, Naruse M. The incidence of gestational hyperthyroidism and postpartum thyroiditis in treated patients with Graves' disease. Thyroid. 2007;17:767–72. https://doi.org/10.1089/thy.2007.0003.

49. Shafi SZ, Alper O, Selvinaz V, Sait MB, Esra C, Yüksel A. Is the measurement of inferior thyroid artery blood flow velocity by color-flow Doppler ultrasonography useful for differential diagnosis between gestational transient thyrotoxicosis and Graves' disease? A prospective study. Clinics (Sao Paulo). 2012;67:125–9. https://doi.org/10.6061/clinics/2012(02)06.
50. Moleti M, Di Mauro M, Sturniolo G, Russo M, Vermiglio F. Hyperthyroidism in the pregnant woman: maternal and fetal aspects. J Clin Transl Endocrinol. 2019;16:100190. https://doi.org/10.1016/j.jcte.2019.100190. Erratum in: J Clin Transl Endocrinol 2020;23:100246. https://doi.org/10.1016/j.jcte.2020.100246.
51. Lee SY, Pearce EN. Testing, monitoring, and treatment of thyroid dysfunction in pregnancy. J Clin Endocrinol Metab. 2021;106:883–92. https://doi.org/10.1210/clinem/dgaa945.
52. Ogawa K, Fujiwara T, Arata N, Sago H. The effects of gestational transient thyrotoxicosis on the perinatal outcomes: a case-control study. Arch Gynecol Obstet. 2017;295:87–93. https://doi.org/10.1007/s00404-016-4219-2.
53. Gross S, Librach C, Cecutti A. Maternal weight loss associated with hyperemesis gravidarum: a predictor of fetal outcome. Am J Obstet Gynecol. 1989;160(906–909) https://doi.org/10.1016/0002-9378(89)90307-4.

Thyroid Storm and Neonatal Hyperthyroidism

Atieh Amouzegar

Introduction

Thyroid storm is a rare but a life-threatening condition which presents with severe clinical signs and symptoms of hyperthyroidism. Hyperthyroidism occurs in 0.1–1% of pregnant women [1, 2] but hyperthyroid pregnant women are more likely to develop a thyroid storm than those who are not pregnant [3]. Thyroid storm can be life-threatening, with a high mortality rate of 10–30% if not recognized immediately and aggressively treated [4]. It can happen in patients with any primary cause of hyperthyroidism which remained undiagnosed or untreated, such as Graves' disease, toxic multinodular goiter, and solitary hyper-functional adenoma, and usually develops by a precipitating factor such as infection, trauma, acute myocardial infarction, surgery, labor, delivery, surgical delivery, or parturition [5]. Diagnosis and treatment of thyroid storm during pregnancy is more critical as it can lead to maternal and fetal mortality. As thyroid storm has a fulminant course and could involve multiple organs including central nervous, thermoregulatory, cardiovascular, and gastrointestinal system, all involved physicians must strive to accurately detail all signs and symptoms to decrease this morbid condition. However, even with early diagnosis, the overall mortality remains high, between 10 and 30% [6].

The diagnosis, pregnancy outcomes, differential diagnosis, treatment, and monitoring of this entity and neonatal hyperthyroidism are reviewed here separately.

A. Amouzegar (✉)
Endocrine Research Center, Research Institute for Endocrine Sciences, Shahid Beheshti University, Tehran, Iran
e-mail: amouzegar@endocrine.ac.ir

F. Azizi, F. Ramezani Tehrani (eds.), *Thyroid Diseases in Pregnancy*,
https://doi.org/10.1007/978-3-030-98777-0_11

Signs and Symptoms, Differential Diagnosis

Clinical findings of thyroid storm are exaggerated form of the usual symptoms of hyperthyroidism including tachycardia with heart beats which can be more than 140 beats/minute and congestive heart failure, hypotension, cardiac arrhythmia, and finally can lead to death from cardiovascular collapse. Agitation, anxiety, delirium, psychosis, stupor, and coma are also common which were considered as main symptoms that make the diagnosis. Gastrointestinal symptoms such as nausea, vomiting, diarrhea, abdominal pain, or even jaundice and liver failure can also occur. Due to decreased peripheral vascular resistance and increased cardiac output during pregnancy compared to non-pregnant periods, developing heart failure is a threat in thyroid storm during pregnancy [7] which occurs in 10% of pregnant women with thyrotoxicosis. Physical examination usually reveals signs of hyperthyroidism such as goiter, ophthalmopathy (if Graves' disease is the diagnosis), lid lag, hand tremor, warm, moist skin, tachycardia, tachypnea, and fever. The clinical signs and symptoms of thyroid storm during pregnancy are the same as non-pregnancy period.

Diagnosis

The diagnosis of thyroid storm is based upon clinical and laboratory findings. There are no universally validated diagnostic criteria for diagnosing thyroid storm but a diagnostic criteria was developed by Burch and Wartofsky based on body temperature, central nervous system effects (agitation, delirium state, psychosis, stupor, seizure, coma), gastrointestinal-hepatic dysfunction (nausea/vomiting, diarrhea, abdominal pain, jaundice), cardiovascular dysfunction (tachycardia, cardiac arrhythmia including atrial fibrillation), heart failure (mild, moderate, severe), and presence or absence of precipitant history. It gives us scores according to the presence of each above symptoms and a score of 45 or more shows that the patient has thyroid storm (Table 1) [8].

Thyroid function tests including TSH, Total T4, free T4, and T3 should be assessed in pregnant patients with clinical suspicion of thyroid storm. During this critical period, other conditions such as mild hyperglycemia, mild hypercalcemia, abnormal liver function tests, abnormal leukocyte count including leukocytosis, or leukopenia should be noticed. Finding the probable causes of thyroid storm is important that can culminate to better prognosis if be treated properly.

Treatment

As thyroid storm is more critical and life-threatening condition during pregnancy, treatment should be initiated promptly targeting all three steps of thyroid hormone formation, release, and action. A multidisciplinary team approach is critical for

Table 1 Diagnostic criteria for thyroid storm

Thermoregulatory dysfunction: temperature, F	**Score**	**Cardiovascular dysfunction: heart rate, bpm**	**Score**
99–99.9	5	90–109	5
100–100.9	10	110–119	10
101–101.9	15	120–129	15
102–102.9	20	130–139	20
103–103.9	25	≥140	25
≥104	30		
Central nervous system dysfunction	**Score**	**Cardiovascular dysfunction: heart failure**	**Score**
Absent	0	Absent	0
Mild (agitation)	10	Mild (pedal edema)	5
Moderate (delirium, psychosis, extreme lethargy)	20	Moderate (bibasilar rales)	10
Severe (seizure, coma)	30	Severe (pulmonary edema)	15
Gastrointestinal and hepatic dysfunction	**Score**	**Cardiovascular dysfunction: atrial fibrillation**	**Score**
Absent	0	Absent	0
Moderate (diarrhea, nausea, abdominal pain)	10	Present	10
Severe (unexplained jaundice)	20		
Precipitant history	Score		
Absent	0		
Present	10		

Adapted from: Burch HB, Wartofsky L. Life-threatening thyrotoxicosis. Thyroid storm. Endocrinol Metab Clin North Am 1993; 22:263. A score of 45 or greater is highly suggestive of thyroid storm: a score of 25 to 44 is suggestive of impending storm, and a score below 25 is unlikely to represent thyroid storm

management of thyroid storm during pregnancy in order to successfully offer the patient all possible therapeutic options. The patient needs to be admitted in an intensive care unit for close monitoring and the implementation of treatment strategies. Therapeutic options should target the thyroid gland in the thyroid hormone synthesis and release and also minimize the adverse effects of circulating thyroid hormone to prevent their action that cause end-organ damage.

The first-line therapy in treating thyroid storm consists of using thionamides (Methimazole, Propylthiouracil), which halt new thyroid hormone production. As these medications inhibit thyroid peroxidase, a key enzyme involved in the formation of T3 and T4 from thyroglobulin, they play a fundamental role in thyroid storm treatment. Both drugs are used to treat hyperthyroidism; however, as PTU has an added benefit of decreasing the peripheral change of T4 to T3, it would be a more favorable treatment option during this critical stage. Secondly, new thyroid hormone synthesis can be blocked by adding nonradioactive iodine which is able to inhibit the organic binding of iodide to thyroglobulin in the thyroid gland by a mechanism known as the Wolff-Chaikoff effect. This effect usually lasts temporary because the thyroid gland eventually finds a way to escape from prolonged iodide excess. Inorganic iodine is suitable to be given orally as a saturated solution of potassium iodine (SSKI). It usually is given 5 drops (equal to 0.25 mL or 250 mg) four times a day or as Lugol's solution with a dose of 8 drops given every 6 h. Be careful that SSKI must be given after thionamides administration in order to prevent worsening of hyperthyroidism as the iodine can be used as a substrate for new thyroid hormone. Using glucocorticoids to reduce T4 to T3 conversion can help in treatment of thyroid storm. Dexamethasone 2 mg every 6 h intravenously can be used in the management of thyroid storm. In addition, it may have effects on underlying autoimmune process, if the thyroid storm is due to Graves' disease, and can be helpful in treating potentially associated low adrenal reserve. General supportive measures, such as giving oxygen, antipyretic drugs, and appropriate cardiovascular monitoring, are also crucial. The perceived underlying cause of precipitating thyroid storm should be treated. Presence of precipitating factors and dehydration, congestive heart failure, dysrhythmia, infection and prevention of adrenal crisis need special attention and must be treated immediately.

Neonatal Hyperthyroidism

Infants born to mothers with Graves' disease may involve with hyperthyroidism. Natural course of the disease shows that it usually is self-limited, but it can be severe, even life-threatening, and may have deleterious effects on neural development.

The prevalence of transient Graves' disease in infants born to these mothers is reported to be up to 20.0% in observational cohort studies with fetal and neonatal hyperthyroidism incidence, between 1 and 5% in all women with active or a past history of Graves' hyperthyroidism [9, 10].

The Value of TRAb and Pathogenesis of Neonatal Hyperthyroidism

Neonatal hyperthyroidism can occur in babies whose mothers have active Graves' disease or who are born to women with a stimulatory TSHR-Ab associated with Hashimoto thyroiditis due to trans-placental passage of the maternal stimulatory TSH receptor antibody (TSHR-Ab) [11], but notice that neonatal hyperthyroidism also can occur in infants of women who do not have active disease during pregnancy but has a history of Graves' hyperthyroidism treated with either thyroidectomy or radioactive iodine in the past and the level of stimulatory TSHR-Ab remained high during pregnancy [12]. The higher the maternal stimulatory TSHR-Ab concentration is during the third trimester, the neonate is at greater risk for developing neonatal Graves' hyperthyroidism. The lowest level of maternal TSHR-Ab leading to neonatal Graves' disease is 4.4 U/L, which corresponded to 3.7 times the upper limit of normal [13]. Neonatal Graves' hyperthyroidism would be expected to occur in 1–5% of infants born to Graves's hyperthyroid mothers, and affects males and females equally [14]. The incidence of neonatal hyperthyroidism is higher in infants who were born to mothers with the higher maternal stimulatory TSHR-Ab concentration during the third trimester of pregnancy. In terms of prevention of neonatal hyperthyroidism, TSHR antibodies should be evaluated even before pregnancy and in pregnant women at risk or have past history of fetal-neonatal hyperthyroidism. Measuring serum TRAb in early pregnancy is a clue in detecting pregnancies at risk of neonatal hyperthyroidism. In hyperthyroid mothers or euthyroid pregnant women who previously received ablative therapy for GD, a TRAb value >5 IU/L or three times the upper limit of normal, during the second and third trimester of pregnancy need close follow-up of the fetus and neonates for fetal/neonatal hyperthyroidism. Mothers who are euthyroid with antithyroid drugs may have high titer of TRAb; but who are euthyroid and remained in euthyroid state, without using antithyroid medication, do not need to be checked for TRAb during pregnancy [15].

Clinical Manifestation of Neonatal Hyperthyroidism

The clinical manifestations of hyperthyroidism in neonates are tachycardia with a bounding pulse, low birth weight for gestational age (SGA) and intrauterine growth restriction (IUGR), premature birth, microcephaly, frontal bossing and triangular face, warm, moist skin, neurological symptoms such as poor sleep, irritability, hyperactivity, and restlessness. Hyperphagia, but poor weight gain, and diarrhea, hepatosplenomegaly, diffuse goiter and sometimes cardiomegaly, cardiac arrhythmias, or heart failure, and abnormal liver function tests (including increase in the levels of AST, ALT, and direct bilirubin) are among the symptoms. Other manifestation such as fetal hydrops and exophthalmos (presumably true Graves' ophthalmopathy) are not common but can occur [16].

Diagnosis

The first step is clinical diagnosis of neonatal hyperthyroidism after reviewing medical reports of the infants and their mothers. In those with a history of Graves' disease with positive TSHR-Ab and also in whom the maternal TSHR-Ab status is unknown measurement of neonates' thyroid function tests including serum TT4 (or FT4), TT3, and TSH is recommended. Having the record of high maternal serum TSHR-Ab during the third trimester helps to diagnosis of neonatal Graves' hyperthyroidism. Elevated FT4, TT4, and total T3, with low TSH, are infamous of neonatal Graves' disease and should be treated until the disease resolves. Infants with normal thyroid function tests are euthyroid but should be followed clinically, with repeat measurements of thyroid function tests if symptoms develop.

Umbilical Cord Blood Sampling, Cordocentesis in Diagnosis of Neonatal Hyperthyroidism

Measurement of TSHR-Ab in cord blood helps to predict the risk of neonatal Graves' disease in the infant. If the mother is known to have positive TSHR-Ab and is or was recently treated with an antithyroid drug, thyroid function tests (FT4, T4, TSH) in cord blood will show the effects on balance of the stimulating antibody and antithyroid drug in utero but do not help the physicians in the prediction of the risk of neonatal hyperthyroidism [17]. So, in this situation, measurement of free T4 and TSH at 2–3 days of life would help more than in cord blood.

Treatment

After diagnosis of neonatal hyperthyroidism, treatment should be initiated promptly. MMI 0.25–1.0 mg/kg per day is the best choice and should be administered every 8 h [17]. Although PTU is also effective, it is not the first choice as it has more frequent and severe side effects, such as a risk of hepatotoxicity. Suppressive action occurs in 1–2 weeks. A beta-adrenergic blocker, such as propranolol in a dose of 2 mg/kg per day every 8 h, can be added to control symptoms of neuromuscular and cardiovascular hyperactivity. Atenolol as a more cardio-specific beta-blocker (1 mg/kg daily) can also be used. Iodine, in the form of Lugol's solution (one drop equal to 8 mg, 126 mg iodine/mL) every 8 h orally or SSKI, one to two drops daily, can be given to inhibit thyroid hormone release. It should be given for short time, 1–2 weeks, and by controlling the disease, it needs to be stopped. Hyperthyroidism is usually controlled within a few weeks using just an antithyroid drug and a beta-blocker. With signs and symptoms of sympathetic hyperactivity, such as tachycardia, hypertension, and poor feeding, a beta-blocker such as propranolol 2 mg/kg per day divided in 2 doses for short period (1–2 weeks) can be added. To prevent thyroid hormone production and peripheral change of T4 to T3, glucocorticoids (prednisolone in 1–2 doses at a dose of 2 mg/kg/day) can also be used in extremely ill infants [17]. It works through inhibiting thyroid hormone secretion and decreasing peripheral conversion of T4 to T3 and controlling inflammation. In a case of heart failure in a severe case, it needs a multidisciplinary approach to control it.

Summary

Although thyroid storm is a rare condition even during pregnancy, it is among endocrine emergencies; even the suspicion of the disease should be treated immediately by a multidisciplinary team in an intensive care setting; otherwise it would accompany with high mortality and morbidity in mothers and their fetus and neonates.

Treatment should address all steps of thyroid hormone production, release, and action, in a well-organized manner besides treating the precipitating factor and providing a supportive care.

Neonatal Graves' disease develops in up to 5% of newborns to mothers with Graves' hyperthyroidism and by the trans-placental passage of maternal TSHR-Ab. Neonatal Graves hyperthyroidism includes premature birth and/or low birth weight for gestational age, hyperactivity, irritability, tachycardia, arrhythmias, microcephaly, and increased frequency of bowel movements, hyperphagia, hepatosplenomegaly, goiter, and stare. Measurement of neonatal thyroid function tests helps in diagnosis of neonatal Graves' disease. Thionamides are the main drugs which can control hyperthyroidism. We expected that the disease improves rapidly and can the neonate be weaned from medication by 3–12 weeks of age. Management of hyperthyroidism during early life needs a multidisciplinary team. Neonatal hyperthyroidism must be recognized promptly and treated adequately; otherwise it can be lead to significant morbidity and mortality.

References

1. Andersen SL, Olsen J, Carle A, Laurberg P. Hyperthyroidism incidence fluctuates widely in and around pregnancy and is at variance with some other autoimmune diseases: a Danish population-based study. J Clin Endocrinol Metab. 2015;100(3):1164–71.
2. Krassas GE, Poppe K, Glinoer D. Thyroid function and human reproductive health. Endocr Rev. 2010;31(5):702–55.
3. Millar LK, Wing DA, Leung AS, Koonings PP, Montoro MN, Mestman JH. Low birth weight and preeclampsia in pregnancies complicated by hyperthyroidism. Obstet Gynecol. 1994;84(6):946–9.
4. Wang HI, Yiang GT, Hsu CW, Wang JC, Lee CH, Chen YL. Thyroid storm in a patient with trauma—a challenging diagnosis for the emergency physician: case report and literature review. J Emerg Med. 2017;52(3):292–8.
5. Waltman PA, Brewer JM, Lobert S. Thyroid storm during pregnancy. A medical emergency. Crit Care Nurse. 2004;24(2):74–9.
6. Chiha M, Samarasinghe S, Kabaker AS. Thyroid storm: an updated review. J Intensive Care Med. 2015;30(3):131–40.
7. Sheffield JS, Cunningham FG. Thyrotoxicosis and heart failure that complicate pregnancy. Am J Obstet Gynecol. 2004;190(1):211–7.
8. Burch HB, Wartofsky L. Life-threatening thyrotoxicosis. Thyroid storm. Endocrinol Metab Clin North Am. 1993;22(2):263–77.
9. Besancon A, Beltrand J, Le Gac I, Luton D, Polak M. Management of neonates born to women with Graves' disease: a cohort study. Eur J Endocrinol. 2014;170(6):855–62.
10. Mitsuda N, Tamaki H, Amino N, Hosono T, Miyai K, Tanizawa O. Risk factors for developmental disorders in infants born to women with Graves disease. Obstet Gynecol. 1992;80(3 Pt 1):359–64.
11. Kiefer FW, Klebermass-Schrehof K, Steiner M, Worda C, Kasprian G, Diana T, et al. Fetal/neonatal thyrotoxicosis in a newborn from a hypothyroid woman with Hashimoto thyroiditis. J Clin Endocrinol Metab. 2017;102(1):6–9.
12. Volpe R, Ehrlich R, Steiner G, Row VV. Graves' disease in pregnancy years after hypothyroidism with recurrent passive-transfer neonatal Graves' disease in offspring. Therapeutic considerations. Am J Med. 1984;77(3):572–8.

13. van Dijk MM, Smits IH, Fliers E, Bisschop PH. Maternal thyrotropin receptor antibody concentration and the risk of fetal and neonatal thyrotoxicosis: a systematic review. Thyroid. 2018;28(2):257–64.
14. McKenzie JM, Zakarija M. Fetal and neonatal hyperthyroidism and hypothyroidism due to maternal TSH receptor antibodies. Thyroid. 1992;2(2):155–9.
15. Alexander EK, Pearce EN, Brent GA, Brown RS, Chen H, Dosiou C, et al. 2017 guidelines of the American Thyroid Association for the diagnosis and management of thyroid disease during pregnancy and the postpartum. Thyroid. 2017;27(3):315–89.
16. Polak M, Legac I, Vuillard E, Guibourdenche J, Castanet M, Luton D. Congenital hyperthyroidism: the fetus as a patient. Horm Res. 2006;65(5):235–42.
17. van der Kaay DC, Wasserman JD, Palmert MR. Management of neonates born to mothers with Graves' disease. Pediatrics. 2016;137(4):e20151878.

Autoimmune Thyroid Disease in Pregnancy

Fahimeh Ramezani Tehrani

Thyroid autoimmunity which is regarded as one of the most prevalent autoimmune disorders is defined as the presence of antibodies against either solely thyroperoxidase (TPOAb), thyroglobulin (TgAb), or thyroid stimulating hormone (TSH) receptor (TRAb), or a combination of them [1]. The first discovery of thyroid autoantibodies is related to detecting higher autoantibodies to thyroglobulin (Tg) in Hashimoto's thyroiditis (the most common cause of hypothyroidism during pregnancy). TSH receptor is a membrane-bound G-protein coupled receptor, being targeted as an antigen by autoantibodies in autoimmune thyroid disease. TSH receptor antibodies (TRAbs) are landmark causative factors for Graves' disease as the most frequent reason of hyperthyroidism during reproductive period. Also, TRAbs induce fetal and neonatal hyperthyroidism [2, 3].

Prevalence

The prevalence of TPOAb and TgAb positivity takes an upward trend with increasing age (in females but not males), representing approximately 9–18% [1]. A long-term follow-up study revealed that thyroid antibodies were developed in 21% of women that reached age 55 and above [4]. Of note, TPOAb and/or TgAb positivity is frequently seen among women during reproductive period with adequate supply of iodine. TPOAb positivity is common in pregnancy and has been linked to several adverse effects. Among pregnant women, the prevalence of TPOAb positivity constitutes approximately 5–12% [5, 6]. On the other hand, seldom do thyroid antibodies present in children, except for post-pubertal girls [7].

F. Ramezani Tehrani (✉)
Reproductive Endocrinology Research Center, Research Institute for Endocrine Sciences, Shahid Beheshti University of Medical Sciences, Tehran, Iran
e-mail: ramezani@endocrine.ac.ir, framezan@post.harvard.edu

F. Azizi, F. Ramezani Tehrani (eds.), *Thyroid Diseases in Pregnancy*,
https://doi.org/10.1007/978-3-030-98777-0_12

Etiology and Influencing Factors

Both Tg and TPO are actively involved in the synthesis and secretion of thyroid hormones. Their expression is highly dependent on growth factors such as IGF-1. Their expression is also stimulated by TSH [8]. Additionally, TSH shows regulatory effect on TPO gene on chromosome 2p25. Having identified the linkage of the chromosome 8q24 locus, containing the Tg gene to the autoimmune thyroiditis, gene polymorphisms was suggested as a landmark factor to induce immune response [9]. Totally, a number of genetic and non-genetic factors have been discussed to be involved in the pathogenesis of thyroid autoimmunity, through which several thyroid antigens, including thyroperoxidase, thyroglobulin and TSH receptor are expressed on the thyrocytes due to thyrocyte damage. Subsequently, antigen-presenting cells (APCs) migrate to lymphoid tissue and induce the activity of $CD4^+$ T cells, leading to B cell activation and increase in the production of antibody [10]. The dominance of autoantibody against TPO and Tg belongs to IgG class [11].

Maternal Adaptations During Pregnancy

During pregnancy, the maternal immune system utilizes several adaptations through local and systemic pathways to establish an immunosuppressive process and hinder the rejection of the fetus, leading to providing an immune tolerance. On the one hand, a number of immunomodulatory molecules and cytokines, secreting from the trophoblast cells of the placenta, lead to decreased $CD4^+$ and reverse the ratio of $CD4^+/CD8^+$ T cells as well as increase the activity of T regulatory cells. On the other hand, changes in the levels of estrogen, progesterone, and corticosteroids lead to the suppression of the B cells activity, reducing the production of antibody [12, 13].

How Thyroid Autoantibodies Negatively Effect on Reproduction and Pregnancy?

Thyroid autoantibodies adversely influenced reproductive status of women and pregnancy outcomes through TSH-dependent and TSH-independent pathways.

TSH-Dependent Pathological Mechanisms

TPOAb positivity leads to lower levels of T3 and T4 and a TSH elevated level in pregnant euthyroid women, reaching its peak to nearly two times higher than those of pregnant women with TPO negative antibody [14] (Fig. 1). The increased TSH

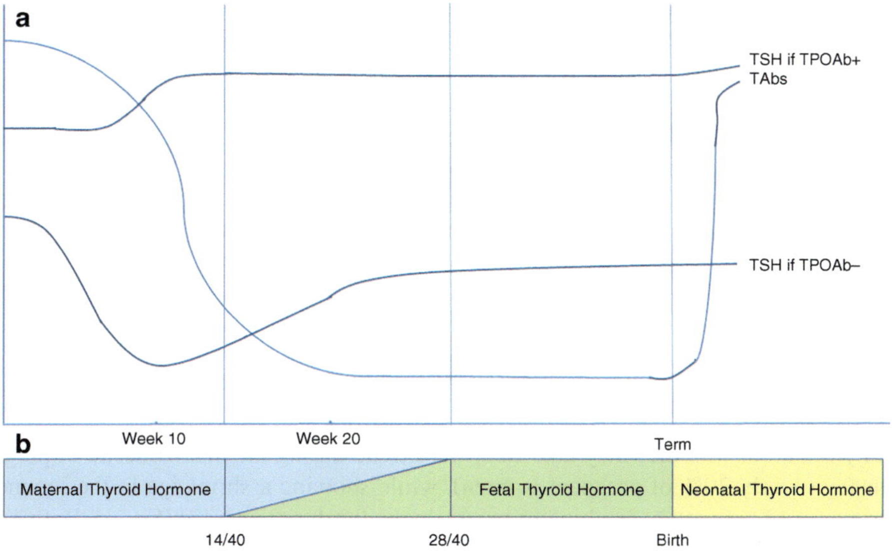

Fig. 1 (**a**) Alterations in TSH and TAbs levels during gestation, considering the status of TPOAb. Generally, immune tolerance leads to a shrinkage in the levels of TAbs in the second trimester of pregnancy, reaching its trough in the third trimester. Pregnant women with TPOAb+ show higher levels of TSH than those with TPOAb−. (**b**) The dependency status of the fetus brain on the supply of maternal TH. During the early stages of pregnancy, the fetal neuronal cells are entirely dependent on the maternal TH for proliferation and migration. After weeks 18–20 of pregnancy, the fetal thyroid gland becomes functionally matured and contributes to the brain development of the fetus. Postnatal brain development is solely dependent on neonatal thyroid hormone production. *TAbs* thyroid antibodies, *TPOAb+* thyroperoxidase antibody positivity, *TPOAb−* thyroperoxidase antibody negativity, *TH* thyroid hormone

contributes to alteration in GnRH pulsatility, leading to the LH response disruption and inadequate function of corpus luteum [15]. Also, thyroid hormones could potentiate FSH effects on granulosa cells, leading to an increase in estrogen production [16]. Furthermore, TSH elevation makes some alteration in the metabolism of estrogen and production of SHBG, leading to changes in the levels of estradiol and testosterone [15]. Additionally, thyroid antibodies through changes in thyroid hormones contribute to decreasing the coagulation factors. All these pathways have significant adverse effect on quality of oocyte and development of placenta; as a result thyroid autoimmunity has been reported to be as a predictor of IVF failure [17].

TSH-Independent Pathological Mechanisms

On the other hand, some negative effects of the thyroid antibodies on fertility are independent of the impacts of TSH. These pathways are as follows: First, T cell-derived cytokine secretion in the women's uteri with antithyroid antibodies and B cell activation (as described in the above sections). Second, thyroid autoimmunity has been strongly linked to endometriosis which is reported in nearly 15% of women during reproductive period and also up to 50% of women with infertility. This disorder negatively affects the process of reproduction as well as the results of IVF [18, 19]. Third, natural killer cells hyperactivity as a known stimulator of immune system occurs in thyroid autoimmunity state via both TSH-dependent and TSH-independent pathways. Noteworthy is that vitamin D deficiency has been reported as a triggering factor for the occurrence of thyroid autoimmunity as well as infertility [20].

Changes of Thyroid Autoantibodies During Pregnancy

Thyroid autoantibodies may take an upward trend during the first trimester of pregnancy (nearly 20% of pregnant women), while showing a shrinkage in the second trimester of pregnancy reaching its trough in the third trimester [3] (Fig. 1). Both Tg and TPO antibodies show similar increasing/deceasing expression trends in various conditions so that they take a downward trend during pregnancy and after antithyroid therapy, while take an upward trend postpartum and after interferon-alpha therapy [3]. While both of these antibodies may predict thyroid dysfunction, TPOAb is more efficient in this prediction [11]. This preference may be partly due to an increase in the prevalence of TPOAb in the community and Graves' disease. Moreover, in the case of serum-positivity for solely one autoantibody, the probability of TPOAb positivity is higher than TgAb positivity. Furthermore, TPOAb is more efficient in predicting postpartum thyroid disease. Finally yet importantly, TgAb alone has not been found to be linked to a disease [3].

Factors that Could Be Associated with the Development of Antibodies

There is uncertainty regarding the exact pathophysiologic aspects of development of antibodies at individual levels; however some possible introduced mechanisms are as follows:

1. An inverse association may exist between the status of exposure to infection and the level of autoimmunity; thyroid antibodies are more observed in towns which their citizens are at less exposure to infection [20].
2. Discontinuation of smoking may contribute to a rise in the level of thyroid autoantibodies [21].
3. Individuals receiving drugs containing iodine such as amiodarone show higher levels of thyroid antibodies [22].

4. Hepatitis C patients receiving interferon alpha and also HIV patients on treatment may show higher levels of thyroid antibodies [23].
5. In patients with thyroid disease, upregulation of thyroid antibodies may occur during postpartum period [24].

Factors Reducing the Levels of Thyroid Autoantibodies [3]

1. The levels of thyroid hormones may be reduced by the time in various situations, including pregnancy, patients receiving antithyroid drugs, patients with Grave's disease receiving prolonged radioiodine therapy, patients with Hashimoto's disease receiving selenium, and by increasing in age.

Reference Interval and Cutoff Value for Thyroid Autoantibodies

According to American Thyroid Association (ATA), reference intervals for thyroid autoantibodies should be determined for each trimester of pregnancy as well as each geographical region [25]. TPOAb cutoffs are not similar in pregnancy and general population. During pregnancy, serum TPOAb levels take an upward trend in the first trimester, whereas showing downward trends in the second and third trimesters [26] (Fig. 1). Of note, the cutoff limits (the 95th percentile) related to TPOAb obtained from various studies and manufacturers belonging to different countries are not comparable, ranging from 0.5 to 143 kU/L. Despite some evidence on clinical significance of increased TPOAb levels, when its levels exceed more than twice the reported upper cutoff value [27], it is suggested that each geographical region identify the trimester-specific reference intervals for TPOAb.

TgAb concentration should be measured in the presence of TSH elevation and TPOAb negativity. In the case of TSH elevation as well as TPOAb and TgAb negativity, thyroid ultrasonography is recommended to detect thyroid texture abnormality and establish the diagnosis of autoimmune thyroiditis [26].

Do Pregnant Women Need to Be Universally Screened for Thyroid Autoimmunity?

Positivity of TPOAb in pregnant women can result in progression to overt hypothyroidism. Although recognition of these autoantibodies as a risk factor for adverse pregnancy outcomes can prevent these complications, it is uncertain whether or not pregnant women should be universally screened [28]. Despite some evidence regarding the cost-effectiveness of the screening of all pregnant women for autoimmune thyroid disease in the first trimester [29], universal screening of thyroid autoantibodies is not recommended due to the lack of sufficient evidence [25], although screening of these autoantibodies is commonly performed in pregnant women identified with overt or subclinical hypothyroidism [30].

What Are the Adverse Fertility and Pregnancy Outcomes of Thyroid Antibodies?

In pregnant women with thyroid autoantibody positivity and normal thyroid hormones, the association between thyroid autoantibodies and abnormal pregnancy outcomes is still unclear and has attracted much attention from researchers worldwide. Although thyroid autoimmunity is regarded as subtle disorder in thyroid function that may result in a small reduction in the thyroxin level during pregnancy, this reduction may be associated with an increase to adverse pregnancy outcomes, including infertility, miscarriage, recurrent spontaneous abortions, preterm delivery, neonatal respiratory distress syndrome, small for gestational age (SGA), low birth weight (LBW), gestational diabetes mellitus (GDM), preeclampsia, cesarean section, placental abruption, depression, and perinatal death [10, 31–39].

The autoantibodies detected in autoimmune diseases can impair fertility through both TSH-dependent and TSH-independent pathways [40]. The association between thyroid antibodies and infertility has not elucidated; however, it has been shown that treatment with low doses of levothyroxine (LT4), which is usually used to treat hypothyroidism, can be considered in such situations [10]. However, ATA recommend the evaluation of serum TSH concentration for all women seeking care for infertility. LT4 therapy is recommended only for infertile women with overt hypothyroidism who seek pregnancy [36]; they revealed that there is not sufficient evidence for prescribing LT4 for euthyroid /SCH TPOAb-positive women seeking fertility treatment.

Thyroid autoimmunity may be associated with reproductive failure including pregnancy loss, either as miscarriage, intrauterine fetal death, or stillbirth [40]. It may be resulted from subtle reduction in thyroid hormones due to the lack of sufficient supply of hormones or may be due to its association with other autoimmune disorders such as anti-phospholipid antibodies [36, 41, 42]; as it presented in a meta-analysis that shows thyroid autoimmunity as a TSH-independent risk for miscarriage [39]. This positive association between thyroid autoantibodies in euthyroid women and miscarriage was reported by Thangaratinam et al. in a meta-analysis including 18 high-qualified studies [43].

Thyroid autoimmunity can also be associated with an increased risk of GDM in women with the higher rate of anti-TPO titers [44, 45]. The potential mechanism for this association could be insulin resistance since serum levels of inflammatory cytokines are increased in patients with thyroid autoimmunity [46]. It has been revealed that similar to patients with impaired glucose tolerance, women with thyroid autoimmunity demonstrate an increased C-reactive protein level which is not modified with their thyroid function status [47, 48]. In line with previous literature, a recent birth cohort concluded that isolated thyroid autoimmunity, represented by positive TPOAb, in early pregnancy were associated with GDM independent of TSH and FT4 [49], finding that needs to confirm by further well-designed prospective studies with a sufficient sample size.

TPOAb positivity may be related to preterm delivery. A recent meta-analysis of 35 cohort studies showed that among pregnant women without overt thyroid disease, subclinical hypothyroidism, isolated hypothyroxinemia, and TPO antibody positivity were significantly associated with higher risk of preterm delivery. They concluded that the association of TPO antibody positivity with preterm delivery did not appear to be related to differences in thyroid function, but was modified by the thyrotropin concentration as exemplified by the higher risk of preterm delivery in TPO antibody-positive women and a thyrotropin concentration above 4.0 mIU/L [32]. It is suggested that TPO antibody positivity may be involved in infectious and inflammatory pathways leading to preterm delivery; however, further studies are recommended to clarify the accurate role of these autoantibodies in the pathogenesis of preterm delivery [50, 51].

Adequate transplacental passage of maternal thyroid hormone is important for normal fetal development and growth [52]. Previous studies revealed that overt maternal hypothyroidism is a well-known risk factor for low birth weight (LBW) [53]. Thyroid autoimmunity may affect fetal birth through thyroid-dependent and thyroid-independent pathways. It has been shown that subclinical hypothyroidism is more common in pregnant women who are positive for thyroperoxidase or thyroglobulin antibodies may be due to a lower thyroid functional capacity [54]. Thyroid hormone regulates different pathways in the mother and fetus throughout gestation. It controls fetal growth by facilitating placentation and the regulation of fetal metabolism; as a result it may directly affect skeletal growth and tissue differentiation. Study revealed a positive association between lipid and protein catabolism and TSH; it resulted in reduction in fetal caloric availability [55]. It has been shown that each 1 SD increase in maternal TSH concentration was associated with a 6 g lower birthweight (−10 to −2; $p = 0.0030$); this adverse effect is more pronounced in those women who are positive for TPOAb (p for interaction = 0.10) [56]. Thyroid autoimmunity may affect fetal birth independent of thyroid hormones and TSH level by increasing placenta vascular resistance that is more prevalent in TPOAb+ women [57].

Despite several studies on thyroid autoimmunity and pregnancy outcomes, there is a controversy regarding the effects of this thyroid dysfunction of pregnancy outcomes in euthyroid women and beneficiary effect of LT4 therapy. There are a limited number of clinical trials on this topic; however they are limited by low sample size, heterogenicities in study population (reporting the results of both SCH and euthyroid TPOAb+ women), lack of assessing iodine status, and lack of assessing all adverse pregnancy outcomes. Further well-designed clinical trials with large enough sample size are highly needed to assess the adverse feto-maternal outcome of thyroid autoimmunity in euthyroid pregnant women and impact of LT4 therapy in this situation.

How Should TPOAb+ Women Be Monitored During Pregnancy?

It is suggested that thyroid autoimmunity during pregnancy can lead to hypothyroidism. Earlier studies have demonstrated that antithyroid Ab titers were highest in the first trimester, although they decreased over the course of gestation [58, 59]. According to ATA guidelines, in women at risk for hypothyroidism, such as euthyroid women with TPOAb+ or TgAb+, an increased surveillance is recommended; this guideline suggests to measure serum TSH level approximately every 4 weeks until mid-gestation and at least once near 30 weeks gestation in these women. Moreover, monitoring and LT4 therapy for TPOAb-positive women with a TSH greater than the pregnancy-specific reference range are recommended [36].

Does Levothyroxine Reduce the Risk of Adverse Pregnancy Outcomes in Euthyroid Women Who Are Thyroid Autoantibody Positive?

Despite several studies assessing thyroid autoimmunity and pregnancy outcomes, most of them have an observational design with a level of weak to moderate-quality evidence [13, 30, 31, 35, 37, 40, 44, 49, 56, 60, 61]. There is a limited number of randomized controlled trials regarding the effect of LT4 therapy on pregnancy outcomes, particularly in euthyroid/SCH women with thyroid autoimmunity. Most of these trials have a low sample size, lack of assessing euthyroid and SCH in the separate groups, lack of evaluating iodine status, and lack of assessing all pregnancy outcomes [34, 59, 62–65]. For women with TPO antibodies who remain euthyroid, treatment with LT4 is controversial. Although some studies have been suggested a lower incidence of some pregnancy adverse outcomes, such as infertility, miscarriage, and preterm delivery, among euthyroid women with thyroid antibodies treated with LT4 than untreated women, results of studies are still inconclusive [59, 62, 64, 65]. Indeed, benefits of LT4 therapy are not clarified for other outcomes, such as GDM, impaired newborn neurodevelopment, SGA, placental abruption, and depression [10]. Although ATA dose not definitively suggest LT4 therapy in all euthyroid pregnant women with positive-thyroid antibodies, 25–50 μg of LT4 as a typical starting dose may be considered for those women with a prior history of pregnancy loss or recurrent miscarriage. However, LT4 therapy for treating euthyroid pregnant women who are thyroid autoantibody positive to prevent preterm delivery is not recommended [36].

Does Levothyroxine Reduce the Risk of Adverse Pregnancy Outcomes in Subclinical Hypothyroid Women Who Are Thyroid Autoantibody Positive?

Despite lack of sufficient data regarding the recommendations for or against routine LT4 therapy during pregnancy in euthyroid thyroid antibody positive women, there are growing bulk of evidence in beneficiary impact of LT4 treatment of SCH thyroid antibody positive women in terms of pregnancy outcomes especially preterm delivery. A prospective study conducted on thyroid peroxidase antibody positive (TPOAb+) women with SCH showed treatment with LT4 decreases the risk of preterm delivery in these women [63]. A recent meta-analysis of 13 studies including 7970 showed the beneficial effects of LT4 therapy on the reduced risks of pregnancy loss and preterm delivery, among pregnant women with SCH [34]. Therefore, ATA recommends an evaluation for TPOAb status in pregnant women with TSH concentrations greater than the pregnancy-specific reference range and LT4 therapy for TPOAb-positive women with SCH [36].

Is Thyroid Autoimmunity Associated with Adverse Neurodevelopmental Outcomes? And Does Levothyroxine Reduce These Adverse Outcomes?

Insufficient data is available regarding the association between maternal TPOAb status and adverse child outcomes, such as neurodevelopmental outcomes. Some studies have been assessed the relationship between maternal thyroid autoimmunity and child development. A case-control study demonstrated lower motor and intellectual development at ages between 25 and 30 months in offspring of euthyroid women with positive TPOAb, compared to children of their TPOAb-negative controls [66]. Another study investigating child neurocognition at age 5.5 years on 97 mothers and their children showed lower perceptual performance and motor scores in children of TgAb-positive mothers, and lower perceptual performance scores noted in children with TgAb-positive cord blood, although no neurodevelopmental outcomes were associated with maternal or infant TPOAb status [67]. There is evidence suggesting an increased risk of sensorineural hearing loss at age 8 in children, lower child intelligence quotient (IQ) at age 4, and externalizing problems in children, especially attention deficit/hyperactivity problems, and autism spectrum in offspring born from TPOAb-positive mothers [56, 61, 68–70]. A few studies have been assessed the efficacy of LT4 therapy for preventing child adverse outcomes. For instance, one study revealed that the mean intelligence quotient (IQ) of children born to SCH TPOAb-positive mothers without LT4 replacement was 7 points lower than the control group [71]. Although a recent meta-analysis of three randomized trials in women with subclinical hypothyroidism diagnosed found no evidence of benefit of LT4 therapy on childhood IQ or neurodevelopmental outcomes, it should be kept in mind that in this meta-analysis one study included women with thyroid peroxidase (TPO) antibodies, one excluded women with TPO antibodies, and the last study did not specify TPO antibody status [72]. Since studies on the association of maternal TPOAb positivity with child neurodevelopment are scarce, further researches are required to confirm these preliminary findings and determine the effects of LT4 therapy on child adverse outcomes.

What Is the Role of Selenium in Treatment of Women with Thyroid Autoimmunity?

There is evidence suggesting selenium therapy for patients with thyroid autoimmunity. This supplementation exerts direct effects on thyroid hormone metabolism and redox processes [73]. In addition to iodine, the thyroid gland depends on selenium for its sufficient functioning [74], and low selenium intake is associated with increased risk of thyroid disease [75].

While some studies conducted on non-pregnant women have demonstrated that selenium can reduce TPOAb concentrations [76–79], the results of randomized controlled trials were heterogenous and conflicting. Dose used of selenium in these studies was 60–200 μg/day [80, 81]. On the other hand, there is evidence suggesting an increased risk of developing type 2 diabetes in patients treated with selenium [82]. Because of insufficient data investigating the risk-benefit of routine selenium supplementation of TPOAb-positive women during pregnancy, ATA does not recommended selenium supplementation for the treatment of TPOAb-positive women during their pregnancy [36].

What Is the Role of Intravenous Immunoglobulin Therapy or Corticosteroid Therapy in Treatment of Women with Thyroid Autoimmunity?

Intravenous immunoglobulins and corticosteroid therapy had been considered as the alternative treatments in women with thyroid autoimmunity [36]. A limited number of clinical trials have been published on the use of intravenous immunoglobulin [83–85] or corticosteroid therapy [86–88] for preventing pregnancy outcomes and treating women with thyroid autoimmunity. One study reported a significant improvement in the rate of live births in pregnant women treated with IVIG, compared to non-treated controls [84]. Another study showed a higher rate of term delivery in women with thyroid autoimmunity treated with LT4 therapy in comparison with IVIG treatment [85]. Moreover, some clinical trials showed the advantages of corticosteroids, such as prednisolone for improving pregnancy outcomes, i.e., pregnancy rate, live birth rate in women euthyroid with thyroid autoimmunity [86–88].

However, due to the existence of insufficient studies in this regard and their limitations, further well-designed randomized controlled trials are required to elucidate the efficacy and side effects of these interventions on pregnancy outcomes. Finally, ATA does not recommend intravenous immunoglobulin and glucocorticoid therapy in euthyroid women with thyroid autoimmunity [36].

Should Euthyroid/Subclinical Hypothyroid TPOAb- Positive Women Be Monitored After Pregnancy?

It is well documented that both pregnancy and the postpartum period have a profound effect on autoimmune thyroid disease [89]. There is an increased risk of development of postpartum thyroid dysfunction among pregnant women with positive anti-TPO in pregnancy [44]. For instance, the highest rates of postpartum thyroiditis occur among women with a prior history of postpartum thyroiditis and in women with positive antithyroid peroxidase (TPO) antibodies who had normal thyroid function during pregnancy [90]. Unfortunately, there are no still obvious recommendation for monitoring euthyroid/ subclinical hypothyroid TPOAb-positive women after pregnancy.

Does Maternal Thyroid Autoimmunity Induce Thyroid Autoimmunity in Offsprings?

Earlier studies have demonstrated that TPO is expressed at gene and protein levels in endometrium and placenta, and the syncytiotrophoblasts and invasive trophoblast cells express TPO protein; however, the study showed no expression of TPO protein in human embryo [57]. It suggested that TPOAb/TgAb in newborn have a maternal origin [67]. Although there is evidence demonstrating that TPOAb can cross the placenta and result in a congenital hypothyroidism through its deteriorative effects on fetus thyroid gland [91, 92], it has been shown that thyroid antibodies do not significantly affect fetal or neonatal thyroid function [93]. However, due to the importance of timely detection of infant hypothyroidism, regardless of maternal thyroid autoimmunity, all newborns should be screened for hypothyroidism by blood spot analysis typically 2–5 days after birth [36].

Summary

Controversies continue regarding beneficial effect of universal screening for detection of thyroid autoimmunity and its treatment in euthyroid women during pregnancy, although monitoring and LT4 therapy for TPOAb-positive women with a

TSH greater than the pregnancy-specific reference range are recommended. Since studies on the association of maternal TPOAb positivity with child neurodevelopment are scarce, further researches are required to determine the effects of LT4 therapy on child adverse outcomes, especially in euthyroid situation.

References

1. Hollowell JG, Staehling NW, Flanders WD, Hannon WH, Gunter EW, Spencer CA, et al. Serum TSH, T4, and thyroid antibodies in the United States population (1988 to 1994): National Health and Nutrition Examination Survey (NHANES III). J Clin Endocrinol Metab. 2002;87(2):489–99.
2. Kahaly GJ, Diana T. TSH receptor antibody functionality and nomenclature. Front Endocrinol. 2017;8:28.
3. Balucan FS, Morshed SA, Davies TF. Thyroid autoantibodies in pregnancy: their role, regulation and clinical relevance. J Thyroid Res. 2013;2013:182472.
4. Chazenbalk GD, Portolano S, Russo D, Hutchison JS, Rapoport B, McLachlan S. Human organ-specific autoimmune disease. Molecular cloning and expression of an autoantibody gene repertoire for a major autoantigen reveals an antigenic immunodominant region and restricted immunoglobulin gene usage in the target organ. J Clin Invest. 1993;92(1):62–74.
5. Shields BM, Knight BA, Hill AV, Hattersley AT, Vaidya B. Five-year follow-up for women with subclinical hypothyroidism in pregnancy. J Clin Endocrinol Metab. 2013;98(12):E1941–5.
6. Nambiar V, Jagtap VS, Sarathi V, Lila AR, Kamalanathan S, Bandgar TR, et al. Prevalence and impact of thyroid disorders on maternal outcome in Asian-Indian pregnant women. J Thyroid Res. 2011;2011:429097.
7. Kaloumenou I, Mastorakos G, Alevizaki M, Duntas LH, Mantzou E, Ladopoulos C, et al. Thyroid autoimmunity in schoolchildren in an area with long-standing iodine sufficiency: correlation with gender, pubertal stage, and maternal thyroid autoimmunity. Thyroid. 2008;18(7):747–54.
8. Clément S, Refetoff S, Robaye B, Dumont JE, Schurmans SP. Low TSH requirement and goiter in transgenic mice overexpressing IGF-I and IGF-I receptor in the thyroid gland. Endocrinology. 2001;142(12):5131–9.
9. Jacobson EM, Tomer Y. The genetic basis of thyroid autoimmunity. Thyroid. 2007;17(10): 949–61.
10. De Leo S, Pearce EN. Autoimmune thyroid disease during pregnancy. Lancet Diabetes Endocrinol. 2018;6(7):575–86.
11. McLachlan SM, Rapoport B. Why measure thyroglobulin autoantibodies rather than thyroid peroxidase autoantibodies? Thyroid. 2004;14(7):510–20.
12. Somerset DA, Zheng Y, Kilby MD, Sansom DM, Drayson MT. Normal human pregnancy is associated with an elevation in the immune suppressive CD25+ CD4+ regulatory T-cell subset. Immunology. 2004;112(1):38–43.
13. Aluvihare VR, Kallikourdis M, Betz AG. Regulatory T cells mediate maternal tolerance to the fetus. Nat Immunol. 2004;5(3):266–71.
14. Pearce EN, Oken E, Gillman MW, Lee SL, Magnani B, Platek D, et al. Association of first-trimester thyroid function test values with thyroperoxidase antibody status, smoking, and multivitamin use. Endocr Pract. 2008;14(1):33–9.
15. Krassas G, Poppe K, Glinoer D. Thyroid function and human reproductive health. Endocr Rev. 2010;31(5):702–55.
16. Maruo T, Hiramatsu S, Otani T, Hayashi M, Mochizuki M. Increase in the expression of thyroid hormone receptors in porcine granulosa cells early in follicular maturation. Eur J Endocrinol. 1992;127(2):152–60.

17. Cramer DW, Sluss PM, Powers RD, McShane P, Ginsburgs ES, Hornstein MD, et al. Serum prolactin and TSH in an in vitro fertilization population: is there a link between fertilization and thyroid function? J Assist Reprod Genet. 2003;20(6):210–5.
18. Hemmings R, Rivard M, Olive DL, Poliquin-Fleury J, Gagné D, Hugo P, et al. Evaluation of risk factors associated with endometriosis. Fertil Steril. 2004;81(6):1513–21.
19. Barnhart K, Dunsmoor-Su R, Coutifaris C. Effect of endometriosis on in vitro fertilization. Fertil Steril. 2002;77(6):1148–55.
20. Twig G, Shina A, Amital H, Shoenfeld Y. Pathogenesis of infertility and recurrent pregnancy loss in thyroid autoimmunity. J Autoimmun. 2012;38(2–3):J275–81.
21. Effraimidis G, Tijssen JG, Wiersinga WM. Discontinuation of smoking increases the risk for developing thyroid peroxidase antibodies and/or thyroglobulin antibodies: a prospective study. J Clin Endocrinol Metab. 2009;94(4):1324–8.
22. Martino E, Bartalena L, Bogazzi F, Braverman LE. The effects of amiodarone on the thyroid. Endocr Rev. 2001;22(2):240–54.
23. Koh LK, Greenspan FS, Yeo PP. Interferon-α induced thyroid dysfunction: three clinical presentations and a review of the literature. Thyroid. 1997;7(6):891–6.
24. Feldt-Rasmussen U, Madsen MH, Rasmussen N, Hegedüs L, Hornnes P. Anti-thyroid peroxidase antibodies during pregnancy and postpartum. Relation to postpartum thyroiditis. Autoimmunity. 1990;6(3):211–4.
25. Stagnaro-Green A, Abalovich M, Alexander E, Azizi F, Mestman J, Negro R, et al. Guidelines of the American Thyroid Association for the diagnosis and management of thyroid disease during pregnancy and postpartum. Thyroid. 2011;21(10):1081–125.
26. Walker JA, Illions EH, Huddleston JF, Smallridge RC. Racial comparisons of thyroid function and autoimmunity during pregnancy and the postpartum period. Obstet Gynecol. 2005;106(6):1365–71.
27. Springer D, Jiskra J, Limanova Z, Zima T, Potlukova E. Thyroid in pregnancy: from physiology to screening. Crit Rev Clin Lab Sci. 2017;54(2):102–16.
28. Aghajanian P, Spencer CA, Wilson ML, Lee RH, Goodwin TM, Mestman JH. Evaluation of risk-factor-based screening for thyroid peroxidase antibody positivity in pregnancy. Clin Endocrinol. 2016;84(3):417–22.
29. Dosiou C, Sanders GD, Araki SS, Crapo LM. Screening pregnant women for autoimmune thyroid disease: a cost-effectiveness analysis. Eur J Endocrinol. 2008;158(6):841–52.
30. Ekinci EI, Chiu WL, Lu ZX, Sikaris K, Churilov L, Bittar I, et al. A longitudinal study of thyroid autoantibodies in pregnancy: the importance of test timing. Clin Endocrinol. 2015;82(4):604–10.
31. Chen L-M, Zhang Q, Si G-X, Chen Q-S, Ye E-l, Yu L-C, et al. Associations between thyroid autoantibody status and abnormal pregnancy outcomes in euthyroid women. Endocrine. 2015;48(3):924–8.
32. Korevaar TI, Derakhshan A, Taylor PN, Meima M, Chen L, Bliddal S, et al. Association of thyroid function test abnormalities and thyroid autoimmunity with preterm birth: a systematic review and meta-analysis. JAMA. 2019;322(7):632–41.
33. Karakosta P, Alegakis D, Georgiou V, Roumeliotaki T, Fthenou E, Vassilaki M, et al. Thyroid dysfunction and autoantibodies in early pregnancy are associated with increased risk of gestational diabetes and adverse birth outcomes. J Clin Endocrinol Metab. 2012;97(12):4464–72.
34. Rao M, Zeng Z, Zhou F, Wang H, Liu J, Wang R, et al. Effect of levothyroxine supplementation on pregnancy loss and preterm birth in women with subclinical hypothyroidism and thyroid autoimmunity: a systematic review and meta-analysis. Hum Reprod Update. 2019;25(3):344–61.
35. Kumru P, Erdogdu E, Arisoy R, Demirci O, Ozkoral A, Ardic C, et al. Effect of thyroid dysfunction and autoimmunity on pregnancy outcomes in low risk population. Arch Gynecol Obstet. 2015;291(5):1047–54.
36. Alexander EK, Pearce EN, Brent GA, Brown RS, Chen H, Dosiou C, et al. 2017 guidelines of the American Thyroid Association for the diagnosis and management of thyroid disease during pregnancy and the postpartum. Thyroid. 2017;27(3):315–89.

37. Han Y, Mao L-J, Ge X, Huang K, Yan S-Q, Ren L-L, et al. Impact of maternal thyroid autoantibodies positivity on the risk of early term birth: Ma'anshan birth cohort study. Endocrine. 2018;60(2):329–38.
38. Huget-Penner S, Feig DS. Maternal thyroid disease and its effects on the fetus and perinatal outcomes. Prenat Diagn. 2020;40(9):1077–84.
39. van den Boogaard E, Vissenberg R, Land JA, van Wely M, van der Post JA, Goddijn M, et al. Significance of (sub) clinical thyroid dysfunction and thyroid autoimmunity before conception and in early pregnancy: a systematic review. Hum Reprod Update. 2011;17(5):605–19.
40. Carp H, Meroni P, Shoenfeld Y. Autoantibodies as predictors of pregnancy complications. Rheumatology. 2008;47(suppl_3):iii6–8.
41. Promberger R, Walch K, Seemann R, Pils S, Ott J. A retrospective study on the association between thyroid autoantibodies with β2-glycoprotein and cardiolipin antibodies in recurrent miscarriage. Iran J Allergy Asthma Immunol. 2017;16(1):72–6.
42. Garrido-Gimenez C, Alijotas-Reig J. Recurrent miscarriage: causes, evaluation and management. Postgrad Med J. 2015;91(1073):151–62.
43. Thangaratinam S, Tan A, Knox E, Kilby MD, Franklyn J, Coomarasamy A. Association between thyroid autoantibodies and miscarriage and preterm birth: meta-analysis of evidence. BMJ. 2011;342:d2616.
44. Konar H, Sarkar M, Roy M. Association of thyroid dysfunction and autoimmunity in pregnant women with diabetes mellitus. J Obstet Gynecol India. 2018;68(4):283–8.
45. Velkoska Nakova V, Krstevska B, Dimitrovski C, Simeonova S, Hadzi-Lega M, Serafimoski V. Prevalence of thyroid dysfunction and autoimmunity in pregnant women with gestational and diabetes type 1. Contributions, Sec Biol Med Sci, MASA, XXXI, 2, p 51–59 (2010). 2010;31(2):51–9.
46. Drugarin D, Negru S, Koreck A, Zosin I, Cristea C. The pattern of a TH1 cytokine in autoimmune thyroiditis. Immunol Lett. 2000;71(2):73–7.
47. Christ-Crain M, Meier C, Guglielmetti M, Huber PR, Riesen W, Staub J-J, et al. Elevated C-reactive protein and homocysteine values: cardiovascular risk factors in hypothyroidism? A cross-sectional and a double-blind, placebo-controlled trial. Atherosclerosis. 2003; 166(2):379–86.
48. Chase HP, Cooper S, Osberg I, Stene LC, Barriga K, Norris J, et al. Elevated C-reactive protein levels in the development of type 1 diabetes. Diabetes. 2004;53(10):2569–73.
49. Huang K, Xu Y, Yan S, Li T, Xu Y, Zhu P, et al. Isolated effect of maternal thyroid-stimulating hormone, free thyroxine and antithyroid peroxidase antibodies in early pregnancy on gestational diabetes mellitus: a birth cohort study in China. Endocr J. 2019;66(3):223–31.
50. Goldenberg RL, Hauth JC, Andrews WW. Intrauterine infection and preterm delivery. N Engl J Med. 2000;342(20):1500–7.
51. De Vito P, Incerpi S, Pedersen JZ, Luly P, Davis FB, Davis PJ. Thyroid hormones as modulators of immune activities at the cellular level. Thyroid. 2011;21(8):879–90.
52. Kim B. Thyroid hormone as a determinant of energy expenditure and the basal metabolic rate. Thyroid. 2008;18(2):141–4.
53. Zhang C, Yang X, Zhang Y, Guo F, Yang S, Peeters RP, et al. Association between maternal thyroid hormones and birth weight at early and late pregnancy. J Clin Endocrinol Metab. 2019;104(12):5853–63.
54. Maraka S, Ospina NMS, O'Keeffe DT, Espinosa De Ycaza AE, Gionfriddo MR, Erwin PJ, et al. Subclinical hypothyroidism in pregnancy: a systematic review and meta-analysis. Thyroid. 2016;26(4):580–90.
55. Belkacemi L, Nelson DM, Desai M, Ross MG. Maternal undernutrition influences placental-fetal development. Biol Reprod. 2010;83(3):325–31.
56. Derakhshan A, Korevaar TI, Taylor PN, Levie D, Guxens M, Jaddoe VW, et al. The association of maternal thyroid autoimmunity during pregnancy with child IQ. J Clin Endocrinol Metab. 2018;103(10):3729–36.

57. Rahnama R, Mahmoudi A-R, Kazemnejad S, Salehi M, Ghahiri A, Soltanghoraee H, et al. Thyroid peroxidase in human endometrium and placenta: a potential target for anti-TPO antibodies. Clin Exp Med. 2021;21(1):79–88.
58. Glinoer D, Riahi M, Grün J-P, Kinthaert J. Risk of subclinical hypothyroidism in pregnant women with asymptomatic autoimmune thyroid disorders. J Clin Endocrinol Metab. 1994;79(1):197–204.
59. Negro R, Formoso G, Mangieri T, Pezzarossa A, Dazzi D, Hassan H. Levothyroxine treatment in euthyroid pregnant women with autoimmune thyroid disease: effects on obstetrical complications. J Clin Endocrinol Metab. 2006;91(7):2587–91.
60. Kashanian M, BozorgzadehVostaKolaei S, Naderi Z, EftekharArdebili M, Sheikhansari N, Javanmanesh F. Evaluation of the relationship between serum anti TPO antibody levels and mood disorders in euthyroid pregnant women. J Matern Fetal Neonatal Med. 2020;33(19):3233–7.
61. Brown AS, Surcel H-M, Hinkka-Yli-Salomäki S, Cheslack-Postava K, Bao Y, Sourander A. Maternal thyroid autoantibody and elevated risk of autism in a national birth cohort. Prog Neuro-Psychopharmacol Biol Psychiatry. 2015;57:86–92.
62. Vissenberg R, Van Dijk M, Fliers E, van der Post J, van Wely M, Bloemenkamp K, et al. Effect of levothyroxine on live birth rate in euthyroid women with recurrent miscarriage and TPO antibodies (T4-LIFE study). Contemp Clin Trials. 2015;44:134–8.
63. Nazarpour S, Ramezani Tehrani F, Simbar M, Tohidi M, Alavi Majd H, Azizi F. Effects of levothyroxine treatment on pregnancy outcomes in pregnant women with autoimmune thyroid disease. Eur J Endocrinol. 2017;176(2):253–65.
64. Wang H, Gao H, Chi H, Zeng L, Xiao W, Wang Y, et al. Effect of levothyroxine on miscarriage among women with normal thyroid function and thyroid autoimmunity undergoing in vitro fertilization and embryo transfer: a randomized clinical trial. JAMA. 2017;318(22):2190–8.
65. Negro R, Schwartz A, Stagnaro-Green A. Impact of levothyroxine in miscarriage and preterm delivery rates in first trimester thyroid antibody-positive women with TSH less than 2.5 mIU/L. J Clin Endocrinol Metabol. 2016;101(10):3685–90.
66. Li Y, Shan Z, Teng W, Yu X, Li Y, Fan C, et al. Abnormalities of maternal thyroid function during pregnancy affect neuropsychological development of their children at 25–30 months. Clin Endocrinol. 2010;72(6):825–9.
67. Williams FL, Watson J, Ogston SA, Visser TJ, Hume R, Willatts P. Maternal and umbilical cord levels of T4, FT4, TSH, TPOAb, and TgAb in term infants and neurodevelopmental outcome at 5.5 years. J Clin Endocrinol Metabol. 2013;98(2):829–38.
68. Wasserman EE, Nelson K, Rose NR, Eaton W, Pillion JP, Seaberg E, et al. Maternal thyroid autoantibodies during the third trimester and hearing deficits in children: an epidemiologic assessment. Am J Epidemiol. 2008;167(6):701–10.
69. Wasserman EE, Pillion JP, Duggan A, Nelson K, Rohde C, Seaberg EC, et al. Childhood IQ, hearing loss, and maternal thyroid autoimmunity in the Baltimore Collaborative Perinatal Project. Pediatr Res. 2012;72(5):525–30.
70. Ghassabian A, Bongers-Schokking JJ, De Rijke YB, Van Mil N, Jaddoe VW, de Muinck Keizer-Schrama SM, et al. Maternal thyroid autoimmunity during pregnancy and the risk of attention deficit/hyperactivity problems in children: the Generation R Study. Thyroid. 2012;22(2):178–86.
71. Haddow JE, Palomaki GE, Allan WC, Williams JR, Knight GJ, Gagnon J, et al. Maternal thyroid deficiency during pregnancy and subsequent neuropsychological development of the child. N Engl J Med. 1999;341(8):549–55.
72. Yamamoto JM, Benham JL, Nerenberg KA, Donovan LE. Impact of levothyroxine therapy on obstetric, neonatal and childhood outcomes in women with subclinical hypothyroidism diagnosed in pregnancy: a systematic review and meta-analysis of randomised controlled trials. BMJ Open. 2018;8(9):e022837.
73. Rayman MP. Selenium and human health. Lancet. 2012;379(9822):1256–68.

74. Schomburg L, Köhrle J. On the importance of selenium and iodine metabolism for thyroid hormone biosynthesis and human health. Mol Nutr Food Res. 2008;52(11):1235–46.
75. Wu Q, Rayman MP, Lv H, Schomburg L, Cui B, Gao C, et al. Low population selenium status is associated with increased prevalence of thyroid disease. J Clin Endocrinol Metabol. 2015;100(11):4037–47.
76. Mazokopakis EE, Papadakis JA, Papadomanolaki MG, Batistakis AG, Giannakopoulos TG, Protopapadakis EE, et al. Effects of 12 months treatment with L-selenomethionine on serum anti-TPO levels in patients with Hashimoto's thyroiditis. Thyroid. 2007;17(7):609–12.
77. Gärtner R, Gasnier BC, Dietrich JW, Krebs B, Angstwurm MW. Selenium supplementation in patients with autoimmune thyroiditis decreases thyroid peroxidase antibodies concentrations. J Clin Endocrinol Metabol. 2002;87(4):1687–91.
78. Fan Y, Xu S, Zhang H, Cao W, Wang K, Chen G, et al. Selenium supplementation for autoimmune thyroiditis: a systematic review and meta-analysis. Int J Endocrinol. 2014;2014:904573.
79. Wichman J, Winther KH, Bonnema SJ, Hegedüs L. Selenium supplementation significantly reduces thyroid autoantibody levels in patients with chronic autoimmune thyroiditis: a systematic review and meta-analysis. Thyroid. 2016;26(12):1681–92.
80. Negro R, Greco G, Mangieri T, Pezzarossa A, Dazzi D, Hassan H. The influence of selenium supplementation on postpartum thyroid status in pregnant women with thyroid peroxidase autoantibodies. J Clin Endocrinol Metabol. 2007;92(4):1263–8.
81. Mao J, Pop VJ, Bath SC, Vader HL, Redman CW, Rayman MP. Effect of low-dose selenium on thyroid autoimmunity and thyroid function in UK pregnant women with mild-to-moderate iodine deficiency. Eur J Nutr. 2016;55(1):55–61.
82. Stranges S, Marshall JR, Natarajan R, Donahue RP, Trevisan M, Combs GF, et al. Effects of long-term selenium supplementation on the incidence of type 2 diabetes: a randomized trial. Ann Intern Med. 2007;147(4):217–23.
83. Kiprov DD, Nachtigall RD, Weaver RC, Jacobson A, Main EK, Garovoy MR. The use of intravenous immunoglobulin in recurrent pregnancy loss associated with combined alloimmune and autoimmune abnormalities. Am J Reprod Immunol. 1996;36(4):228–34.
84. Stricker RB, Steinleitner A, Bookoff CN, Weckstein LN, Winger EE. Successful treatment of immunologic abortion with low-dose intravenous immunoglobulin. Fertil Steril. 2000;73(3):536–40.
85. Vaquero E, De Carolis C, Valensise H, Romanini C, Lazzarin N, Moretti C. Mild thyroid abnormalities and recurrent spontaneous abortion: diagnostic and therapeutical approach. Am J Reprod Immunol. 2000;43(4):204–8.
86. Litwicka K, Arrivi C, Varricchio MT, Mencacci C, Greco E. In women with thyroid autoimmunity, does low-dose prednisolone administration, compared with no adjuvant therapy, improve in vitro fertilization clinical results? J Obstet Gynaecol Res. 2015;41(5):722–8.
87. Turi A, Giannubilo SR, Zanconi S, Mascetti A, Tranquilli AL. Preconception steroid treatment in infertile women with antithyroid autoimmunity undergoing ovarian stimulation and intrauterine insemination: a double-blind, randomized, prospective cohort study. Clin Ther. 2010;32(14):2415–21.
88. Michael AE, Papageorghiou AT. Potential significance of physiological and pharmacological glucocorticoids in early pregnancy. Hum Reprod Update. 2008;14(5):497–517.
89. Weetman AP. Immunity, thyroid function and pregnancy: molecular mechanisms. Nat Rev Endocrinol. 2010;6(6):311.
90. Nicholson WK, Robinson KA, Smallridge RC, Ladenson PW, Powe NR. Prevalence of postpartum thyroid dysfunction: a quantitative review. Thyroid. 2006;16(6):573–82.
91. Tanda M, Cusini C, Colombo A, Premoli P, Rosetti S, Cromi A, et al. Iodine supplementation in women of reproductive age: a survey of clinical practice among Italian gynecologists and midwives. J Endocrinol Invest. 2019;42(3):353–5.
92. Pop VJ, de Vries E, van Baar AL, Waelkens J, De Rooy H, Horsten M, et al. Maternal thyroid peroxidase antibodies during pregnancy: a marker of impaired child development? J Clin Endocrinol Metabol. 1995;80(12):3561–6.
93. Panth P, Guerin G, DiMarco NM. A review of iodine status of women of reproductive age in the USA. Biol Trace Elem Res. 2019;188(1):208–20.

Thyroid Nodules and Thyroid Cancer in the Pregnant Woman

Trevor E. Angell

Introduction

A thyroid nodule is defined as a discrete lesion within the thyroid gland that can be seen as radiologically distinct from the surrounding thyroid tissue [1]. Thyroid nodules are common in the adult population, and are found more frequently in women [2–5]. Although the presence of thyroid nodules increases with age, the burden of disease on young women remains substantial [6], and the first identification of a thyroid nodule may be during pregnancy. The purpose of thyroid nodule evaluation is to detect possible thyroid cancer. Ideally, the management approach reduces the health risk posed by thyroid cancer while balancing the potential harm of diagnostic and therapeutic interventions and minimizing patient distress. These principles are perhaps most evident when thyroid nodules or cancer are discovered in a pregnant woman. The risks and potential contraindications associated with any intervention performed during pregnancy must be taken into account. Pregnancy has a profound influence on thyroid physiology, and thus the impact of gestation upon nodule formation, malignant transformation, and cancer behavior must also be considered. This chapter will focus on the detection, evaluation, and treatment of thyroid nodules and thyroid cancer during pregnancy.

T. E. Angell (✉)
Division of Endocrinology and Diabetes, Keck School of Medicine of the University of Southern California, Los Angeles, CA, USA
e-mail: trevor.angell@med.usc.edu

F. Azizi, F. Ramezani Tehrani (eds.), *Thyroid Diseases in Pregnancy*,
https://doi.org/10.1007/978-3-030-98777-0_13

Thyroid Nodules During Pregnancy

The estimated prevalence of a palpable thyroid nodule is approximately 5–6% in adult women, while up to 68% of adults may have a thyroid nodule detectable by imaging, such as computed tomography (CT), magnetic resonance (MR), or ultrasound [5, 7]. While the occurrence of nodules (both solitary and multiple) is more frequent with advancing age, thyroid nodules may be first detected in younger women during pregnancy. Most frequently this is by palpation of the neck and may be influenced by the greater contact with medical care women receive when pregnant or receiving pregnancy-related care. However, given the indolent nature of thyroid nodule growth [8, 9], it is likely that most thyroid nodules detected at this time were present before pregnancy. Studies using ultrasonographic evaluation have suggested the prevalence of thyroid nodules in pregnant women to be 3–21% with higher mean age in women with nodules compared to women without nodules [10–12], though the fact that these populations were from areas of mild to moderate iodine-deficiency may limit the generalizability of these data. Because of the increased incidence of thyroid nodules with age and current trends in the United States of America (USA) and elsewhere of increasing average maternal age [13], the frequency of thyroid nodules among women during pregnancy is likely to be higher in the future than has been historically noted.

Many of the physiologic effects of pregnancy may impact the formation and/or growth of thyroid nodules. The stimulatory effects of human chorionic gonadotropin (hCG) as well as changes in serum thyroid hormone binding and iodine status are known to have effects on the function of the thyroid gland during pregnancy [14, 15]. In addition, in vitro study of thyroid progenitor cells demonstrated expression of estrogen receptor alpha (ERα) and beta (ERβ), and the addition of 17b-estradiol stimulated thyroid cell growth [16]. Iodine excess, as defined by high urinary iodine to creatinine ratio, also has been associated with an increased risk of thyroid nodule formation in pregnant women [17].

Consistent with this, previous studies have reported both nodule formation and enlargement during pregnancy. In a case-control study from Iran, in which 298 women in the first trimester of pregnancy and 290 matched nonpregnant women without known thyroid disease were evaluated by ultrasound and compared for the presence of thyroid nodules. The percentage of women with thyroid nodules was similar between the two groups (16.4% vs. 16.6%; $p = 0.85$), as was the average number of nodules per subject [18], suggesting that gestational effects on thyroid nodules are not observed early in pregnancy. Looking longitudinally over pregnancy, Kung et al. [11] evaluated 221 newly pregnant women using serial ultrasound examinations from the first trimester to the third trimester. This study found that the proportion of women with a thyroid nodule increased by 10%, though most of these new nodules measured <5 mm in largest dimension. Additionally, in a case-control study by Karger et al. [19], the authors demonstrated that compared to nulliparous controls, there was an increased prevalence of thyroid nodules in women with prior pregnancy. Finally, an analysis of 26 pregnant women from an iodine-deficient area by Sahin et al. showed a significant but minimal increase in the largest nodule diameter from the first to the third trimester (11.9 ± 4.8 mm vs. 12.6 ± 5.4 mm; $p = 0.002$) but no increase in nodule formation [20]. Together these data suggest that pregnancy may exert an impact on thyroid nodule formation and/or growth during pregnancy, but that such change will usually be of little to no clinical impact. Consistent with this conclusion, there is currently no recommendation for routine screening evaluation for thyroid nodules in pregnant women, nor serial or increased frequency of monitoring of existing nonmalignant nodules during pregnancy [21].

Evaluation and Diagnosis

Similar to the case in nonpregnant individuals, the identification of a possible thyroid nodule during pregnancy is typically made through palpable during physical examination of the thyroid or incidentally on an imaging study obtained for an unrelated indication. The evaluation of thyroid nodules that are diagnosed during pregnancy should in general proceed similarly to nodules found in nonpregnant patients. Pregnant women for whom there is an initial suspicion of a thyroid nodule should have ultrasound evaluation of the thyroid and cervical neck lymph nodes and measurement of serum thyroid stimulating hormone (TSH), also known as thyrotropin [1]. In conjunction with these assessments, history and physical examination should be performed to assess any increased risk for malignancy. Historical details to obtain include any childhood radiation exposures or radiation therapy to the head, neck, or mantle regions, and significant family history of medullary or non-medullary thyroid cancer, as well as hereditary syndromes that carry an increased risk of thyroid tumors, such as familial adenomatosis polyposis, PTEN hamartoma syndrome, multiple endocrine neoplasia syndrome, or Carney complex. Additionally, a symptom history of neck pain, rapidly enlarging masses, or persistent hoarse of voice would raise the possibility of more aggressive thyroid cancer. The physical examination should focus not only on identifying any thyroid nodules, but on recognizing findings that raise suspicion for thyroid cancer, such as very hard and fixed nodules, the presence of lymphadenopathy, or hoarse voice, that may not have been noted by the patient.

Thyroid ultrasound does not utilize ionizing radiation and is safe during pregnancy. Ultrasonographic evaluation can provide important cancer risk stratification, not only by describing the size and location of a thyroid nodule, but by evaluating features associated with malignancy, such as solid versus cystic contents, parenchymal echogenicity, the presence and type of calcifications, margins, and abnormal cervical lymph nodes [22]. Several systems for classifying nodules have emerged [1, 23], and while there are limitations in both the accuracy of ultrasonographic features and the reproducibility of their reporting [24, 25], they are valuable for providing an estimate of cancer risk and providing recommendations on when further diagnostic assessment with ultrasound-guided fine needle aspiration biopsy (FNAB) should be performed [1, 23, 26].

Assessment of TSH in the setting of a thyroid nodule is performed to detect a suppressed TSH that may might indicate an autonomously functioning nodule, which would portend a greatly reduced risk of malignancy [2, 21]. The physiologic reduction in TSH due to the effect of hCG during pregnancy can mimic that which would be seen with a functioning nodule, but the inability to employ radioactive iodine (RAI) uptake testing during pregnancy complicates confirmation of autonomous nodule function. This has led to recommendations that when a suppressed TSH is noted beyond 16 weeks gestational age, further evaluation may be deferred until after pregnancy when TSH can be accurately repeated [1, 21]. When clear clinical manifestations of hyperthyroidism are present management with antithyroid drugs may be used to prevent adverse pregnancy consequences. In contrast, women with subclinical hyperthyroidism should be monitored closely for the emergence of overt hypothyroidism during pregnancy. Measurement of serum TSH in those with abnormal thyroid exam or imaging findings may also facilitate identification of thyroid dysfunction (especially hypothyroidism) that should be addressed to optimize pregnancy outcome.

The criteria for performing further thyroid nodule assessment with FNAB are the same as for nonpregnant women, but individualized decision-making is important to consider [1, 21]. Primarily, which thyroid nodules should undergo FNAB is now guided by sonographic risk and may be based on one of a number of stratification systems current available. Many of these systems, including those from the USA [1, 23], do not recommend FNAB for intrathyroidal nodules <1 cm without evidence of metastases. Otherwise, for thyroid nodules with a sonographic appearance highly suspicious for malignancy, FNAB is performed for nodules ≥1 cm, whereas for thyroid nodules with lower risk appearance aspiration biopsy is recommended only at larger sizes (1.5–2.5 cm). There are also thyroid nodules that have features strongly correlated with a benign etiology, including those with a so-called "spongiform" appearance and purely cystic nodules, for which no biopsy may be required.

The decision to perform FNAB during pregnancy should be guided by providing optimal patient-centered care, and must balance potential risks and expected benefits. FNAB, including use of subcutaneous lidocaine analgesia, is considered safe during pregnancy [27–29]. Expected side effects from FNAB include mild procedural discomfort and bruising and serious side effects are fortunately extremely rare [30]. Performing FNAB, including the common practice of using subcutaneous lidocaine, is a safe procedure during pregnancy [31]. Pregnancy does not appear to have an effect of the cytologic interpretation or results from thyroid FNA [31, 32], though there are no high-quality prospective data in this regard.

The primary benefit of FNAB is the acquisition of a cytologic diagnosis, which can significantly improve thyroid cancer risk assessment [1, 4, 33, 34]. The Bethesda system for reporting thyroid cytopathology introduced in 2009, and revised in 2017, is increasingly used in the around the world and is recommended in the USA for cytologic classification of FNAB aspiration [1]. In general populations with thyroid nodules, the expected distribution of cytologic results (and risk of malignancy estimated by the result) would be approximately: 2–20% nondiagnostic/unsatisfactory (5–10%); 60–70% a benign (0–3%); 5–10% malignant (94–99%); and finally,

15–30% with and indeterminate result (6–75% depending on specific category) for which possible malignancy is suggested but not confirmed [30, 34]. Since most thyroid nodules in pregnant patients were present prior to pregnancy, the distribution of cytologic findings and risk of malignancy are expected to be similar to nonpregnant women, but specific data in pregnancy are lacking. Previous data have indicated the overall cancer risk in pregnant women with a thyroid nodule to be 12–43%. In a study of 57 pregnancy women, the risk of malignancy was 50% for nodules with indeterminate cytology nodules, 75% for those with malignant cytology, and no cancers were found in nodules with benign cytology results [31]. Similarly, in a separate study of 40 pregnant women who underwent FNA, 100% of nodules with malignancy were cancerous, 33% of nodules with indeterminate cytology, and 0% of benign cytology nodules [32]. However, current data are limited by small sample size, likely selection bias for patients undergoing FNAB, and description prior to current sonographic risk assessment and use of the Bethesda classifications.

Management with active observation is preferred for benign thyroid disease over diagnostic resection, especially during pregnancy. Confirmed malignant nodules, on the other hand, may benefit surgical resection at some point. Thyroid nodules with indeterminate cytology after FNAB represent a diagnostic dilemma because the presence of malignancy, and thus optimal management, remains uncertain [1, 35]. The use of additional adjuvant testing of these nodules to improve cancer risk stratification has been the topic of numerous studies. One emerging modality that continues to grow in application in nonpregnant patients is molecular diagnostic testing that analyzes the genomic material from thyroid tissue collected by FNAB [35, 36]. In nonpregnant women, molecular diagnostic testing of cytologically indeterminate thyroid nodules can improve pre-operative cancer risk assessment [36–38]. Though generally uncommon in nodules with indeterminate cytology, the *BRAF* gene mutation leading to the BRAFV600E mutated protein almost proves the presence of thyroid cancer [1, 36, 37]. Similarly, *RET/PTC* fusions are highly specific for thyroid cancer, but are found only rarely in patients without specific radiation exposure. Other gene mutations that occur more frequently, such as those in the *RAS* genes, may be found in both benign and malignant thyroid nodules and are not well correlated with aggressive tumor behavior [39, 40]. Commercially available, clinically validated molecular diagnostic tests now evaluate changes in DNA and/or RNA expression from thyroid nodule aspiration material to improve the prediction of benign or malignant pathology [41–43]. Although it is unknown if the results of these molecular tests would be affected by pregnancy, these tests are not currently recommended in pregnant women because of a lack of data for test performance in this population.

After the diagnostic assessment to determine the probability of malignancy within a thyroid nodule, management options can be considered. Benign thyroid nodules that are otherwise asymptomatic do not require specific surveillance during pregnancy [21]. For confirmed or suspected malignant nodules, the usual prompt surgical resection typically considered for nonpregnant patients may not be the preferred approach during pregnancy. Uncommon aggressive forms of thyroid cancer, such as medullary or anaplastic carcinomas, will require prompt management. The majority of thyroid cancers, however, represent differentiated thyroid cancers that behave in a relatively indolent fashion, including during pregnancy. In such differentiated thyroid cancers, investigations have not confirmed greater harm when treatment is deferred until after pregnancy [44]. Moreover, for indeterminate thyroid nodules, malignancies are more likely to be less aggressive variants of thyroid carcinoma [45]. Additionally, risks of thyroid surgery in pregnant women may be higher than in nonpregnant women [46–48]. This balance for benefits and risks should be considered and a conservative approach to cytologically indeterminate or malignant nodules can be considered. Indeed, performing FNAB during pregnancy should be an informed, patient-centered decision, recognizing the downstream risks of possible surgery, as well as the possibility of substantial worry on the part of the pregnant patient at the time of diagnosis and during the remainder of the pregnancy if surgical intervention is deferred.

For suspicious nodules that do not undergo FNAB, or nodules with indeterminate cytology, that are observed during pregnancy, repeat sonographic monitoring performed in the early second trimester may be used to detect clinically significant growth or invasion that would lead to surgical intervention during gestation, while the management of nodules without concerning change at this point can be delayed to the postpartum period. When FNA biopsy confirms the presence of differentiated thyroid cancer, a conservative management approach may still be warranted and is discussed further below.

Evaluation and Management of Thyroid Cancer During Pregnancy

Incidence

The incidence of a thyroid cancer diagnosed during pregnancy or during the first 12 months postpartum has been estimated at 14.4–21.7 cases per 100,000 pregnancies [49–51]. Using data from 4,846,505 obstetric patients linked to the California Cancer Registry from 1991–1999, Smith et al. found a papillary thyroid cancer incidence of 14.4/100,000 pregnancies [49]. A somewhat higher incidence was reported by Lee et al., in a population-based study from Australia including data from 781,907 women who gave birth from 1994–2008 [50]. In this study, the incidence of thyroid and other endocrine cancers was 17.4 per 100,000 pregnancies, of which most (14.2 cases/100,000) were diagnosed in the first year postpartum compared to 3.2 cases/100,000 during gestation. In a more recent study of health plan and registry data, Cottreau et al. investigated pregnancy-associated cancer (PAC) incidence per 100,000 pregnancies in the United States [51]. Analyzing 775,709 pregnancies from 2001 to 2013, thyroid cancer represented 20% of all observed PAC events and was the second most common cancer site after breast (25%). The incidence of thyroid cancer was found to be 21.7 cases per 100,000 pregnancies, with approximately

20% of thyroid cancers diagnosed during pregnancy, while 80% were diagnosed in the 12 months after delivery. Differences in these data may be attributable to the distinct registries used and the populations represented. Since early pregnancy abortions (for any reason) were not included in these datasets, cancer incidence could be underestimated if diagnosis early in pregnancy led to pregnancy termination; the extent to which this would have occurred in women diagnosed with thyroid cancer is not known. Despite their limitations, these studies provide a basis for estimating the incidence of pregnancy-associated thyroid cancers.

Prognosis

Determining the prognosis of thyroid cancer diagnosed during pregnancy has been the subject of ongoing investigations. Seminal population-based studies in the United States evaluating the prognosis of women diagnosed with differentiated thyroid cancer (DTC) around the time of pregnancy have provided general reassurance regarding the natural history of this disease. Moosa and Mazzaferri [44] reported the outcomes of 61 women diagnosed with DTC during pregnancy compared to 528 age-matched control women who were not pregnant, with a median follow-up of roughly 20 years. The two groups did not differ significantly in initial pathologic findings with respect to tumor size, lymph node metastasis, stage, or distant metastatic disease. Recurrence of DTC was also similar, and was observed in 15% of the pregnancy group compared to 23% of the control group. Importantly, this study also compared women who had surgical intervention for DTC during pregnancy (23% of the cohort with average time from diagnosis to surgery of 1.1 ± 1.0 months) to women who had surgery after pregnancy (77% of the cohort with average time from diagnosis to surgery of 16.1 ± 19.7 months). Despite this delay, pathologic findings and rates of recurrence and distant metastases were similar, indicating the safety of deferring surgery until after completion of pregnancy. A separate study of women aged 18–46 years old with DTC from the New Mexico Tumor Registry from 1970 to 1991 [52]. The authors compared the outcomes of 464 nonpregnant women with DTC to 22 women diagnosed with DTC during pregnancy, 16 of whom had surgery delayed until after pregnancy, and found similar survival between these groups.

Using data linked to the California Cancer Registry, Yasmeen et al. [53] analyzed 595 cases of DTC diagnosis from 9 month prior to pregnancy to 12 months postpartum compared to 2270 age-matched nonpregnant women with DTC and found similar survival was observed between groups. Women diagnosed in association with pregnancy were noted to be younger and more frequently had private insurance, which may also influence the prognosis observed in this group. Nevertheless, these data further support earlier results of similar thyroid cancer prognosis compared to nonpregnant female patients. An analysis of the linked date registries from 1999 to 2012 by Chen et al. included 301 women with DTC diagnosed between 5 years before and 9 months after a pregnancy [54]. The median time from pregnancy to DTC diagnosis was 2.62 years and the median follow-up after cancer diagnosis was

7.92 years. Compared to the control group of 903 nonpregnant women with DTC, no significant differences in tumor size, presence of extrathyroidal extension, rate of metastatic disease, or tumor stage were found between groups, and a similar 5-year disease-specific survival was 99.5% in both groups.

Together these studies describe the natural history of DTC diagnosed during pregnancy as similar to that of nonpregnant patients with respect to survival or clinical evidence of recurrent disease. It should be noted that older data did not utilize modern modalities for thyroid cancer surveillance, such as high-resolution ultrasound of the neck and thyroglobulin (Tg) measurement, and despite these reassuring findings, some data have raised concern regarding more aggressive behavior of DTC diagnosed during pregnancy. In a single-center study by Vannucchi et al., the data from 123 women who were <45 years old who had had total thyroidectomy for DTC were retrospective analyzed [55]. Patients were divided into three groups: (1) women diagnosed more than 1 year after completing pregnancy; (2) women diagnosed during pregnancy or within 1 year postpartum; or (3) women diagnosed before pregnancy or who were nulliparous. In contrast to the studies highlighted above, the definition or persistent disease utilized current biochemical criteria involving elevated thyroglobulin and/or thyroglobulin antibody, in addition to structural disease identified pathologically or radiographically. In Group 2 women with DTC related to pregnancy, 9/15 (60%) had disease persistence (two-thirds of which were based on biochemical criteria), compared to 4.2% and 13.1% in groups 1 and 3, respectively. A higher rate of lymph node metastases was observed in women with DTC related to pregnancy (Group 2). Interestingly, when patient tumors were evaluated for estrogen receptor alpha (ERα) positivity by immunohistochemistry, DTC tumors from women diagnosed during pregnancy showed significantly higher ERα (87.5%) than those of women in the other two groups. In a similarly designed study by Messuti et al. [56], among the included 340 women with DTC who underwent total thyroidectomy and radioactive iodine, patients diagnosed with DTC during or within 2 years of pregnancy had a higher rate of persistent disease (10.5%) compared to women with DTC diagnosed >2 years after delivery (1.3%) or nulliparous women (4.7%). In this study however, DTC diagnosed during pregnancy was not associated with either lymph node metastases or ERα positive status. In a subsequent study of nonpregnant patients, ERα and progesterone receptor (PR) status was evaluated by immunohistochemistry on PTC tumors from 182 male or female patients [57]. Though ERα or PR positivity was associated with larger tumor size and BRAFV600E mutation, there was no correlation with lymph node metastasis, extrathyroidal extension, or persistent disease after treatment. Comparing 24 women diagnosed with PTC to 30 nonpregnancy women treated at the University of Sydney, Australia, Lee et al. found that PTC diagnosed during or within 12 months of pregnancy was associated with larger tumor size (22.8 vs 13.7 mm), and a greater percentage of resected lymph nodes with metastasis (32% vs. 15%) but no difference in disease-free survival during a mean follow-up of 44 months [50].

Relatively few data directly evaluate the degree of thyroid cancer progression when observed by ultrasound. Oh et al. [58] studied 19 patients diagnosed with PTC "just before" pregnancy or before 20 weeks of gestation with ultrasound evaluation.

The median tumor size was 0.91 cm with 64.8% being ≤1 cm. The median ultrasound interval was 9.5 months and 26% of primary PTC tumors showed a significant increase in tumor volume. Of 3 patients who had cervical lymph nodes seen on baseline ultrasound, two showed an increase in metastatic lymph node size, but no patient without abnormal lymph node findings developed clinical lymph node metastases during monitoring during pregnancy. As part of the long-term observational data of active surveillance of papillary thyroid microcarcinoma (PMC) at Kuma Hospital, Japan, Ito et al. identified 50/1549 women with PMC who went through pregnancy. PMC lesions remained stable in 90% of cases. Only four PMC tumors increased by ≥3 mm during pregnancy and did not grow further in two patients who continued to be observed without surgical resection [59].

In summary, the evidence current suggests similar survival outcomes for DTC associated with pregnancy compared to DTC unrelated to pregnancy. Evidence for more aggressive pathologic features or higher rates of persistent disease after initial surgery have been inconsistent and require further validation. Additional aspects of treatment that would influence the observed associations, such as extent of initial surgery and follow-up strategies, should be considered. There remains no clear evidence that delaying surgical intervention until after pregnancy for the majority of DTC has a negative effect on outcomes.

Surgical Treatment During Pregnancy

In most cases, DTC diagnosed in early pregnancy is amenable to conservative management, in which sonographic monitoring for evidence of highly aggressive behavior is performed and resection considered if there is evidence of significant growth, invasion, or lymph node metastases, ideally before 24–26 weeks gestational age to minimize obstetric complications of surgery [1]. As stated above, an exception to these recommendations is the rare findings of a more aggressive thyroid malignancy, including medullary, poorly differentiated, or anaplastic carcinomas, as well as clinically aggressive DTC. In such circumstances, immediate therapy is often warranted during pregnancy.

Sosa and colleagues [46] conducted a retrospective cross-sectional study of pregnant women who underwent thyroid ($n = 165$) or parathyroid ($n = 36$) surgery during pregnancy (data from the Health Care Utilization Projection Nationwide Inpatient Sample (HCUP-NIS) from 1999 to 2005). Ninety-two patients (46%) underwent surgery for thyroid cancer and procedures included total and partial thyroidectomy. Patients in the cohort were compared to 31,155 contemporary nonpregnant patients undergoing the same procedures. The authors compared rates of endocrine complications, including maternal hypoparathyroidism, hypocalcemia, tetany, and recurrent laryngeal nerve injury, and general surgical complications, such as cardiovascular and infectious or wound events. Pregnant patients had higher endocrine and general surgical complications (15.9 vs 8.1% and 11.4 vs 3.6%, $p = 0.001$ for both), longer length of hospital stay (2 days vs 1 day; $p = 0.001$), and higher hospital costs (\$6873 vs \$5963; $p = 0.007$). Pregnancy remained a significant predictor of these worse clinical outcomes in a multivariate regression analysis. Other independent predictors of worse clinical outcomes were lower surgeon volume, non-White race, Charlson comorbidity score ≥2, and non-private insurance. A thyroid cancer diagnosis (vs benign thyroid disease or hyperparathyroidism) was not a predictor of maternal or fetal complications, but was an independent predictor of surgical complications. Performance of the operation by a high-volume surgeon, defined as one in the ≥75th percentile, was associated with decreased maternal (0% vs 12%, $p = 0.002$) and fetal (1.2% vs 12%, $p = 0.01$) among pregnant patients.

Two smaller studies have also evaluated surgical outcomes in pregnant patients with differentiated thyroid cancer [47, 48]. Ureno et al. [47] compared outcomes of patients with papillary thyroid cancer who underwent thyroid surgery during pregnancy (second trimester, $n = 24$) versus the year following delivery ($n = 21$). Patients were similar in age (median 32 years in both groups) and tumor characteristics with well-differentiated pathology, moderate rates of lymph node metastases (14/24, 58% in pregnant vs 14/21, 66% in postpartum surgery patients), rare extrathyroidal extension (1/24, 4% vs 2/21, 9.5%), and no distant metastases. Among pregnant patients, most underwent lobectomy (21/24, 87.5% vs 17/21, 80.9% in postpartum surgery group) with lymph node dissection (24/24, 100% vs 21/21, 100% postpartum group) during the second trimester (19/24, 79.2%). The authors reported no surgical complications, such as postoperative bleeding, hoarseness, hypoparathyroidism, or anaphylactic reactions, in either group. Operative and anesthesia times were similar between groups, with a trend toward increased blood loss in pregnant patients (102.5 mL, range 20–497 mL vs 70 mL, range 14–436 mL; $p = 0.05$). Regarding maternal-fetal outcomes, all infants were delivered at ≥40 weeks gestation with no significant difference in mode of delivery or peri-natal complications or fetal birth weight. There were no miscarriages in either group. Boucek and colleagues [48] evaluated maternal and obstetric outcomes of well-differentiated thyroid cancer in a cohort of 35 women who were pregnant or became pregnant during thyroid cancer treatment. Patients were identified from the International Network on Cancer, Infertility, and Pregnancy registry in Europe from 2004 to 2016. Twenty-nine of 35 (83%) underwent surgery for thyroid cancer during pregnancy, and 6 delayed surgical treatment until after delivery. Of surgeries, 24/29 (83%) had total thyroidectomy and 4/29 (14%) had lobectomy including LN dissection in 6 of these patients; 1 additional patient underwent only LN resection without primary thyroid surgery. Surgery was performed for most patients in the second trimester. All women had Stage 1 (AJCC8) disease without distant metastasis, and 22 of 29 went on to receive radioactive iodine therapy after delivery. Surgical outcomes were not reported in this study. Regarding maternal-fetal outcomes, three pregnancies were electively terminated. Two patients elected for termination in the first trimester following a diagnosis of DTC with lymph node metastasis, and one pregnancy was terminated in the second trimester for congenital malformations of the fetus unrelated to thyroid cancer diagnosis. Of remaining pregnant patients, the mean gestational age at delivery was 40 weeks and there were not preterm deliveries. The study reported no other fetal or maternal complications. Several other case series of pregnant patients who underwent surgery for thyroid cancer have been reported in the literature with fewer than ten cases each and are reviewed elsewhere [46].

Taken together, these data suggest that surgery for thyroid cancer performed during the second trimester may carry an increased risk of surgical complications, as well as maternal-fetal complications. These risks are reduced, though perhaps not to the level expected in nonpregnant patients, when the surgery is performed by a high-volume thyroid surgeon. Furthermore, data from Asia [47] suggests that when thyroid cancer surgery is performed during pregnancy, partial thyroidectomy is associated with a lower rate of surgical complications, as is generally recognized for nonpregnant patients. It is important to note that these data derive primarily from patients with DTC, which has an overall excellent prognosis [60]. The risk of delayed surgery for patients with more aggressive forms of thyroid cancer during pregnancy, including poorly differentiated and anaplastic thyroid cancer, is likely greater and requires a patient-specific assessment and approach.

Management of Preexisting Thyroid Cancer During Pregnancy

The relatively high incidence of thyroid cancer in reproductive aged women combined with its excellent prognosis means that many women with a previous diagnosis of thyroid cancer may become pregnant. The monitoring of women with preexisting thyroid carcinoma remains ongoing during any pregnancies, though the decision to perform noninvasive and/or invasive evaluations should balance the likelihood of detecting disease that would be treated during pregnancy against the risks of testing.

A maternal serum Tg concentration <2 ng/dL supports the absence of active thyroid malignancy. In contrast, Tg ≥2 IU/L or rising concentrations over time [1, 61] suggest recurrence or progression of disease, though precise cut-offs predicting disease in patients who have not undergone RAI therapy are less well defined. Approximately 20% of thyroid cancer patients harbor antibodies to Tg (TgAb), which can interfere with Tg measurement and cause falsely low Tg values [61, 62]. TgAb assessment should be performed when assessing Tg, and if TgAb is present, any Tg result should be cautiously interpreted given the possibility of interpretation interference. For patients in whom Tg or TgAb suggests persistent thyroid cancer, a thorough physical examination and neck ultrasound should be performed to identify an anatomic source. Whole body diagnostic radioactive iodine scanning must not be performed due to the ability for iodine to cross the placenta and radiation exposure. Other high-energy imaging modalities such as CT, positron emission tomography (PET), or MRI to search for metastatic disease is complicated by contraindications that exist during pregnancy and the need for such testing should be individualized.

Studies investigating the influence that pregnancy may exert on thyroid cancer have generally found no effect on progression [63–66], but may have consequences in some populations [63, 64, 67]. In a retrospective study of 235 women with previous DTC who went through pregnancy, Rakhlin et al. found that no woman who had excellent, indeterminate, or biochemically incomplete response to thyroid according to the American Thyroid Association criteria [1] developed structural recurrence [63]. In a separate study by Hirsch et al. [64], 63 women with a previous diagnosis of PTC were followed through a pregnancy at a median time after diagnosis of 5.08 ± 4.39 years after cancer treatment and no progression of PTC was noted in women who were considered disease-free prior to pregnancy. Contrary to these reassuring findings, thyroid cancer progression may be a concern in patients with persistent cancer at the time of pregnancy. Of the 13 women with persistent PTC pre-pregnancy in the study by Hirsch et al., six showed either structural or biochemical progression [64]. Of the 38 women with preexisting structurally incomplete response to therapy in Rakhlin et al. [63], 11 (29%) had progression during gestation, though new treatment recommendations were only considered necessary in 8% of cases. Recently, Xi et al. collected data on 124 women 16–25 years old who underwent thyroidectomy and RAI for DTC who had lung metastases and compared 37 patients who had a gestation >6 months after treatment to 87 controls without pregnancy [65]. Disease recurrence was defined as identification of progression on imaging or a ≥25% increase in Tg or TgAb. Progression-free survival between the pregnancy and nonpregnancy groups was similar at 5 years (94.5% vs. 89.8%) and 10 years (63.2% vs. 58.1%). 5-year and 10-year overall survival was also similar between groups. Reports from individual cases, however, demonstrate that disease progression can result in clinical worsening of disease and morbidity [67].

Monitoring of thyroid hormone status and degree of TSH suppression is also essential to the ongoing management of women with DTC during pregnancy. During pregnancy, thyroid hormone production by the thyroid would typically increase substantially due to the physiologic effects of hCG and other gestational changes [68, 69]. Previous thyroidectomy and reliance on exogenous levothyroxine supplementation results in an inability to endogenously augment thyroid hormone supply and maternal hypothyroidism will frequently result with an increase in the dose of levothyroxine provided. This demand for greater amounts of thyroid hormone begins early in gestation and increases until approximately 16–20 weeks of gestation, after which the increased demand remain stable until returning to pre-pregnancy requirements [69]. For women with a diagnosis of thyroid cancer, before or during the pregnancy, The TSH goal should reflect the goal for TSH suppression that would otherwise be recommended for thyroid cancer management based on the underlying risk of recurrence and response to therapy, while avoiding clinical evidence of thyroid hormone excess [1]. Even mild suppression (0.5–2.0 mIU/L) advocated for patients at very low risk of DTC recurrence provides sufficient thyroid hormone to minimize the risks to pregnancy [21].

In summary, progression of DTC during pregnancy rarely occurs in women who do not have evidence of disease prior to pregnancy. For women who have persistent DTC, particularly if there is known structural disease in lymph nodes or at distant metastatic sites such as the lungs, there is an increased risk of observable progression, but often this will not be symptomatic or require new intervention during pregnancy. During pregnancy, TSH should be maintained at stable levels through proactive monitoring and adjustment of levothyroxine therapy. Of note, Tg concentrations may rise during pregnancy due potentially to the stimulatory effects of hCG on the TSH receptor. In euthyroid women from an iodine-sufficient population thyroglobulin concentration at 8 weeks gestation was significantly greater than pre-pregnancy levels and returned to baseline postpartum [70]. While historically, DTC patients lacked any thyroid tissue due to total thyroidectomy and radioactive iodine (RAI) ablation, women who become pregnant after treatment without use of RAI or after lobectomy alone could have increased Tg from normal thyroid tissue that should not be automatically construed as a sign of disease progression.

Pregnancy and Radioactive Iodine

Many women with DTC will have received treatment with radioactive iodine (RAI) after initial surgery, which may impact future pregnancy planning. The results of large studies [71] and systemic review [72] from more than a decade ago assessing of fertility outcomes in patients with thyroid cancer who received RAI therapy provided reassuring findings that there was not an increased risk of infertility, miscarriage, birth defects, or other adverse maternal-fetal outcomes. Results from newer studies have conflicted, with some showing lower rates of pregnancy in DTC women who received RAI [73, 74] and another finding no associated risk [75]. A current meta-analysis of 22 studies by Piek et al. focusing on the effects of RAI on fertility did not find that RAI therapy was associated with an increased risk of not having a pregnancy [76].

Several studies have investigated the effect of RAI treatment on concentration of anti-Mullerian Hormone (AMH), which is a marker of ovarian reserve and potentially reproductive capacity. While results have varied, numerous data suggest significant reduction in AMH levels in the 12 months following RAI treatment for DTC [77–80], though not confirmed in all studies [81, 82] and lower AMH levels have not been specifically linked to infertility. In the analysis by Van Velsen et al. [80], AMH decline was more pronounced in women ≥35 years old and the analysis of women with DTC in the California Cancer Registry by Wu et al. [73] found a significantly lower birth rate in women aged 35–39 years who received RAI compared to those who did not.

These data suggest that RAI does not have a consistently detectable deleterious effect on fertility, but more careful consideration should be given more cautious to use and lower dosing in women ≥35 years old who desire fertility. Existing data often lack granularity with respect to other variables that may affect fertility, such as TSH levels, burden of disease, and patient desire for fertility. Indeed, treatment with RAI may alter a woman's pregnancy desire [80] and influence observed birth rates.

The timing of pregnancy after RAI for DTC should also be considered. RAI therapy is often used following surgical resection [1], but is contraindicated during gestation due to direct radiation-related risk of teratogenicity or effects on fetal thyroid tissue after placental transfer of RAI into the fetal circulation. If RAI therapy is indicated, treatment must be delayed until after pregnancy, and ideally until after the conclusion of lactation because of the potential for high RAI concentrations in breast milk. Preparation for RAI treatment may lead to unstable thyroid hormone levels that may require medication adjustments and monitoring. Because of the possible deleterious effects of abnormal thyroid hormone status on fertility and pregnancy, as well as concerns regarding direct effects of residual radiation on fetal tissue, recommendations have maintained that women should refrain from attempting pregnancy for at least 6 months after receiving therapeutic radioactive iodine treatment [21].

Summary

The identification of thyroid nodules occurs frequently during pregnancy. Assessment with TSH, ultrasound, and FNAB when indicated can be safely performed during pregnancy and provide cancer risk assessment. In rare, high-risk scenarios thyroidectomy during pregnancy is necessary, reinforcing the need for careful initial diagnostic evaluation. But most thyroid cancers detected during pregnancy do not pose an immediate risk during gestation and outcomes are similar when surgery is deferred until the postpartum. Therefore, the approach to thyroid nodules and cancer during pregnancy should be generally more conservative and decisions to pursue evaluation and thyroidectomy should be individualized, weighing the risks and benefits of interventions against those of the condition itself.

Disclosures Dr. Angell (none).

References

1. Haugen BR, Alexander EK, Bible KC, Doherty GM, Mandel SJ, Nikiforov YE, Pacini F, Randolph GW, Sawka AM, Schlumberger M, Schuff KG, Sherman SI, Sosa JA, Steward DL, Tuttle RM, Wartofsky L. 2015 American Thyroid Association management guidelines for adult patients with thyroid nodules and differentiated thyroid cancer: the American Thyroid Association guidelines task force on thyroid nodules and differentiated thyroid cancer. Thyroid. 2016;26:1–133.
2. Burman KD, Wartofsky L. Clinical practice. Thyroid nodules. N Engl J Med. 2015;373:2347–56.
3. Frates MC, Benson CB, Doubilet PM, Kunreuther E, Contreras M, Cibas ES, Orcutt J, Moore FD Jr, Larsen PR, Marqusee E, Alexander EK. Prevalence and distribution of carcinoma in patients with solitary and multiple thyroid nodules on sonography. J Clin Endocrinol Metab. 2006;91:3411–7.
4. Yassa L, Cibas ES, Benson CB, Frates MC, Doubilet PM, Gawande AA, Moore FD Jr, Kim BW, Nosé V, Marqusee E, Larsen PR, Alexander EK. Long-term assessment of a multidisciplinary approach to thyroid nodule diagnostic evaluation. Cancer. 2007;111:508–16.
5. Guth S, Theune U, Aberle J, Galach A, Bamberger CM. Very high prevalence of thyroid nodules detected by high frequency (13 MHz) ultrasound examination. Eur J Clin Invest. 2009;39:699–706.

6. Kwong N, Medici M, Angell TE, Liu X, Marqusee E, Cibas ES, Krane JF, Barletta JA, Kim MI, Larsen PR, Alexander EK. The influence of patient age on thyroid nodule formation, multinodularity, and thyroid cancer risk. J Clin Endocrinol Metab. 2015;100:4434–40.
7. Tunbridge WM, Evered DC, Hall R, Appleton D, Brewis M, Clark F, Evans JG, Young E, Bird T, Smith PA. The spectrum of thyroid disease in a community: the Whickham survey. Clin Endocrinol. 1977;7:481–93.
8. Durante C, Costante G, Lucisano G, Bruno R, Meringolo D, Paciaroni A, Puxeddu E, Torlontano M, Tumino S, Attard M, Lamartina L, Nicolucci A, Filetti S. The natural history of benign thyroid nodules. JAMA. 2015;313:926–35.
9. Angell TE, Vyas CM, Medici M, Wang Z, Barletta JA, Benson CB, Cibas ES, Cho NL, Doherty GM, Doubilet PM, Frates MC, Gawande AA, Heller HT, Kim MI, Krane JF, Marqusee E, Moore FD Jr, Nehs MA, Zavacki AM, Larsen PR, Alexander EK. Differential growth rates of benign vs. malignant thyroid nodules. J Clin Endocrinol Metab. 2017;102:4642–7.
10. Struve CW, Haupt S, Ohlen S. Influence of frequency of previous pregnancies on the prevalence of thyroid nodules in women without clinical evidence of thyroid disease. Thyroid. 1993;3:7–9.
11. Kung AW, Chau MT, Lao TT, Tam SC, Low LC. The effect of pregnancy on thyroid nodule formation. J Clin Endocrinol Metab. 2002;87:1010–4.
12. Glinoer D, Soto MF, Bourdoux P, Lejeune B, Delange F, Lemone M, Kinthaert J, Robijn C, Grun JP, de Nayer P. Pregnancy in patients with mild thyroid abnormalities: maternal and neonatal repercussions. J Clin Endocrinol Metab. 1991;73:421–7.
13. Martin JA, Hamilton BE, Osterman MJK, Driscoll AK. National vital statistics report, vol 70(2). 2021. https://www.cdc.gov/nchs/data/nvsr/nvsr70/nvsr70-02-508.pdf.
14. Krassas GE, Poppe K, Glinoer D. Thyroid function and human reproductive health. Endocr Rev. 2010;31:702–55.
15. Hershman JM. The role of human chorionic gonadotropin as a thyroid stimulator in normal pregnancy. J Clin Endocrinol Metab. 2008;93:3305–6.
16. Xu S, Chen G, Peng W, Renko K, Derwahl M. Oestrogen action on thyroid progenitor cells: relevant for the pathogenesis of thyroid nodules? J Endocrinol. 2013;218:125–33.
17. Gao M, Chen W, Sun H, Fan L, Wang W, Du C, Chen Y, Lin L, Pearce EN, Shen J, Cheng Y, Wang C, Zhang W. Excessive iodine intake is associated with formation of thyroid nodules in pregnant Chinese women. Nutr Res. 2019;66:61–7.
18. Shokri S, Hekmatnia A, Farghadani M, Aminorroaya A, Amini M, Kianpour M, Akbari M, Hekmatnia F. Thyroid volume and nodular and diffuse thyroid diseases by ultrasonography in pregnant women: a case-control study. J Res Med Sci. 2020;25:13.
19. Karger S, Schötz S, Stumvoll M, Berger F, Führer D. Impact of pregnancy on prevalence of goitre and nodular thyroid disease in women living in a region of borderline sufficient iodine supply. Horm Metab Res. 2010;42:137–42.
20. Sahin SB, Ogullar S, Ural UM, Ilkkilic K, Metin Y, Ayaz T. Alterations of thyroid volume and nodular size during and after pregnancy in a severe iodine-deficient area. Clin Endocrinol. 2014;81:762–8.
21. Alexander EK, Pearce EN, Brent GA, Brown RS, Chen H, Dosiou C, Grobman WA, Laurberg P, Lazarus JH, Mandel SJ, Peeters RP, Sullivan S. 2017 guidelines of the American Thyroid Association for the diagnosis and management of thyroid disease during pregnancy and the postpartum. Thyroid. 2017;27:315–89.
22. Moon HJ, Sung JM, Kim EK, Yoon JH, Youk JH, Kwak JY. Diagnostic performance of gray-scale US and elastography in solid thyroid nodules. Radiology. 2012;262:1002–13.
23. Grant EG, Tessler FN, Hoang JK, Langer JE, Beland MD, Berland LL, Cronan JJ, Desser TS, Frates MC, Hamper UM, Middleton WD, Reading CC, Scoutt LM, Stavros AT, Teefey SA. Thyroid ultrasound reporting Lexicon: white paper of the ACR Thyroid Imaging, Reporting and Data System (TIRADS) Committee. J Am Coll Radiol. 2015;12:1272–9.
24. Hoang JK, Middleton WD, Farjat AE, Teefey SA, Abinanti N, Boschini FJ, Bronner AJ, Dahiya N, Hertzberg BS, Newman JR, Scanga D, Vogler RC, Tessler FN. Interobserver vari-

ability of sonographic features used in the American College of Radiology thyroid imaging reporting and data system. AJR Am J Roentgenol. 2018;211:162–7.
25. Grani G, Lamartina L, Cantisani V, Maranghi M, Lucia P, Durante C. Interobserver agreement of various thyroid imaging reporting and data systems. Endocr Connect. 2018;7:1–7.
26. Yang R, Zou X, Zeng H, Zhao Y, Ma X. Comparison of diagnostic performance of five different ultrasound TI-RADS classification guidelines for thyroid nodules. Front Oncol. 2020;10:598225.
27. Belfiore A, La Rosa GL. Fine-needle aspiration biopsy of the thyroid. Endocrinol Metab Clin North Am. 2001;30:361–400.
28. Goellner JR, Gharib H, Grant CS, Johnson DA. Fine needle aspiration cytology of the thyroid, 1980 to 1986. Acta Cytol. 1987;31:587–90.
29. Choe W, McDougall IR. Thyroid cancer in pregnant women: diagnostic and therapeutic management. Thyroid. 1994;4:433–5.
30. Angell TE, Maurer R, Wang Z, Kim MI, Alexander CA, Barletta JA, Benson CB, Cibas ES, Cho NL, Doherty GM, Doubilet PM, Frates MC, Gawande AA, Krane JF, Marqusee E, Moore FD, Nehs MA, Larsen PR, Alexander EK. A cohort analysis of clinical and ultrasound variables predicting cancer risk in 20,001 consecutive thyroid nodules. J Clin Endocrinol Metab. 2019;104:5665–72.
31. Marley EF, Oertel YC. Fine-needle aspiration of thyroid lesions in 57 pregnant and postpartum women. Diagn Cytopathol. 1997;16:122–5.
32. Tan GH, Gharib H, Goellner JR, van Heerden JA, Bahn RS. Management of thyroid nodules in pregnancy. Arch Intern Med. 1996;156:2317–20.
33. Bongiovanni M, Crippa S, Baloch Z, Piana S, Spitale A, Pagni F, Mazzucchelli L, Di Bella C, Faquin W. Comparison of 5-tiered and 6-tiered diagnostic systems for the reporting of thyroid cytopathology: a multi-institutional study. Cancer Cytopathol. 2012;120:117–25.
34. Cibas ES, Ali SZ. The 2017 Bethesda system for reporting thyroid cytopathology. Thyroid. 2017;27:1341–6.
35. Durante C, Grani G, Lamartina L, Filetti S, Mandel SJ, Cooper DS. The diagnosis and management of thyroid nodules: a review. JAMA. 2018;319:914–24.
36. Tumino D, Grani G, Di Stefano M, Di Mauro M, Scutari M, Rago T, Fugazzola L, Castagna MG, Maino F. Nodular thyroid disease in the era of precision medicine. Front Endocrinol (Lausanne). 2020;10:907.
37. Nikiforov YE, Ohori NP, Hodak SP, Carty SE, LeBeau SO, Ferris RL, Yip L, Seethala RR, Tublin ME, Stang MT, Coyne C, Johnson JT, Stewart AF, Nikiforova MN. Impact of mutational testing on the diagnosis and management of patients with cytologically indeterminate thyroid nodules: a prospective analysis of 1056 FNA samples. J Clin Endocrinol Metab. 2011;96:3390–7.
38. Alexander EK, Schorr M, Klopper J, Kim C, Sipos J, Nabhan F, Parker C, Steward DL, Mandel SJ, Haugen BR. Multicenter clinical experience with the Afirma gene expression classifier. J Clin Endocrinol Metab. 2014;99:119–25.
39. Angell TE. RAS-positive thyroid nodules. Curr Opin Endocrinol Diabetes Obes. 2017; 24:372–6.
40. Medici M, Kwong N, Angell TE, Marqusee E, Kim MI, Frates MC, Benson CB, Cibas ES, Barletta JA, Krane JF, Ruan DT, Cho NL, Gawande AA, Moore FD Jr, Alexander EK. The variable phenotype and low-risk nature of RAS-positive thyroid nodules. BMC Med. 2015;13:184.
41. Steward DL, Carty SE, Sippel RS, Yang SP, Sosa JA, Sipos JA, Figge JJ, Mandel S, Haugen BR, Burman KD, Baloch ZW, Lloyd RV, Seethala RR, Gooding WE, Chiosea SI, Gomes-Lima C, Ferris RL, Folek JM, Khawaja RA, Kundra P, Loh KS, Marshall CB, Mayson S, McCoy KL, Nga ME, Ngiam KY, Nikiforova MN, Poehls JL, Ringel MD, Yang H, Yip L, Nikiforov YE. Performance of a multigene genomic classifier in thyroid nodules with indeterminate cytology: a prospective blinded multicenter study. JAMA Oncol. 2019;5:204–12.
42. Patel KN, Angell TE, Babiarz J, Barth NM, Blevins T, Duh QY, Ghossein RA, Harrell RM, Huang J, Kennedy GC, Kim SY, Kloos RT, LiVolsi VA, Randolph GW, Sadow PM, Shanik

MH, Sosa JA, Traweek ST, Walsh PS, Whitney D, Yeh MW, Ladenson PW. Performance of a genomic sequencing classifier for the preoperative diagnosis of cytologically indeterminate thyroid nodules. JAMA Surg. 2018;153:817–24.
43. Lupo MA, Walts AE, Sistrunk JW, Giordano TJ, Sadow PM, Massoll N, Campbell R, Jackson SA, Toney N, Narick CM, Kumar G, Mireskandari A, Finkelstein SD, Bose S. Multiplatform molecular test performance in indeterminate thyroid nodules. Diagn Cytopathol. 2020;48:1254–64.
44. Moosa M, Mazzaferri EL. Outcome of differentiated thyroid cancer diagnosed in pregnant women. J Clin Endocrinol Metab. 1997;82:2862–6.
45. Liu X, Medici M, Kwong N, Angell TE, Marqusee E, Kim MI, Larsen PR, Cho NL, Nehs MA, Ruan DT, Gawande A, Moore F Jr, Barletta J, Krane JF, Cibas ES, Yang T, Alexander EK. Bethesda categorization of thyroid nodule cytology and prediction of thyroid cancer type and prognosis. Thyroid. 2016;26:256–61.
46. Kuy S, Roman SA, Desai R, Sosa JA. Outcomes following thyroid and parathyroid surgery in pregnant women. Arch Surg. 2009;144:399–406; discussion 406.
47. Uruno T, Shibuya H, Kitagawa W, Nagahama M, Sugino K, Ito K. Optimal timing of surgery for differentiated thyroid cancer in pregnant women. World J Surg. 2014;38:704–8.
48. Boucek J, de Haan J, Halaska MJ, Plzak J, Van Calsteren K, de Groot CJM, Dahl Steffensen K, Fruscio R, Massolt ET, Klaritsch P, Zola P, Amant F, International Network on Cancer, Infertility, and Pregnancy. Maternal and obstetrical outcome in 35 cases of well-differentiated thyroid carcinoma during pregnancy. Laryngoscope. 2018;128:1493–500.
49. Smith LH, Danielsen B, Allen ME, Cress R. Cancer associated with obstetric delivery: results of linkage with the California cancer registry. Am J Obstet Gynecol. 2003;189:1128–35.
50. Lee JC, Zhao JT, Clifton-Bligh RJ, Gill AJ, Gundara JS, Ip J, Sywak MS, Delbridge LW, Robinson BG, Sidhu SB. Papillary thyroid carcinoma in pregnancy: a variant of the disease? Ann Surg Oncol. 2012;19:4210–6.
51. Cottreau CM, Dashevsky I, Andrade SE, Li DK, Nekhlyudov L, Raebel MA, Ritzwoller DP, Partridge AH, Pawloski PA, Toh S. Pregnancy-associated cancer: a U.S. population-based study. J Womens Health (Larchmt). 2019;28:250–7.
52. Herzon FS, Morris DM, Segal MN, Rauch G, Parnell T. Coexistent thyroid cancer and pregnancy. Arch Otolaryngol Head Neck Surg. 1994;120:1191–3.
53. Yasmeen S, Cress R, Romano PS, Xing G, Berger-Chen S, Danielsen B, Smith LH. Thyroid cancer in pregnancy. Int J Gynaecol Obstet. 2005;91:15–20.
54. Chen AC, Livhits MJ, Du L, Wu JX, Kuo EJ, Yeh MW, Leung AM. Recent pregnancy is not associated with high-risk pathological features of well-differentiated thyroid cancer. Thyroid. 2018;28:68–71.
55. Vannucchi G, Perrino M, Rossi S, Colombo C, Vicentini L, Dazzi D, Beck-Peccoz P, Fugazzola L. Clinical and molecular features of differentiated thyroid cancer diagnosed during pregnancy. Eur J Endocrinol. 2010;162:145–51.
56. Messuti I, Corvisieri S, Bardesono F, Rapa I, Giorcelli J, Pellerito R, Volante M, Orlandi F. Impact of pregnancy on prognosis of differentiated thyroid cancer: clinical and molecular features. Eur J Endocrinol. 2014;170:659–66.
57. Vannucchi G, De Leo S, Perrino M, Rossi S, Tosi D, Cirello V, Colombo C, Bulfamante G, Vicentini L, Fugazzola L. Impact of estrogen and progesterone receptor expression on the clinical and molecular features of papillary thyroid cancer. Eur J Endocrinol. 2015;173:29–36.
58. Oh HS, Kim WG, Park S, Kim M, Kwon H, Jeon MJ, Lee JH, Baek JH, Song DE, Kim TY, Shong YK, Kim WB. Serial neck ultrasonographic evaluation of changes in papillary thyroid carcinoma during pregnancy. Thyroid. 2017;27:773–7.
59. Ito Y, Miyauchi A, Kudo T, Ota H, Yoshioka K, Oda H, Sasai H, Nakayama A, Yabuta T, Masuoka H, Fukushima M, Higashiyama T, Kihara M, Kobayashi K, Miya A. Effects of pregnancy on papillary microcarcinomas of the thyroid re-evaluated in the entire patient series at Kuma hospital. Thyroid. 2016;26:156–60.

60. Lechner MG, Bernardo AC, Lampe A, Praw SS, Tam SH, Angell TE. Changes in stage distribution and disease-specific survival in differentiated thyroid cancer with transition to American Joint Committee on Cancer 8th edition: a systematic review and meta-analysis. Oncologist. 2021;26(2):e251–60.
61. Webb RC, Howard RS, Stojadinovic A, Gaitonde DY, Wallace MK, Ahmed J, Burch HB. The utility of serum thyroglobulin measurement at the time of remnant ablation for predicting disease-free status in patients with differentiated thyroid cancer: a meta-analysis involving 3947 patients. J Clin Endocrinol Metab. 2012;97:2754–63.
62. Spencer CA, Takeuchi M, Kazarosyan M, Wang CC, Guttler RB, Singer PA, Fatemi S, LoPresti JS, Nicoloff JT. Serum thyroglobulin autoantibodies: prevalence, influence on serum thyroglobulin measurement, and prognostic significance in patients with differentiated thyroid carcinoma. J Clin Endocrinol Metab. 1998;83:1121–7.
63. Rakhlin L, Fish S, Tuttle RM. Response to therapy status is an excellent predictor of pregnancy-associated structural disease progression in patients previously treated for differentiated thyroid cancer. Thyroid. 2017;27:396–401.
64. Hirsch D, Levy S, Tsvetov G, Weinstein R, Lifshitz A, Singer J, Shraga-Slutzky I, Grozinski-Glasberg S, Shimon I, Benbassat C. Impact of pregnancy on outcome and prognosis of survivors of papillary thyroid cancer. Thyroid. 2010;20:1179–85.
65. Xi C, Zhang Q, Song HJ, Shen CT, Zhang GQ, Sun JW, Qiu ZL, Luo QY. Pregnancy does not affect the prognoses of differentiated thyroid cancer patients with lung metastases. J Clin Endocrinol Metab. 2021;106(8):e3185–97.
66. Budak A, Gulhan I, Aldemir OS, Ileri A, Tekin E, Ozeren M. Lack of influence of pregnancy on the prognosis of survivors of thyroid cancer. Asian Pac J Cancer Prev. 2013;14:6941–3.
67. Nguyen CT, Singer PA. A challenging case of progression of persistent structural disease in pregnancy. In: the 89th annual meeting of the American Thyroid Association. 10/30/2019-11/3/2019. Chicago, IL.
68. Korevaar TIM, Medici M, Visser TJ, Peeters RP. Thyroid disease in pregnancy: new insights in diagnosis and clinical management. Nat Rev Endocrinol. 2017;13:610–22.
69. Alexander EK, Marqusee E, Lawrence J, Jarolim P, Fischer GA, Larsen PR. Timing and magnitude of increases in levothyroxine requirements during pregnancy in women with hypothyroidism. N Engl J Med. 2004;351:241–9.
70. Zhang X, Li C, Mao J, Wang W, Xie X, Peng S, Wang Z, Han C, Zhang X, Wang D, Fan C, Shan Z, Teng W. Gestation-specific changes in maternal thyroglobulin during pregnancy and lactation in an iodine-sufficient region in China: a longitudinal study. Clin Endocrinol. 2017;86:229–35.
71. Garsi JP, Schlumberger M, Rubino C, Ricard M, Labbé M, Ceccarelli C, Schvartz C, Henri-Amar M, Bardet S, de Vathaire F. Therapeutic administration of 131I for differentiated thyroid cancer: radiation dose to ovaries and outcome of pregnancies. J Nucl Med. 2008;49: 845–52.
72. Sawka AM, Lakra DC, Lea J, Alshehri B, Tsang RW, Brierley JD, Straus S, Thabane L, Gafni A, Ezzat S, George SR, Goldstein DP. A systematic review examining the effects of therapeutic radioactive iodine on ovarian function and future pregnancy in female thyroid cancer survivors. Clin Endocrinol. 2008;69:479–90.
73. Wu JX, Young S, Ro K, Li N, Leung AM, Chiu HK, Harari A, Yeh MW. Reproductive outcomes and nononcologic complications after radioactive iodine ablation for well-differentiated thyroid cancer. Thyroid. 2015;25:133–8.
74. Ko KY, Yen RF, Lin CL, Cheng MF, Huang WS, Kao CH. Pregnancy outcome after I-131 therapy for patients with thyroid cancer: a nationwide population-based cohort study. Medicine (Baltimore). 2016;95:e2685.
75. Anderson C, Engel SM, Weaver MA, Zevallos JP, Nichols HB. Birth rates after radioactive iodine treatment for differentiated thyroid cancer. Int J Cancer. 2017;141:2291–5.
76. Piek MW, Postma EL, van Leeuwaarde R, de Boer JP, Bos AME, Lok C, Stokkel M, Filipe MD, van der Ploeg IMC. The effect of radioactive iodine therapy on ovarian function and

fertility in female thyroid cancer patients: a systematic review and meta-analysis. Thyroid. 2021;31:658–68.
77. Acıbucu F, Acıbucu DO, Akkar ÖB, Dokmetas HS. Evaluation of ovarian reserve with AMH level in patients with well-differentiated thyroid cancer receiving radioactive iodine ablation treatment. Exp Clin Endocrinol Diabetes. 2016;124:593–6.
78. Evranos B, Faki S, Polat SB, Bestepe N, Ersoy R, Cakir B. Effects of radioactive iodine therapy on ovarian reserve: a prospective pilot study. Thyroid. 2018;28:1702–7.
79. Yaish I, Azem F, Gutfeld O, Silman Z, Serebro M, Sharon O, Shefer G, Limor R, Stern N, Tordjman KM. A single radioactive iodine treatment has a deleterious effect on ovarian reserve in women with thyroid cancer: results of a prospective pilot study. Thyroid. 2018;28:522–7.
80. van Velsen EFS, Visser WE, van den Berg SAA, Kam BLR, van Ginhoven TM, Massolt ET, Peeters RP. Longitudinal analysis of the effect of radioiodine therapy on ovarian reserve in females with differentiated thyroid cancer. Thyroid. 2020;30:580–7.
81. Giusti M, Mittica M, Comite P, Campana C, Gay S, Mussap M. Anti-Müllerian hormone in pre-menopausal females after ablative radioiodine treatment for differentiated thyroid cancer. Endocrine. 2018;60:516–23.
82. Mittica M, Dotto A, Comina M, Teliti M, Monti E, Giusti M. Cross-sectional and prospective study on anti-Müllerian hormone changes in a cohort of pre-menopausal women with a history of differentiated thyroid cancer. Thyroid Res. 2020;13:1.

Postpartum Thyroiditis: Diagnosis and Management

Caroline T. Nguyen

Definition

In 1948, Roberton first reported on the frequent occurrence of hypothyroidism in the postpartum period [1]. However, it was not until the 1970s when physicians increasingly reported the observation of postpartum thyroid dysfunction in the literature [2, 3]. In 1982, the seminal paper by Amino et al. drew attention to the entity of postpartum thyroiditis (PPT), defined as transient new onset thyroid dysfunction occurring in the first year postpartum with the majority of patients returning to a euthyroid state by the end of the first postpartum year. The authors reported a 5% prevalence and speculated that PPT had to do with the immunologic changes associated with pregnancy [4].

Epidemiology

More than two decades and several studies later, the prevalence of PPT ranges from 1 to 22% in the literature, but is generally accepted to be about 5%. Such variation in prevalence is due to factors such as study design, definition of PPT, hormone assay methodology, and frequency of screening [5–9]. Affecting 1 in 20 women in the postpartum period, PPT is one of the most common endocrine conditions affecting women.

C. T. Nguyen (✉)
Division of Endocrinology, Diabetes, and Metabolism, Keck School of Medicine, University of Southern California, Los Angeles, CA, USA
e-mail: Caroline.Nguyen@med.usc.edu

F. Azizi, F. Ramezani Tehrani (eds.), *Thyroid Diseases in Pregnancy*,
https://doi.org/10.1007/978-3-030-98777-0_14

Etiology

The data suggests PPT is most likely an autoimmune-mediated destructive thyroiditis [10]. There is a strong association with thyroid antibody positivity, both thyroid peroxidase antibody (TPOAb) as well as thyroglobulin antibody (TgAb) [11] with higher antibody levels being associated with an increased risk [5, 12]. A pregnant woman with TPO Ab+ in early pregnancy has up to a 50% chance of developing PPT [12–14]. There is an association between PPT and HLA haplotypes consistent with autoimmune thyroid disease [15–17]. Furthermore, PPT occurs in the postpartum period, a time of immune reconstitution and rise of antibody titers after immune suppression during pregnancy. PPT has been associated with both humoral and cellular immune reactions including lymphocyte changes, complement activation, dynamic changes in TPO IgG subtypes, and increased natural killer (NK) and cytotoxic T cells [18–23]. Histologically, PPT is similar to Hashimoto's thyroiditis, characterized by chronic lymphocytic infiltration and tissue injury [24].

Clinical Presentation

While PPT typically occurs in the early postpartum period, PPT can occur after a spontaneous or induced abortion as well [2, 25, 26]. The immunologic changes that occur after a termination of a pregnancy are similar to those during the postpartum period. Furthermore, women taking levothyroxine therapy (LT4) for mild hypothyroidism [27–29] can develop PPT if there is sufficient functional parenchymal thyroid tissue remaining. Women with a history of Graves' disease (GD) prior to pregnancy or during pregnancy can also develop PPT [30].

Similar to other types of thyroiditis, PPT may present in approximately 25% of cases with a classic biphasic presentation consisting of transient thyrotoxicosis occurring rather abruptly between 2 and 4 months postpartum due to release of preformed thyroid hormone from the gland, followed by a hypothyroid phase 4–6 months postpartum with eventual restoration to a euthyroid state by 7–12 months postpartum. The most common presentation which occurs in 50% of cases of PPT consists of a transient hypothyroid phase occurring between 3 and 7 months. The remainder of patients present with isolated transient thyrotoxicosis beginning between 2 and 4 months postpartum (Fig. 1) [5]. Most patients with PPT will return to a euthyroid state by the end of 12 months [32, 33]. However, the incidence of persistent hypothyroidism at 12 months has ranged from 0.1 to 50% in the literature [18, 32, 34].

Patients presenting with thyrotoxicosis may have a non-tender goiter and symptoms such as fatigue, palpitations, heat-intolerance, or increased irritability [5, 8, 35]. The symptoms tend to be relatively mild. Symptoms of hypothyroidism can include fatigue, impaired memory or concentration, dry skin, muscle aches, cold intolerance, hair changes, and difficulty losing weight and may be more clinically significant [35].

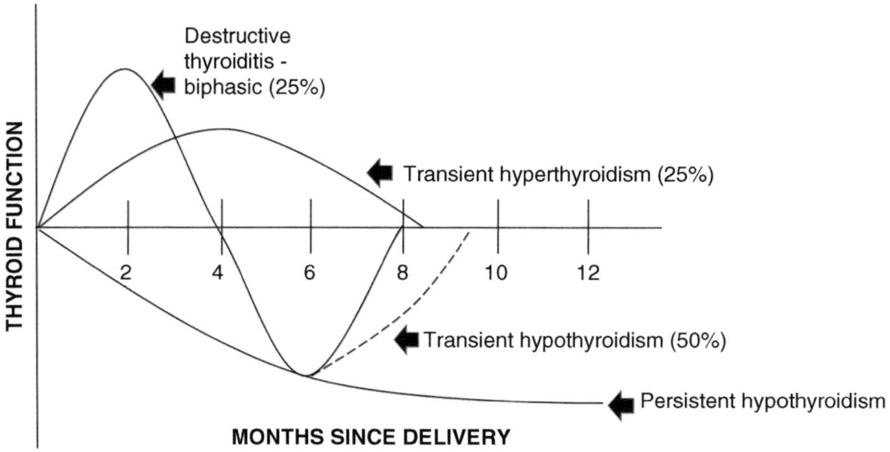

Fig. 1 The varying clinical courses of postpartum thyroiditis. Roughly 50% present with transient hypothyroidism, 25% with transient hyperthyroidism, and 25% with biphasic destructive thyroiditis [31]

PPT and Postpartum Depression

The relationship between PPT and postpartum depression remains unclear. The symptoms for PPT can overlap with those for postpartum depression. While some studies have shown an increased prevalence of depression in women with PPT compared to controls [36–38], other studies have not shown an association [8, 39, 40]. In a recent population-based study of over 300,000 people, the rate of first-onset psychiatric disorders was higher in women with first-onset autoimmune thyroid disease postpartum compared to those without postpartum autoimmune disease (RR 1.88 CI 1.25–2.81). The study reported that the comorbidity index, or likelihood of co-occurrence of these two events was 2.26 times as common than if they were independent events [41]. Treatment with LT4 in a prospective randomized control study did not show an effect on the rate of postpartum depression in patients with TPOAb+ [42]. All patients with depression should be screened for thyroid dysfunction [32].

Thyroid Dysfunction and Breastfeeding

Hyperthyroidism and hypothyroidism can potentially impact milk letdown and inhibit successful breastfeeding. The data is sparse consisting mainly of case studies. Nevertheless, thyroid function should be evaluated in women experiencing poor lactation as the general recommendation is to treat women with hypothyroidism.

While antithyroid drugs (ATDs) are safe in lactating women [43, 44], ATDs are not used in the treatment of the thyrotoxic phase of PPT as it is a destructive thyroiditis [32].

Laboratory Studies

Thyroid function tests correspond to the phase of PPT and are helpful in making the diagnosis. During the thyrotoxic phase, TSH is suppressed with moderately elevated thyroxine (T4) levels. During the hypothyroid phase, T4 and triiodothyronine (T3) are low. TSH may "lag" and remain suppressed in the hypothyroid phase before rising. In addition, TSH can be suppressed with normal T4 and T3 during the transition between the thyrotoxic and hypothyroid phases in the biphasic course [45]. TPOAb is positive in the majority of patients. TgAb may also be positive. Third-generation TSH-receptor antibody (TRAb) assay or thyroid-stimulating immunoglobulin (TSI), involved in the pathogenesis of GD are not generally present in PPT unless the patient had a prior history of GD. Levels of thyroglobulin (Tg), a protein made by thyroid follicular cells and a substrate for the synthesis of thyroid hormones, may be elevated during the thyrotoxic phase although is not typically used in the diagnosis of PPT.

Ultrasound

The diagnosis of PPT is generally made using the history and physical along with the laboratory findings. However, ultrasound (US) findings have been described that may be helpful [46]. The thyroid blood flow in PPT will typically be low [47]. Hypoechogenicity has been associated with PPT. In one study, hypoechogenicity was present in 98.5% of patients with PPT compared to 7% in the control group ($p < 0.001$). Mean thyroid volume at the time of diagnosis was 77% greater in those with PPT than in the control group [48]. In another study evaluating women who did not have detectable antibodies, US revealed evidence of thyroiditis in 60% of women who developed PPT compared to 21% in those who did not develop PPT [6].

Differential Diagnosis

The thyrotoxic phase of PPT can present similarly to thyrotoxicosis due to GD, which can recur or present for the first time in the postpartum period. However, the frequency of GD in the postpartum period is significantly lower than that of PPT, affecting 0.54% of the population [49]. Nevertheless, diagnosis is challenging because PPT can affect patients with a history of GD [30]. Distinguishing between

Table 1 Graves' disease compared to postpartum thyroiditis (PPT)

	Graves' disease	Postpartum thyroiditis (PPT)
Onset	3–12 months	1–6 months
Physical exam	Goiter Thyroid bruit Graves' ophthalmopathy	Goiter +/–
Symptoms	Moderate/Severe	Mild
Labs	Total T3/total T4 > 20 FT3/FT4 > 2.8 TSH-receptor antibody +	<20 FT3/FT4 < 2.8 TSH-receptor antibody –
Thyroid blood flow	High	Low
Radioactive iodine uptake	High	Low

PPT and GD is important because the clinical course and management of the two conditions differ (Table 1). Patients with GD will require treatment with antithyroid drugs (ATDs) and possible definitive treatment with radioactive iodine or surgery. Patients with PPT may require no treatment at all.

The timing of onset of symptoms may be helpful. In one study, 86% of patients who presented with thyrotoxicosis within the first 3 months had PPT while all patients who developed thyrotoxicosis symptoms after 6.5 months had GD [47]. The symptoms of hyperthyroidism are generally more mild in PPT compared to GD. Physical exam findings diagnostic of GD include Graves' ophthalmopathy or visible goiter with thyroid bruit.

As stated above, TRAb or TSI titers are elevated in patients with GD and typically undetectable in patients with PPT. A T3:T4 ratio <20 is more suggestive of PPT, which consists of release of preformed thyroid hormone compared to GD where T3 is preferentially elevated [50]. The use of FT3:FT4 is less well established. In one study the FT3:FT4 ratio of those with PPT was statistically lower than those with GD, with all patients with PPT having a ratio <3.2 [30]. FT3:FT4 <2.8 has also been used [18].

Thyroid blood flow on ultrasonography is high in patients with GD and low in PPT [47]. If the diagnosis remains unclear, a radioactive iodine uptake (RAIU) can help establish the diagnosis although this is rarely necessary with the current sensitive and specific TRAB/TSI assays. If a RAIU is performed, the uptake will be low in PPT compared to normal or elevated in women with GD. Women who receive ^{123}-I or technetium (Tc-99m) scans should discard breastmilk for several days after the study [32]. ^{131}-I is contraindicated in women who are breastfeeding.

Permanent Hypothyroidism

The prevalence of permanent hypothyroidism 12 months after delivery ranges from 2 to 54% [6, 34, 51]. Long-term data of permanent hypothyroidism has been more consistent [51–54]. At 3–12 years postpartum, the incidence of permanent hypothyroidism is 30–50% [45, 55]. Higher titers of thyroid antibodies and TSH levels during the initial hypothyroid phase, greater maternal age, multiparity, history of pregnancy loss, and greater degree of thyroid hypoechogenicity on ultrasound have been associated with an increased risk for developing permanent hypothyroidism [5, 51–54, 56].

Treatment

While most cases of PPT resolve spontaneously, treatment may be indicated for symptomatic patients for symptom relief. B-blockers such as propranolol or metoprolol are effective at controlling adrenergic symptoms. In women who are breastfeeding, the lowest dose necessary to alleviate symptoms should be used. Atenolol is avoided as it is more highly protein-bound and may concentrate in breast milk. At high doses, atenolol has been associated with bradycardia and hypoglycemia in infants [57]. ATDs are not effective to treat the thyrotoxicosis phase of PPT which is due to a destructive thyroiditis and the release of preformed thyroid hormone rather than increased thyroid hormone production. In patients who become euthyroid after the thyrotoxic phase, TSH should be checked in 4–8 weeks to screen for hypothyroidism [32].

Women with significant hypothyroid symptoms or women attempting pregnancy or breastfeeding should be treated with levothyroxine (LT4) 50–100 mcg/day and adjusted as needed for symptom relief. Treatment can then be gradually weaned at approximately 12 months to see whether patients have had resolution of the thyroiditis and return to a euthyroid state [5]. Treatment should not be weaned if a patient is attempting pregnancy or is again pregnant. Women who are successfully weaned off of LT4 should have their TSH checked annually as the rate for permanent hypothyroidism is high several years after PPT as reported above. In addition, women with subclinical hypothyroidism in the postpartum period should also be followed closely as they are at increased risk for permanent hypothyroidism as well [45].

One paper has suggested T3 as a treatment alternative. The premise is to use a submaximal dose of triiodothyronine (T3) that will provide symptom relief but enable FT4 levels to rise, signifying spontaneous recovery of thyroid function [18]. There are no randomized controlled trials assessing treatment options for PPT. At this time, the data on using T3 is sparse. If the patient is not treated with thyroid hormone, thyroid function should be checked periodically until euthyroidism is restored and women should be counseled on use of contraception until euthyroid.

Risk Factors

As stated above, 30–50% of TPOAb+ women will develop PPT with higher TPOAb titers in the first trimester associated with greater risk of development [12, 58]. Two studies from Italy report rates as high as 60–70% [6, 9]. Accordingly, the majority of women who develop PPT have positive TPOAb [7]. However, in one study 15% of women who develop PPT had isolated TgAb and 5% may have neither TPOAb or TgAb [6].

The incidence of PPT is higher in women with autoimmune diseases. Women with Type 1 diabetes mellitus (T1DM) have incidence rates 3–4 times that of women in the general population [59–61]. The incidence of PPT is also higher in women with systemic lupus erythematous [62], Sjogren's syndrome [63], and chronic viral hepatitis [64]. The prevalence of PPT in women who have a prior history of GD is reported to be 44% [30]. Interestingly, an increased incidence of PPT has also been described in patients with gestational diabetes compared to healthy pregnant women 19.6% vs 10.2% respectively [65].

As stated above, PPT can occur in women who have hypothyroidism on treatment antedating pregnancy. In a recent study by Moleti et al. women with Hashimoto's disease (HD) who were euthyroid on no treatment in the first trimester compared to women with HD who were hypothyroid on levothyroxine in the first trimester had four times higher risk of PPT. This suggest that the risk of PPT depends on the amount of thyroid gland that is unaffected by HD [29].

A study evaluating recurrent episodes of PPT found that women who have had an episode of PPT have a 70% chance of developing PPT in subsequent pregnancies. Women who were TPO Ab+ and euthyroid after their first pregnancy still have a 25% risk of developing PPT in a future pregnancy [66].

Prevention

Treatment with levothyroxine or iodine during pregnancy or in the postpartum period have not been effective at reducing the incidence of PPT as demonstrated by two randomized placebo-controlled trials [67, 68]. One randomized controlled study showed that selenium supplementation of 200 mg daily reduced TPOAb levels and the incidence of PPT and hypothyroidism in women treated compared to those taking placebo [69]. Mantovani et al. showed selenium decreased TPOAb levels [70]. However, a smaller randomized controlled study did not show that low dose selenium of 60 mg per day had any effect on TPOAb levels throughout pregnancy compared to placebo [71]. The latter two studies looked at TPOAb status but not PPT incidence. Currently, the data is insufficient to recommend routine selenium supplementation during pregnancy especially because treatment may not be harmless. Selenium use has been associated with an increased risk of DM2 [72, 73].

Vitamin D supplementation has been shown in one study to decrease antibody titers in women with a history of PPT with either normal or deficient vitamin D levels [74]. However, whether vitamin D supplementation can reduce the risk of PPT or permanent hypothyroidism remains to be studied. Another study found that consuming oily fish high in omega-3 compared to larger predator fish such as swordfish was associated with lower TPOAb levels. The authors speculated that it may have to do with larger fish having higher levels of immunotoxicants such as mercury and other pollutants [75]. The incidence of PPT was not measured in this study.

Conclusion

PPT is a common endocrine condition that can be easily missed. PPT can occur in women with no history of thyroid disease and symptoms of thyroid dysfunction can overlap with new motherhood or postpartum depression. However, diagnosis is important because effectively treating women who are symptomatic will help them feel better during a critical time in their lives. In addition, women with a history of PPT should have their thyroid function monitored as they are at high risk to develop permanent hypothyroidism and recurrence of PPT in future pregnancies. Distinguishing between PPT and GD is key as the latter requires treatment with ATD while ATD are not helpful in treating PPT. By being aware of the risk factors, clinical course, and progression of PPT, a physician can provide symptom relief, avoid unnecessary use of ATD, and counsel patients in order to optimize thyroid function for future pregnancies.

Summary

Physicians caring for patients who are pregnant or have a desire to become pregnant need to be aware of risk factors for postpartum thyroiditis (PPT) such as + TPO Ab status, history of autoimmune disease, and history of hypothyroidism not on full replacement levothyroxine. By understanding the clinical course, which can vary from hyperthyroidism to hypothyroidism and span a year's time, a physician can help counsel the patient in regard to expectations and appropriate monitoring. Patients with a history of PPT need to be counseled on the increased risk of subsequent episodes with future pregnancies and have their thyroid hormone levels checked prior to future pregnancy as some may remain hypothyroid. Although PPT affects 5% of women, the diagnosis is missed because signs and symptoms are often attributed to new motherhood. All mothers with symptoms of postpartum depression should be evaluated for thyroid dysfunction. Educating patients on the signs and symptoms of PPT and encouraging them to speak to their physicians will facilitate early diagnosis and symptomatic treatment if needed.

References

1. Hew R. Lassitude, coldness, and hair changes following pregnancy, and their response to treatment with thyroid extract. Br Med J. 1948;2 Suppl:2275–6.
2. Amino N, Miyai K, Kuro R, Tanizawa O, Azukizawa M, Takai S, et al. Transient postpartum hypothyroidism: fourteen cases with autoimmune thyroiditis. Ann Intern Med. 1977;87(2):155–9.
3. Ginsberg J, Walfish PG. Post-partum transient thyrotoxicosis with painless thyroiditis. Lancet. 1977;1(8022):1125–8.

4. Amino N, Mori H, Iwatani Y, Tanizawa O, Kawashima M, Tsuge I, et al. High prevalence of transient post-partum thyrotoxicosis and hypothyroidism. N Engl J Med. 1982;306(14):849–52.
5. Stagnaro-Green A. Approach to the patient with postpartum thyroiditis. J Clin Endocrinol Metab. 2012;97(2):334–42.
6. Benvenga S, Di Bari F, Vita R, Le Donne M, Triolo O, Granese R, et al. Relatively high rate of postpartum thyroiditis in the straits of Messina area. Predictivity of both postpartum thyroiditis and permanent hypothyroidism by performing, in the first trimester of gestation, thyroid ultrasonography and measurement of serum thyroperoxidase and thyroglobulin autoantibodies. J Clin Transl Endocrinol. 2019;15:12–8.
7. Nicholson WK, Robinson KA, Smallridge RC, Ladenson PW, Powe NR. Prevalence of postpartum thyroid dysfunction: a quantitative review. Thyroid. 2006;16(6):573–82.
8. Walfish PG, Meyerson J, Provias JP, Vargas MT, Papsin FR. Prevalence and characteristics of post-partum thyroid dysfunction: results of a survey from Toronto, Canada. J Endocrinol Invest. 1992;15(4):265–72.
9. Filippi U, Brizzolara R, Venuti D, Cesarone A, Maritati VA, Podestà M, et al. Prevalence of post-partum thyroiditis in Liguria (Italy): an observational study. J Endocrinol Invest. 2008;31(12):1063–8.
10. Weetman AP. Immunity, thyroid function and pregnancy: molecular mechanisms. Nat Rev Endocrinol. 2010;6(6):311–8.
11. Muller AF, Drexhage HA, Berghout A. Postpartum thyroiditis and autoimmune thyroiditis in women of childbearing age: recent insights and consequences for antenatal and postnatal care. Endocr Rev. 2001;22(5):605–30.
12. Premawardhana LD, Parkes AB, John R, Harris B, Lazarus JH. Thyroid peroxidase antibodies in early pregnancy: utility for prediction of postpartum thyroid dysfunction and implications for screening. Thyroid. 2004;14(8):610–5.
13. Lazarus JH. Prediction of postpartum thyroiditis. Eur J Endocrinol. 1998;139(1):12–3.
14. Weetman AP. Prediction of post-partum thyroiditis. Clin Endocrinol. 1994;41(1):7–8.
15. Jansson R, Säfwenberg J, Dahlberg PA. Influence of the HLA-DR4 antigen and iodine status on the development of autoimmune postpartum thyroiditis. J Clin Endocrinol Metab. 1985;60(1):168–73.
16. Pryds O, Lervang HH, Kristensen HP, Jakobsen BK, Svejgaard A. HLA-DR factors associated with postpartum hypothyroidism: an early manifestation of Hashimoto's thyroiditis? Tissue Antigens. 1987;30(1):34–7.
17. Vargas MT, Briones-Urbina R, Gladman D, Papsin FR, Walfish PG. Antithyroid microsomal autoantibodies and HLA-DR5 are associated with postpartum thyroid dysfunction: evidence supporting an autoimmune pathogenesis. J Clin Endocrinol Metab. 1988;67(2):327–33.
18. Amino N, Arata N. Thyroid dysfunction following pregnancy and implications for breastfeeding. Best Pract Res Clin Endocrinol Metab. 2020;34(4):101438.
19. Stagnaro-Green A, Roman SH, Cobin RH, el-Harazy E, Wallenstein S, Davies TF. A prospective study of lymphocyte-initiated immunosuppression in normal pregnancy: evidence of a T-cell etiology for postpartum thyroid dysfunction. J Clin Endocrinol Metab. 1992;74(3):645–53.
20. Shi X, Li C, Li Y, Guan H, Fan C, Teng Y, et al. Circulating lymphocyte subsets and regulatory T cells in patients with postpartum thyroiditis during the first postpartum year. Clin Exp Med. 2009;9(4):263–7.
21. Teng D, Li C, Teng Y, Ouyang Y, Li Y, Teng W. Dynamic changes of IgG subtypes of thyroid peroxidase antibody in patients with postpartum thyroiditis. Gynecol Obstet Invest. 2010;69(1):24–9.
22. Kuijpens JL, De Hann-Meulman M, Vader HL, Pop VJ, Wiersinga WM, Drexhage HA. Cell-mediated immunity and postpartum thyroid dysfunction: a possibility for the prediction of disease? J Clin Endocrinol Metab. 1998;83(6):1959–66.
23. Amino N, Tada H, Hidaka Y. Postpartum autoimmune thyroid syndrome: a model of aggravation of autoimmune disease. Thyroid. 1999;9(7):705–13.

24. Mizukami Y, Michigishi T, Nonomura A, Hashimoto T, Nakamura S, Tonami N, et al. Postpartum thyroiditis. A clinical, histologic, and immunopathologic study of 15 cases. Am J Clin Pathol. 1993;100(3):200–5.
25. Stagnaro-Green A. Post-miscarriage thyroid dysfunction. Obstet Gynecol. 1992;80(3 Pt 2):490–2.
26. Marqusee E, Hill JA, Mandel SJ. Thyroiditis after pregnancy loss. J Clin Endocrinol Metab. 1997;82(8):2455–7.
27. Caixàs A, Albareda M, García-Patterson A, Rodríguez-Espinosa J, de Leiva A, Corcoy R. Postpartum thyroiditis in women with hypothyroidism antedating pregnancy? J Clin Endocrinol Metab. 1999;84(11):4000–5.
28. Sergi M, Tomlinson G, Feig DS. Changes suggestive of post-partum thyroiditis in women with established hypothyroidism: incidence and predictors. Clin Endocrinol. 2015;83(3):389–93.
29. Moleti M, Mauro MD, Alibrandi A, Vita R, Benvenga S, Vermiglio F. Postpartum thyroiditis in women with euthyroid and hypothyroid Hashimoto's thyroiditis antedating pregnancy. J Clin Endocrinol Metab. 2020;105(7):dgaa197.
30. Tagami T, Hagiwara H, Kimura T, Usui T, Shimatsu A, Naruse M. The incidence of gestational hyperthyroidism and postpartum thyroiditis in treated patients with Graves' disease. Thyroid. 2007;17(8):767–72.
31. Nguyen CT, Mestman JH. Postpartum thyroiditis. Clin Obstet Gynecol. 2019;62(2):359–64.
32. Alexander EK, Pearce EN, Brent GA, Brown RS, Chen H, Dosiou C, et al. 2017 guidelines of the American Thyroid Association for the diagnosis and management of thyroid disease during pregnancy and the postpartum. Thyroid. 2017;27(3):315–89.
33. Pearce EN, Farwell AP, Braverman LE. Thyroiditis. N Engl J Med. 2003;348(26):2646–55.
34. Stagnaro-Green A, Schwartz A, Gismondi R, Tinelli A, Mangieri T, Negro R. High rate of persistent hypothyroidism in a large-scale prospective study of postpartum thyroiditis in southern Italy. J Clin Endocrinol Metab. 2011;96(3):652–7.
35. Lazarus JH. Clinical manifestations of postpartum thyroid disease. Thyroid. 1999;9(7):685–9.
36. Harris B, Fung H, Johns S, Kologlu M, Bhatti R, McGregor AM, et al. Transient post-partum thyroid dysfunction and postnatal depression. J Affect Disord. 1989;17(3):243–9.
37. Hayslip CC, Fein HG, O'Donnell VM, Friedman DS, Klein TA, Smallridge RC. The value of serum antimicrosomal antibody testing in screening for symptomatic postpartum thyroid dysfunction. Am J Obstet Gynecol. 1988;159(1):203–9.
38. Pop VJ, de Rooy HA, Vader HL, van der Heide D, van Son M, Komproe IH, et al. Postpartum thyroid dysfunction and depression in an unselected population. N Engl J Med. 1991;324(25):1815–6.
39. Kent GN, Stuckey BG, Allen JR, Lambert T, Gee V. Postpartum thyroid dysfunction: clinical assessment and relationship to psychiatric affective morbidity. Clin Endocrinol. 1999;51(4):429–38.
40. Lucas A, Pizarro E, Granada ML, Salinas I, Sanmartí A. Postpartum thyroid dysfunction and postpartum depression: are they two linked disorders? Clin Endocrinol. 2001;55(6):809–14.
41. Bergink V, Pop VJM, Nielsen PR, Agerbo E, Munk-Olsen T, Liu X. Comorbidity of autoimmune thyroid disorders and psychiatric disorders during the postpartum period: a Danish nationwide register-based cohort study. Psychol Med. 2018;48(8):1291–8.
42. Harris B, Oretti R, Lazarus J, Parkes A, John R, Richards C, et al. Randomised trial of thyroxine to prevent postnatal depression in thyroid-antibody-positive women. Br J Psychiatry. 2002;180:327–30.
43. Azizi F, Khoshniat M, Bahrainian M, Hedayati M. Thyroid function and intellectual development of infants nursed by mothers taking methimazole. J Clin Endocrinol Metab. 2000;85(9):3233–8.
44. Azizi F, Bahrainian M, Khamseh ME, Khoshniat M. Intellectual development and thyroid function in children who were breast-fed by thyrotoxic mothers taking methimazole. J Pediatr Endocrinol Metab. 2003;16(9):1239–43.

45. Azizi F. The occurrence of permanent thyroid failure in patients with subclinical postpartum thyroiditis. Eur J Endocrinol. 2005;153(3):367–71.
46. Pedersen OM, Aardal NP, Larssen TB, Varhaug JE, Myking O, Vik-Mo H. The value of ultrasonography in predicting autoimmune thyroid disease. Thyroid. 2000;10(3):251–9.
47. Ide A, Amino N, Kang S, Yoshioka W, Kudo T, Nishihara E, et al. Differentiation of postpartum Graves' thyrotoxicosis from postpartum destructive thyrotoxicosis using antithyrotropin receptor antibodies and thyroid blood flow. Thyroid. 2014;24(6):1027–31.
48. Shahbazian HB, Sarvghadi F, Azizi F. Ultrasonographic characteristics and follow-up in postpartum thyroiditis. J Endocrinol Invest. 2005;28(5):410–2.
49. Hidaka Y, Tamaki H, Iwatani Y, Tada H, Mitsuda N, Amino N. Prediction of post-partum Graves' thyrotoxicosis by measurement of thyroid stimulating antibody in early pregnancy. Clin Endocrinol. 1994;41(1):15–20.
50. Amino N, Yabu Y, Miki T, Morimoto S, Kumahara Y, Mori H, et al. Serum ratio of triiodothyronine to thyroxine, and thyroxine-binding globulin and calcitonin concentrations in Graves' disease and destruction-induced thyrotoxicosis. J Clin Endocrinol Metab. 1981;53(1):113–6.
51. Sarvghadi F, Hedayati M, Mehrabi Y, Azizi F. Follow up of patients with postpartum thyroiditis: a population-based study. Endocrine. 2005;27(3):279–82.
52. Tachi J, Amino N, Tamaki H, Aozasa M, Iwatani Y, Miyai K. Long term follow-up and HLA association in patients with postpartum hypothyroidism. J Clin Endocrinol Metab. 1988;66(3):480–4.
53. Lucas A, Pizarro E, Granada ML, Salinas I, Roca J, Sanmartí A. Postpartum thyroiditis: long-term follow-up. Thyroid. 2005;15(10):1177–81.
54. Othman S, Phillips DI, Parkes AB, Richards CJ, Harris B, Fung H, et al. A long-term follow-up of postpartum thyroiditis. Clin Endocrinol. 1990;32(5):559–64.
55. Stuckey BG, Kent GN, Ward LC, Brown SJ, Walsh JP. Postpartum thyroid dysfunction and the long-term risk of hypothyroidism: results from a 12-year follow-up study of women with and without postpartum thyroid dysfunction. Clin Endocrinol. 2010;73(3):389–95.
56. Premawardhana LD, Parkes AB, Ammari F, John R, Darke C, Adams H, et al. Postpartum thyroiditis and long-term thyroid status: prognostic influence of thyroid peroxidase antibodies and ultrasound echogenicity. J Clin Endocrinol Metab. 2000;85(1):71–5.
57. American Academy of Pediatrics Committee on Drugs. Transfer of drugs and other chemicals into human milk. Pediatrics. 2001;108(3):776–89.
58. Kuijpens JL, Pop VJ, Vader HL, Drexhage HA, Wiersinga WM. Prediction of post partum thyroid dysfunction: can it be improved? Eur J Endocrinol. 1998;139(1):36–43.
59. Gerstein HC. Incidence of postpartum thyroid dysfunction in patients with type I diabetes mellitus. Ann Intern Med. 1993;118(6):419–23.
60. Alvarez-Marfany M, Roman SH, Drexler AJ, Robertson C, Stagnaro-Green A. Long-term prospective study of postpartum thyroid dysfunction in women with insulin dependent diabetes mellitus. J Clin Endocrinol Metab. 1994;79(1):10–6.
61. Gallas PR, Stolk RP, Bakker K, Endert E, Wiersinga WM. Thyroid dysfunction during pregnancy and in the first postpartum year in women with diabetes mellitus type 1. Eur J Endocrinol. 2002;147(4):443–51.
62. Stagnaro-Green A, Akhter E, Yim C, Davies TF, Magder L, Petri M. Thyroid disease in pregnant women with systemic lupus erythematosus: increased preterm delivery. Lupus. 2011;20(7):690–9.
63. Gudbjörnsson B, Karlsson-Parra A, Karlsson E, Hällgren R, Kämpe O. Clinical and laboratory features of Sjögren's syndrome in young women with previous postpartum thyroiditis. J Rheumatol. 1994;21(2):215–9.
64. Elefsiniotis IS, Vezali E, Pantazis KD, Saroglou G. Post-partum thyroiditis in women with chronic viral hepatitis. J Clin Virol. 2008;41(4):318–9.
65. Maleki N, Tavosi Z. Evaluation of thyroid dysfunction and autoimmunity in gestational diabetes mellitus and its relationship with postpartum thyroiditis. Diabet Med. 2015;32(2):206–12.

66. Lazarus JH, Ammari F, Oretti R, Parkes AB, Richards CJ, Harris B. Clinical aspects of recurrent postpartum thyroiditis. Br J Gen Pract. 1997;47(418):305–8.
67. Nøhr SB, Jørgensen A, Pedersen KM, Laurberg P. Postpartum thyroid dysfunction in pregnant thyroid peroxidase antibody-positive women living in an area with mild to moderate iodine deficiency: is iodine supplementation safe? J Clin Endocrinol Metab. 2000;85(9):3191–8.
68. Kämpe O, Jansson R, Karlsson FA. Effects of L-thyroxine and iodide on the development of autoimmune postpartum thyroiditis. J Clin Endocrinol Metab. 1990;70(4):1014–8.
69. Negro R, Greco G, Mangieri T, Pezzarossa A, Dazzi D, Hassan H. The influence of selenium supplementation on postpartum thyroid status in pregnant women with thyroid peroxidase autoantibodies. J Clin Endocrinol Metab. 2007;92(4):1263–8.
70. Mantovani G, Isidori AM, Moretti C, Di Dato C, Greco E, Ciolli P, et al. Selenium supplementation in the management of thyroid autoimmunity during pregnancy: results of the "SERENA study", a randomized, double-blind, placebo-controlled trial. Endocrine. 2019;66(3):542–50.
71. Mao J, Pop VJ, Bath SC, Vader HL, Redman CW, Rayman MP. Effect of low-dose selenium on thyroid autoimmunity and thyroid function in UK pregnant women with mild-to-moderate iodine deficiency. Eur J Nutr. 2016;55(1):55–61.
72. Stranges S, Marshall JR, Natarajan R, Donahue RP, Trevisan M, Combs GF, et al. Effects of long-term selenium supplementation on the incidence of type 2 diabetes: a randomized trial. Ann Intern Med. 2007;147(4):217–23.
73. Rayman MP. Selenium and human health. Lancet. 2012;379(9822):1256–68.
74. Krysiak R, Kowalcze K, Okopien B. The effect of vitamin D on thyroid autoimmunity in non-lactating women with postpartum thyroiditis. Eur J Clin Nutr. 2016;70(5):637–9.
75. Benvenga S, Vigo MT, Metro D, Granese R, Vita R, Le Donne M. Type of fish consumed and thyroid autoimmunity in pregnancy and postpartum. Endocrine. 2016;52(1):120–9.

Postpartum Thyrotoxicosis

Fereidoun Azizi

Introduction

Profound alterations in the immune system, in particular protective mechanisms of the placenta and systemic immune response, occur during pregnancy [1, 2]. In the postpartum period, these specific immune responses are slowly lost and may be accompanied by "a period of exacerbation" of autoimmune activity, 3–12 months following delivery [3], which may cause beginning, relapse, or worsening of autoimmune thyroid disorders, namely postpartum thyroiditis and Graves' disease. Thyrotoxicosis phase of postpartum thyroiditis and hyperthyroidism caused by Graves' disease are the most frequent causes of hyperthyroid state during postpartum period [4]. However, other causes of thyrotoxicosis such as painless sporadic thyrotoxicosis, subacute painful thyroiditis, toxic nodular goiter, and iodine-induced and iatrogenic thyrotoxicosis may also be seen in the first year after delivery [5].

The objective of this article is to discuss changes of thyroid antibodies during postpartum period and to review causes, clinical presentations, diagnosis, management, and monitoring of postpartum thyrotoxicosis.

Postpartum Alterations of Thyroid Antibodies

Several changes occur in the immune system following conception. These are categorized as cell immune mediated response by T helper 1 (Th1) and humoral reaction by T helper 2 (Th2). Due to possibility of adverse effects from Th1 cytokine on the fetus, during pregnancy a shift in T cell physiology from Th1 to Th2 immune

F. Azizi (✉)
Endocrine Research Center, Research Institute for Endocrine Sciences,
Shahid Beheshti University of Medical Sciences, Tehran, Iran
e-mail: azizi@endocrine.ac.ir

F. Azizi, F. Ramezani Tehrani (eds.), *Thyroid Diseases in Pregnancy*,
https://doi.org/10.1007/978-3-030-98777-0_15

response may be observed [6, 7]. In addition, helper/suppressor (CD4/CD8) ratio is increased during the first trimester of pregnancy, which will decline in the second and third trimesters [3].

Following delivery, the immune suppression present during pregnancy is gradually lost; this will be followed by a period of exacerbation of autoimmunity between 3 and 12 months postpartum, before its return to complete normal status [8–10]. Therefore, women with autoimmune thyroid disorders, i.e., Hashimoto's thyroiditis or Graves' disease, may experience recurrence or worsening of their illness. In addition, postpartum period may be the first appearance of these disorders due to exacerbation of already present autoimmune disarrangement [9].

Postpartum thyroid dysfunction (PPTD) is distinguished by the occurrence of transient or permanent thyroid dysfunction in the postpartum period. PPTD is a common autoimmune disease with a prevalence of 1.1–11.4%, mean 7% [11–16] in women worldwide and as high as 18–25% in women with other autoimmune disease, such as type 1 diabetes [17, 18]. This disease may present as hypo- or hyperthyroidism or may have a course of both presentations. Symptoms and signs of thyrotoxicosis commonly occur between 1 and 6 months, mostly at 3 months postpartum [19]. In about 30% of women with PPTD, the thyrotoxic phase is not clinically recognized because of lack of symptoms of hyperthyroidism. It has been reported that 20–30% of PPTD patients experience only hyperthyroid phase and other 40–50% may develop hypothyroidism following thyrotoxic state [19, 20].

The incidence of Graves' disease in the postpartum period is 0.2% [21]. This is 10–20 times lower than the incidence of thyrotoxicosis due to PPTD [9, 22]. Women with a history of Graves' hyperthyroidism, in particular in the first trimester of pregnancy, are more prone to exacerbation or relapse of disease after delivery [8–10]. Few weeks after delivery. There is a rise in TSH receptor antibodies (TRAb) titer following postpartum autoimmune response, which stimulates thyroid hormone synthesis, production, and release by binding to TSH receptors of thyrocytes [23]. The TRAb production is suppressed during late pregnancy, which explains remission or improvement of Graves' hyperthyroid manifestations in the third trimester of pregnancy. Less frequently, hyperthyroidism may occur as a first presentation in woman with Graves' disease during postpartum period [20, 21].

Clinical Presentation

Symptoms of hyperthyroidism may be mild and resemble those of the normal puerperium experience. Irritability, palpitation, increased sweating, heat intolerance, mood swings, tremor, and anxiety are usually present in women with postpartum thyrotoxicosis and may overlap with normal postpartum symptoms [22]. However, some patients may experience excessive fatigue, sleepiness, or manic behavior in this period [23].

In postpartum thyrotoxicosis caused by Graves' disease signs of tachycardia, weight loss, tremor, and thyroid eye disease often are present, while in patients with thyrotoxic phase of PPTD, symptoms and signs of hyperthyroidism are milder and may even be partly or totally absent [9, 22].

Laboratory Findings

In overt hyperthyroidism, there is increase in serum free T4 (fT4) and/or T3 and suppressed or undetectable serum TSH [24]. A combination of serum TSH less than 0.4 mU/L and normal serum fT4 and T3 concentration denotes diagnosis of subclinical hyperthyroidism. Elevated serum T3 with normal fT4 titer and suppressed serum TSH denotes T3 toxicosis. It is noteworthy that low serum TSH may be present in central hypothyroidism, postpartum hypophysitis, and non-thyroidal illness, as well. The differential diagnosis of an elevated fT4 includes non-thyroidal illness, familial dysalbuminemic hyperthyroxinemia, and consumption of high doses of propranolol, oral cholecystographic agents, amiodarone and amphetamine abuse [8, 20].

Etiology

Thyrotoxic phase of PPTD and Graves' hyperthyroidism are two most common causes of postpartum thyrotoxicosis. Rarely other causes such as painless sporadic thyroiditis, subacute painful thyroiditis and very rarely iatrogenic thyrotoxicosis, toxic nodular goiter and iodine-induced thyrotoxicosis may occur during postpartum period. Table 1 summarizes clinical and laboratory findings of various causes of postpartum thyrotoxicosis.

PPTD: Women may have mild symptoms of hyperthyroidism or may be asymptomatic. During pregnancy and postpartum period these women have higher prevalence of positive TPOAb titers, and exaggerated autoimmune response, with lesser changes in T helper/suppressor ratio [25]. In PPTD women the state of hyperthyroidism occurs between 2 and 6 months after delivery. This phase is self-limited and subsides without any treatment. Either euthyroidism or hypothyroid state may follow the thyrotoxic state in PPTD. Coexistence of Graves' disease and PPTD may rarely complicate the diagnosis [26].

Graves' disease: Postpartum Graves' disease occurs during the first year, in particular 1–3 months after delivery; this period is associated with a greater frequency of the relapse, exacerbation, or onset of Graves' hyperthyroidism. 12–40% of Graves' hyperthyroidism in women of childbearing age may occur in the postpartum period [27], where there is a significant rise in serum TRAb, fT4, T3, and fT3/fT4 ratio [28].

Table 1 Clinical and laboratory characteristics of main causes of postpartum thyrotoxicosis[a]

Characteristic	Graves' disease	Postpartum thyroiditis	Painless sporadic thyroiditis	Painful subacute thyroiditis
Frequency	Common	Most common	Rare	Rare
Timing	4–7 months postpartum	2–6 months postpartum	Any time	Any time (seasonal)
Symptoms	Hyperthyroidism	Mild hyperthyroidism	None	Fever, malaise
Signs	Goiter, exophthalmos, hyperthyroidism	Goiter	Goiter	Tender goiter, mild hyperthyroidism
Etiology	Autoimmune	Autoimmune	Autoimmune	Unknown
Erythrocyte sedimentation rate	Normal	Normal	Normal	High
Radioiodine uptake	High	Low	Low	Low
Triiodothyronine/ thyroxine ratio	High	Low	Low	Variable
Thyroid peroxidase antibodies	High	High	High	Low or absent
Thyrotropin receptor-stimulating antibodies (TRAb)	Present	Absent	Absent	Absent

[a]Rare etiologies are toxic nodular goiter, iodine-induced and iatrogenic thyrotoxicosis

Painless sporadic thyroiditis: Clinical and laboratory characteristics and management of this rare autoimmune disorder are similar to those of the PPTD. Patients have no or very mild symptoms with the presence of a small diffuse goiter in about half of the patients [29].

Subacute painful thyroiditis: It may rarely occur during the postpartum period and is not related to autoimmune alteration of this period. Patient often presents with pain in the region of the thyroid and constitutional symptoms. Elevated erythrocyte sedimentation rate and a low radioiodine thyroid uptake (RAIU) confirm the diagnosis of subacute thyroiditis. Serum TSH is usually suppressed and FT4 and T3 may mildly be increased [29].

Other causes: Iodine-indued thyrotoxicosis and toxic nodular goiter may also occur in the postpartum period. Iatrogenic thyrotoxicosis may complicate very rarely the differential diagnosis of thyrotoxicosis in a young mother. The diagnosis is confirmed by the absence of goiter, a low RAIU, and low serum thyroglobulin [30].

Differential diagnosis: Diagnosis of the cause of hyperthyroidism may be possible based on history and physical examination. Presence of thyroid eye disease in Graves' disease and a painful thyroid in subacute thyroiditis are the most helpful clinical findings in differential diagnosis.

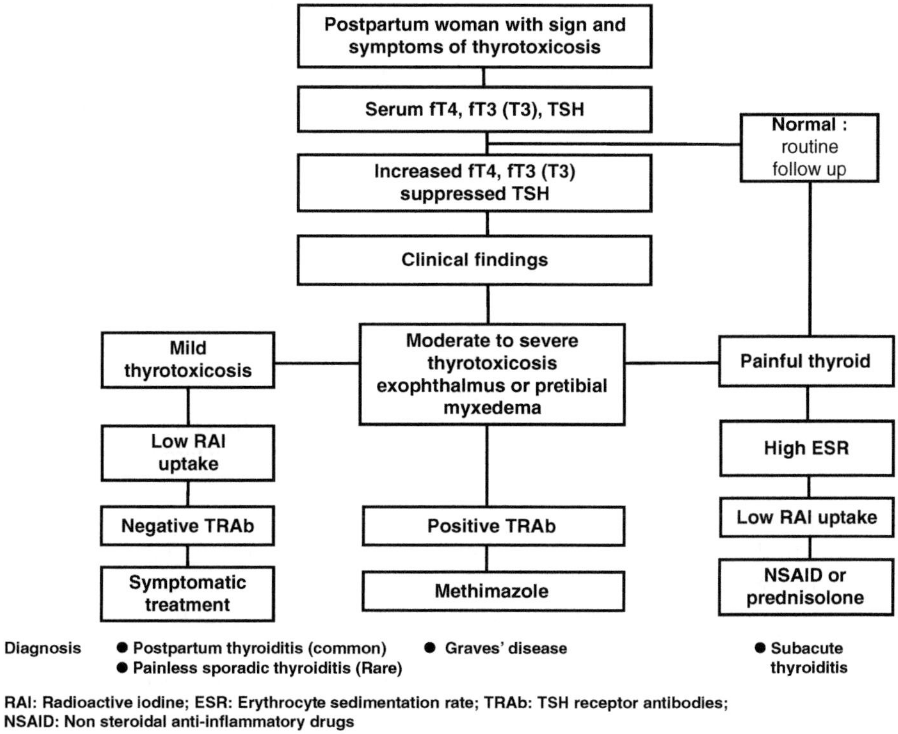

Fig. 1 Proposed evaluation and management schema for postpartum thyrotoxicosis

The major task of physician is differentiation of thyrotoxic phase of PPTD from Graves' disease [31]. Goiter usually occurs in both diseases but is often more prominent in the latter. The RAIU is always low in PPT, elevated or normal in Graves'; TRAb titer is elevated in Graves' and negative in PPT. Serum triiodothyronine/thyroxine ratio and FT3/FT4 ratio are increased in Graves' and decreased in most patients with destructive thyroiditis, iatrogenic, or iodine-induced thyrotoxicosis. Figure 1 demonstrates workup of women with thyrotoxicosis in the postpartum period.

Various types of thyroiditis are accompanied by a low RAIU because inflammatory changes in the thyroid result in suppressed TSH and an inability to iodine concentration [32]. While RAIU is increased in Graves' disease where hyperthyroidism is caused by excessive thyroid hormone synthesis and release. Low thyroid RAIU is also detected in exogenous thyroid hormone ingestion, struma ovarii, and iodine-induced thyrotoxicosis.

An elevated thyroglobulin is accompanied by increase in FT4 and FT3 in Graves' disease, while in PPTD, increase in serum thyroglobulin concentrations precedes the onset of thyrotoxicosis [21].

Subacute thyroiditis is differentiated from PPTD by the presence of systematic symptoms, thyroid pain, increased erythrocyte sedimentation rate, and C-reactive protein. In addition, TPOAb titers are elevated in PPTD [33, 34]. Thyroid blood flow in Doppler ultrasonography is increased in Graves' disease, while it is low in PPTD [35].

Management

Patients in the thyrotoxic phase of PPT have relatively few symptoms lasting only a few weeks and do not need any treatment. Antithyroid drugs are not indicated because the biosynthesis is not increased and etiology of hyperthyroidism is excessive release of thyroid hormones [36]. Sodium ipodate remarkably inhibits the peripheral deiodination of T4 to generate T3 and may be administered 500 mg daily in severe thyrotoxicosis caused by destruction-induced thyrotoxicosis [37].

Antithyroid drug (methimazole) is the treatment of choice of postpartum Graves' hyperthyroidism [10, 36]. The doses, duration, and follow-up management of hyperthyroidism with antithyroid drugs are the same as those for patients with Graves' who are not in the postpartum period. Continuing antithyroid drugs for 12–18 months is recommended followed by appropriate monitoring for detection of relapse.

Radioiodine administration is one therapeutic modality for postpartum Graves'; however, infant care for up to 7 days or longer according to radiation safety instructions may be very difficult for the mother; likewise, radioiodine treatment is contraindicated in the breast-feeding mother [9].

If the mother is not breast-feeding, radioiodine therapy becomes the treatment of choice when there is contraindication for antithyroid drugs or in women who develop side effects during medical treatment. For the occasional patient who develops side effects of antithyroid drugs and avoids radioiodine treatment, subtotal thyroidectomy would be advisable, following careful control of hyperthyroidism [20, 21]. Subacute painful thyroiditis may be treated with β-blockers. Non-steroidal anti-inflammatory agents or prednisolone may be considered for women with moderate to severe signs and symptoms.

Management of Breast-Feeding Women

Breast-feeding women with thyrotoxicosis require special considerations both in diagnosis and management of hyperthyroidism. Radioiodine therapy should not be given to breast-feeding women, because it is secreted in the milk. Ingestion of as low as 5–10 μCi doses of ^{123}I and ^{131}I for thyroid uptake test requires discontinuation of nursing for 2 days and few weeks, respectively [37]. Use of thyroid RAIU test for the differential diagnosis of thyrotoxicosis should be avoided; in special cases, ^{123}I should be used because of its extremely short physical half-life of 13 h, compared to the 8-day half-life of ^{131}I.

It has been shown that the thyroid function and physical and intellectual development of children breast-fed by thyrotoxic mothers on antithyroid drugs remain unaffected [38]. Treatment of breast-feeding mothers for up to 1 year with daily doses of 20 and 30 mg MMI at initiation with following titration method to maintenance dose does not disturb the thyroid function of breast-fed infants [38–40]. Furthermore, thyroid function tests and physical and intellectual growth of these children remain normal [39, 41]. It is estimated that peak concentration of milk MMI after a dose of 40 mg is 0.72 ± 0.07 μg/mL, and that following ingestion of a single 20 mg dose of MMI by mother, the breast-fed infant receives approximately 50 μg MMI (7 μg/kg for a 5-month-old infant). Serum MMI concentration of breast-fed infants whose mothers received 20–30 mg MMI daily was in safe range of less than 0.03 μg/mL [39, 41]. Therefore, no routine screening of thyroid function in breast-fed infants is recommended unless abnormal growth or cognition is observed [20, 38].

Monitoring and follow-Up

Follow-up of patients with postpartum thyrotoxicosis differs depending on the etiology of disease. The thyrotoxic phase of PPTD is self-limited; however, patient should be carefully followed in the second half of postpartum year for the occurrence of hypothyroidism, which may require levothyroxine treatment, for at least 1 year [4]. Permanent hypothyroidism may occur in long-term follow-up of PPTD, even those with original presentation of subclinical hypothyroidism [42].

Patients with postpartum Graves' disease should be treated with MMI for 12–18 months. It has been shown that TRAb titers were lower in these patients compared to MMI-treated non-postpartum hyperthyroidism after 12 months of MMI treatment [43]. Recurrence rate of hyperthyroidism after MMI withdrawal is much lower than women with non-postpartum hyperthyroidism (21 vs 68%, $p = 0.002$). This difference is probably due to peculiar immunologic aggravation after delivery which lasts up to 12 months and is followed by a restoration of the pre-pregnancy immune balance [44]. This phenomenon may synergize with the MMI effect in immune modulation and reduction of circulating thyroid antibodies [45].

Summary

Thyrotoxicosis during postpartum period must be looked for and careful management should be given for proper health of mother and neonate. Physicians should carefully precede with proper differential diagnosis, in particular that of PPTD and Graves' disease, and deliver appropriate care to postpartum women and ensure that correct management will improve the quality of life of mothers and their infants in this important period of life.

References

1. Amino N, Tada H, Hidaka Y. Autoimmune thyroid disease and pregnancy. J Endocrinol Invest. 1996;19:59–70.
2. King A, Loke YW, Chaouat G. NK cells and reproduction. Immunol Today. 1997;18:64–6.
3. Lazarus JH, Ludgate ME. Prevention and treatment of postpartum Graves' disease. Bailliere Clin Endocrinol Metab. 1997;11:549–60.
4. Stagnaro-Green A, Abalovich M, Alexander E, Azizi F, Mestman J, Negro R, et al. Guidelines of the American Thyroid Association for the diagnosis and management of thyroid disease during pregnancy and postpartum. Thyroid. 2011;21:1–45.
5. Azizi F. Postpartum thyroid disorders. Ann Thyroid. 2018;3:75–83.
6. Wegmann TG, Lin H, Guilbert L, Mosmann TR. Bidirectional cytokine interactions in the maternal-fetal relationship: is successful pregnancy a TH2 phenomenon? Immunol Today. 1993;14:353–6.
7. Powrie F, Menon S, Coffman RL. Interleukin-4 and interleukin-10 synergize to inhibit cell-mediated immunity in vivo. Eur J Immunol. 1993;23:3043–9.
8. Stagnaro-Green A, Abalovich M, Alexander E, Azizi F, Mestman J, Negro R, et al. Guidelines of the American Thyroid Association for the diagnosis and management of thyroid disease during pregnancy and postpartum. Thyroid. 2011;21:1081–125.
9. Azizi F, Braverman L. Management of postpartum thyrotoxicosis. Curr Opin Endocrinol Diabetes. 2005;12:471–6.
10. Azizi F. Treatment of post-partum thyrotoxicosis. J Endocrinol Invest. 2006;29:244–7.
11. Nikolai TF, Turney SL, Roberts RC. Postpartum lymphocytic thyroiditis. Prevalence, clinical course, and long-term follow-up. Arch Intern Med. 1987;147:221–4.
12. Premawardhana LD, Parkes AB, Ammari F, John R, Darke C, Adams H, et al. Postpartum thyroiditis and long-term thyroid status: prognostic influence of thyroid peroxidase antibodies and ultrasound echogenicity. J Clin Endocrinol Metab. 2000;85:71–5.
13. Roti E, Bianconi L, Gardini E, Minelli R, De Franco ML, Bacchi Modena A, et al. Postpartum thyroid dysfunction in an Italian population residing in an area of mild iodine deficiency. J Endocrinol Invest. 1991;14:669–74.
14. Shahbazian HB, Sarvghadi F, Azizi F. Prevalence and characteristics of postpartum thyroid dysfunction in Tehran. Eur J Endocrinol. 2001;145:397–401.
15. Roti E, Uberti E. Post-partum thyroiditis—a clinical update. Eur J Endocrinol. 2002;146:275–9.
16. Stagnaro-Green A. Postpartum thyroiditis. Best Pract Res Clin Endocrinol Metab. 2004;18:303–16.
17. Benvenga S, Pintaudi B, Vita R, Di Vieste G, Di Benedetto A. Serum thyroid hormone autoantibodies in type 1 diabetes mellitus. J Clin Endocrinol Metab. 2015;100:1870–8.
18. Di Bari F, Granese R, Le Donne M, Vita R, Benvenga S. Autoimmune abnormalities of postpartum thyroid diseases. Front Endocrinol. 2017;8:166.
19. Othman S, Phillips DI, Parkes AB, Richards CJ, Harris B, Fung H, et al. A long-term follow-up of postpartum thyroiditis. Clin Endocrinol. 1990;32:559–64.
20. Alexander EK, Pearce EN, Brent GA, Brown RS, Chen H, Dosiou C, et al. 2017 guidelines of the American Thyroid Association for the diagnosis and management of thyroid disease during pregnancy and the postpartum. Thyroid. 2017;27:315–89.
21. De Groot L, Abalovich M, Alexander EK, Amino N, Barbour L, Cobin RH, et al. Management of thyroid dysfunction during pregnancy and postpartum: an Endocrine Society clinical practice guideline. J Clin Endocrinol Metab. 2012;97:2543–65.
22. Freeman R, Rosen H, Thysen B. Incidence of thyroid dysfunction in an unselected postpartum population. Arch Intern Med. 1986;146:1361–4.
23. Greene MF, Creasy RK, Resnik R, Iams JD, Lockwood CJ, Moore T. Creasy and Resnik's maternal-fetal medicine: principles and practice. E-Book: Elsevier Health Sciences; 2008.
24. Goldstein AL. New-onset Graves' disease in the postpartum period. J Midwifery Womens Health. 2013;58:211–4.

25. Stagnaro-Green A, Roman SH, Cobin RH, el-Harazy E, Wallenstein S, Davies TF. A prospective study of lymphocyte-initiated immunosuppression in normal pregnancy: evidence of a T-cell etiology for postpartum thyroid dysfunction. J Clin Endocrinol Metab. 1992;74:645–53.
26. Yoshida S, Takamatsu J, Kuma K, Ohsawa N. Thyroid-stimulating antibodies and thyroid stimulation-blocking antibodies during the pregnancy and postpartum period: a case report. Thyroid. 1992;2:27–30.
27. Amino N, Tanizawa O, Mori H, Iwatani Y, Yamada T, Kurachi K, et al. Aggravation of thyrotoxicosis in early pregnancy and after delivery in Graves' disease. J Clin Endocrinol Metab. 1982;55:108–12.
28. Gonzalez-Jimenez A, Fernandez-Soto ML, Escobar-Jimenez F, et al. Thyroid function parameters and TSH-receptor antibodies in healthy subjects and Graves' disease patients: a sequential study before, during and after pregnancy. Thyroidology. 1993;5:13–20.
29. Pearce EN, Farwell AP, Braverman LE. Thyroiditis. N Engl J Med. 2003;348:2646–55.
30. Ross DS, Burch HB, Cooper DS, Greenlee C, Lauberg P, Luiza Maia A, et al. 2016 American Thyroid Association guidelines for diagnosis and management of hyperthyroidism and other causes of thyrotoxicosis. Thyroid. 2016;26:1343–21.
31. Momotani N, Noh J, Ishikawa N, Ito K. Relationship between silent thyroiditis and recurrent Graves' disease in the postpartum period. J Clin Endocrinol Metab. 1994;79:285–9.
32. Ross DS. Syndromes of thyrotoxicosis with low radioactive iodine uptake. Endocrinol Metab Clin N Am. 1998;27:169–85.
33. Tozzoli R, Bagnasco M, Giavarina D, Bizzaro N. TSH receptor autoantibody immunoassay in patients with Graves' disease: improvement of diagnostic accuracy over different generations of methods. Autoimmune Rev. 2012;12:107–13.
34. Ide A, Amino N, Kang S, Yoshioka W, Kudo T, Nishihara E, et al. Differentiation of postpartum Graves' thyrotoxicosis from postpartum destructive thyrotoxicosis using antithyrotropin receptor antibodies and thyroid blood flow. Thyroid. 2014;24:1027–31.
35. Ota H, Amino N, Morita S, Kobayashi K, Kubota S, Fukata S, et al. Quantitative measurement of thyroid blood flow for differentiation of painless thyroiditis from Graves' disease. Clin Endocrinol. 2007;67:41–5.
36. Mestman J. Thyroid and parathyroid diseases in pregnancy. Obstetrics: normal and problem pregnancies. 5th ed. London: Churchill Livingstone; 2007. p. 1023–9.
37. Mountford PJ, Coakley AJ. A review of the secretion of radioactivity in human breast milk: data, quantitative analysis and recommendations. Nucl Med Commun. 1989;10:15–27.
38. Azizi F, Khoshniat M, Bahrainian M, Hedayati M. Thyroid function and intellectual development of infants nursed by mothers taking methimazole. J Clin Endocrinol Metab. 2000;85:3233–8.
39. Azizi F, Hedayati M. Thyroid function in breast-fed infants whose mothers take high doses of methimazole. J Endocrinol Invest. 2002;25:493–6.
40. Azizi F. Effect of methimazole treatment of maternal thyrotoxicosis on thyroid function in breast-feeding infants. J Pediatr. 1996;128:855–8.
41. Azizi F, Bahrainian M, Khamseh ME, Khoshniat M. Intellectual development and thyroid function in children who were breast-fed by thyrotoxic mothers taking methimazole. J Pediatr Endocrinol Metab. 2003;16:1239–43.
42. Azizi F. The occurrence of permanent thyroid failure in patients with subclinical postpartum thyroiditis. Eur J Endocrinol. 2005;153:367–71.
43. Rotondi M, Capelli V, Coperchini F, et al. Postpartum and non-post-partum relapsing Graves' hyperthyroidism display different response to anti-thyroid drugs. Eur J Endocrinol. 2021;178:589–94.
44. Amino N, Tada H, Hidaka Y. Postpartum autoimmune thyroid syndrome: a model of aggravation of autoimmune disease. Thyroid. 1999;9:705–13.
45. Weetman AP. The immunomodulatory effects of antithyroid drugs. Thyroid. 1994;4:145–6.

Thyroid and Infertility

Gesthimani Mintziori

Introduction

Infertility is defined as the failure to achieve a clinical pregnancy after at least 12 months of regular unprotected sexual intercourse [1]. Infertility which can be either attributed to male factor, female factor, or both, while in some cases the cause is not detected (idiopathic infertility), represents an ongoing challenge globally [2].

Thyroxine is essential in early pregnancy and crucial for fetal brain development and growth and thyroid dysfunction and/or autoimmunity are quite common in women of reproductive age, as reported in previous chapters. Apart from that, it is now well reported that the hypothalamus-pituitary-thyroid axis interacts with the hypothalamus-pituitary-gonads axis in various levels and ways. Recent evidence suggests that on top of these interactions, a local action of thyroid hormones in reproductive tissues is highly probable. Thyroid hormone and TSH receptors (TRs and TSHRs respectively) have been detected in the granulosa cells, the follicular fluid, and the endometrium; and deiodinases 2 and 3 have been detected in the ovaries [3]. Interestingly TRs that are located in the endometrium seem to cross talk with the estrogen receptors (ERs) and are expressed differently during the different phases of menstrual cycle [4]. According to experimental data, TRα1 and TRβ1are expressed in mid-luteal phase. An increase has been reported during secretory phase, followed by a decrease [4]. This is clinically interested as it has been suggested that TR and TSHR expression is related to human endometrium receptivity [5].

TR and TSHR are also found in granulosa and ovarian stromal cells [6]. TR α1 and TR β1 are found in the epithelium, but the receptors are differently distributed in the oocytes and granulosa cells at the different developmental stages of the follicle. The presence of the thyroid and TSH receptors in the reproductive tissues

G. Mintziori (✉)
Medical School, Aristotle University of Thessaloniki, Thessaloniki, Greece

F. Azizi, F. Ramezani Tehrani (eds.), *Thyroid Diseases in Pregnancy*,
https://doi.org/10.1007/978-3-030-98777-0_16

implies a local action of thyroid hormone and TSH, respectively. It is already known that T_3 inhibits aromatase activity in granulosa cells and that, together with FSH, enhances granulosa cells proliferation and inhibits granulosa cells apoptosis by the PI3K/Akt pathway [7].

Hypothyroidism and Infertility

Hypothyroidism, including subclinical hypothyroidism, is a common disease in women of reproductive age. Subclinical hypothyroidism is defined as an elevated serum TSH with a normal serum free thyroxine concentrations. Both overt and subclinical hypothyroidism have been linked to infertility, higher miscarriage rate, lower live birth rate, preterm deliveries, and low birthweight for gestational age (Fig. 1). Hypothyroidism per se can cause ovulatory disorders that in turn can comprise a challenge to fertility.

According to an observational cohort study involving women desiring pregnancy with history of miscarriage or subfertility from 49 hospitals across the UK [8], overt hypothyroidism, defined as having a TSH > 4.50 mIU/L and fT4 < 10 pmol/L, was diagnosed in 0.2% of women (95% CI, 0.1–0.3) and overt hyperthyroidism, defined as having a TSH < 0.44 mIU/L and fT4 > 21 pmol/L, in 0.3% (95% CI, 0.2–0.3) of the women. Interestingly, only 2.4% (95% CI, 2.1–2.6) of the women were diagnosed with subclinical hypothyroidism, defined as having a TSH > 4.50 mIU/L. Of course, if the cutoff for TSH is lowered to 2.50 mIU/L, then subclinical hypothyroidism would have been diagnosed in 19.9% (95% CI, 19.3–20.5) of the women. TPOAb were detected in 9.5% of the women. A retrospective study that involved 2279 women with normal thyroid function and 289 with subclinical hypothyroidism has shown that subclinical hypothyroidism is linked to lower AMH concentrations (median: 2.05 vs. 2.51 ng/mL, $p = 0.015$) and lower antral follicle counts (median: 10.0 vs. 11.0, $p = 0.013$) in comparison to euthyroidism [9]. A Cochrane meta-analysis with the aim to evaluate levothyroxine replacement in subfertile women with either subclinical hypothyroidism or euthyroidism with thyroid autoimmunity

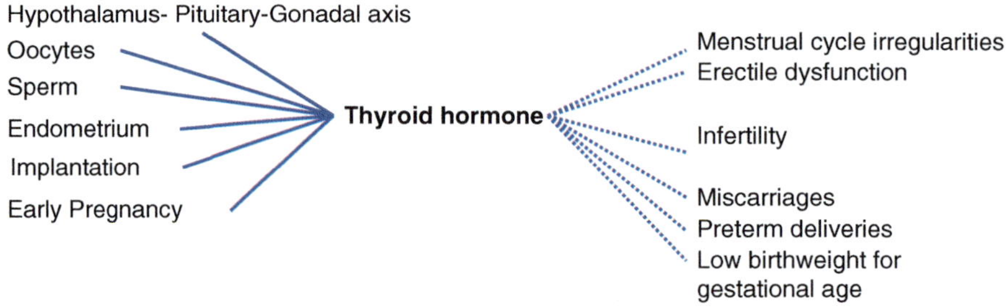

Fig. 1 Targets of thyroid hormone actions and reproduction-related symptoms of thyroid dysfunction

undergoing assisted reproduction was unable to draw strong conclusions mainly because of the low quality of the available evidence [10]. Another meta-analysis on the same topic though had suggested that LT_4 supplementation may be recommended for women with subclinical hypothyroidism or euthyroidism with thyroid autoimmunity undergoing IVF/ICSI, mainly as a protection from miscarriages [11].

According to the 2021 European Thyroid Association (ETA) guidelines [12] all women planning assisted reproduction should be screened for TSH and TPOAb/and TPOAb concentrations. Treatment with LT4 should be discussed in infertile women with TAI and serum TSH >2.5 mIU/L. In fact, as infertility per se is a risk factor of thyroid dysfunction, all women with infertility should be screened for thyroid dysfunction and autoimmunity.

Among infertile men subclinical hypothyroidism may affect up to 7.4%. It has been suggested that in men with hypothyroidism the increased oxidative stress in the testis may be the main trigger for sperm abnormalities reported in these men [13]. Though the effects of overt hypothyroidism in the male reproductive system have been thoroughly described (abnormal sperm parameters including morphology and motility) less is known about subclinical hypothyroidism. In specific, hypothyroidism seems to decrease both the activity of glutathione reductase and catalase transcript expression and activity [14]. This is believed to cause a reduction in sperm mitochondrial activity and acrosome integrity [15]. Regarding the erectile function, there is evidence to support that this is strongly affected by thyroid hormone concentrations. It has been reported that untreated hypothyroidism may lead to delayed ejaculation [16].

It has been suggested that men with subclinical hypothyroidism may have deteriorated reproductive outcomes after assisted reproduction technology (ART) in comparison to euthyroid men [17]. However, it seems that this is the case for men older than 35 years [17]. In any case, according to the 2021 ETA guidelines all men with impaired sperm parameters should be screened for thyroid disease [12].

To sum up, all infertile women as well as infertile men with impaired sperm parameters should be screened for thyroid dysfunction. Thyroid supplementation, if necessary. Should start at the earliest convenience, as thyroid function is crucial for the normal development of the pregnancy.

Hyperthyroidism and Infertility

Hyperthyroidism both men and women has been linked to compromised reproductive outcomes. Hyperthyroidism is defined as an excess of thyroid hormone production and is commonly symptomatic. Similar to hypothyroidism, hyperthyroidism can be either overt or subclinical (TSH below the reference range, T3 and fT4 within the normal range). Thyrotoxicosis is another entity, defined as an excess of thyroid hormone concentration (and not necessarily production). Graves' disease is the leading cause of hyperthyroidism in both men and women. Other causes of hyperthyroidism and/or thyrotoxicosis include toxic multinodular goiter, thyroid toxic adenoma, iodine-induced hyperthyroidism (Jod-Basedow phenomenon), de Quervain, postpartum, and factitious thyroiditis. Main symptoms include fatigue, excessive sweating and tremor, palpitations, anxiety, heat intolerance, and diarrhea. Menstrual irregularities in women are not uncommon, and sometimes they comprise the main presenting symptom. It has been suggested that 5.8% of hyperthyroid women may be infertile [18].

Men with hyperthyroidism may experience symptoms related to decreased libido, gynecomastia, and/or premature ejaculation. Their sperm parameters may be strongly affected (sperm motility and morphology) [3]. As such infertility can be caused by hyperthyroidism either due to decreased libido, erectile dysfunction, or impaired spermatogenesis.

Hyperthyroid women commonly present with symptoms related to menstrual irregularities, including amenorrhea, oligomenorrhea, and hypomenorrhea [3]. It has been reported that in women with hyperthyroidism testosterone, Δ4-androstenedione but also estradiol and sex hormone binding globulin (SHBG) are all increased. Luteinizing hormone (LH) response to gonadotropin-releasing hormone (GnRH) is also higher in women with hyperthyroidism than those in euthyroid state. In any case, the effects of hyperthyroidism in fertility potential seem to be magnified when thyroid autoimmunity is also present, the latter being a common clinical scenario. Indeed, the presence of anti-TSH antibodies have specifically been associated with infertility (both primary and secondary).

According to a multi-center observational cohort study from 49 centers in the UK, overt hyperthyroidism (TSH < 0.44 mIU/L, fT4 > 21 pmol/L) was present in 0.3% (95% CI 0.2–0.3) of the 19,213 infertile women studied [8]. However, the rates of thyroid dysfunction may be underestimated in this study due to its study design. Older studies have calculated the prevalence of clinical and subclinical hyperthyroidism to be 2.1% in infertile women [18]. Vice versa, it has been suggested that infertility is present in 5.8% of women with hyperthyroidism [19].

In conclusion, both men and women with infertility and hyperthyroidism (subclinical and clinical) may present with symptoms and signs that will lead to the hyperthyroidism diagnosis. When treated hyperthyroidism, in both men and women, reproductive plans should be discussed as they may affect the hyperthyroidism treatment options.

Thyroid Autoimmunity and Infertility

Thyroid autoimmunity (TAI) is defined as the presence of Anti-TPO and/or anti-Tg antibodies and comprises the most common endocrine disease in women of reproductive age, with a prevalence between 5 and 20% [20]. It is now evident that when TAI is present, the relative risk for female infertility increases. On top of that, women with recurrent miscarriages have a higher incidence of Tg- and/or TPO-abs, amounting as high as 25% [20].

According to a meta-analysis involving nine studies and a total of 4396 women, live birth rate (LBR) of women with TAI is lower in comparison to that of those without TAI [odds ratio (OR): 0.73, 95% CI: 0.54–0.99, $p = 0.04$; I^2: 41%)] [21].

Various theories have been put forward to explain how TAI may influence female fertility: According to the first theory, it is not TAI per se, but the abnormal autoimmune background that results in the negative impact on fertility. A recent registry-based retrospective study from Taiwan demonstrated that women with Hashimoto thyroiditis had a 2.40-fold higher risk of premature ovarian failure than those without Hashimoto thyroiditis with a hazard ratio (HR) of 2.40 (95% confidence interval (CI) = 1.02–5.68) [22]. According to another theory on the same direction, TAI is not a cause, just a confounding factor, with age being the main cause that results in detrimental effects on female fertility [3]. The presence of TAI does increase with age anyway. Another theory however suggests that TAI results in a relative deficiency in thyroid hormone. Thus, women with TAI have a diminished "reservoir" of thyroid hormone. Lastly it has been suggested that TAI may have a cytotoxic reaction in the follicle fluid damaging the oocyte and, thus, can lead to poorer oocyte quality and decreased developmental potential [3]. Thyroid antibodies have been indeed detected in the follicular fluid and recent evidence demonstrates decreased T cell cytotoxicity in women with repeated implantation failure and TAI in comparison to those without TAI [23]. Anyway, TAI has been directly linked with other causes of infertility, such as endometriosis, ovarian failure, and polycystic ovarian syndrome [3].

According to the guidelines of ETA all women with infertility should be screened for thyroid function and presence of thyroid autoimmunity (anti-TPO and/or antiTG) [12]. In these guidelines, the presence of thyroid autoimmunity has a significant impact on the decision of providing thyroid hormone supplementation as this is suggested for women with TSH levels >2.5 mIU/L and thyroid autoimmunity, whereas this is not the case for those with same TSH values without thyroid autoimmunity [12].

Summary

Thyroid dysfunction and/or autoimmunity are quite common in women of reproductive age and thyroxine is essential in early pregnancy and crucial for fetal brain development and growth. Thyroid disease in women (including hypothyroidism and hyperthyroidism (both subclinical and overt) and/or thyroid autoimmunity have been linked to adverse reproductive outcomes. Similarly thyroid dysfunction in men is associated with erectile dysfunction and disturbances is sperm parameters. Early detection of thyroid disorders and thyroid hormone supplementation, when needed, is crucial for the improvement of fertility potential of both men and women.

References

1. World Health Organization (WHO). International classification of diseases, 11th revision (ICD-11) Geneva: WHO; 2018.
2. Inhorn MC, Patrizio P. Infertility around the globe: new thinking on gender, reproductive technologies and global movements in the 21st century. Hum Reprod Update. 2015;21(4):411–26.
3. Mintziori G, Goulis DG. In vitro fertilization/intracytoplasmic insemination and thyroid function: reviewing the evidence. Metabolism. 2018;86:44–8.
4. Aghajanova L, Stavreus-Evers A, Lindeberg M, Landgren BM, Sparre LS, Hovatta O. Thyroid-stimulating hormone receptor and thyroid hormone receptors are involved in human endometrial physiology. Fertil Steril. 2011;95:230–7.
5. Colicchia M, Campagnolo L, Baldini E, Ulisse S, Valensise H, Moretti C. Molecular basis of thyrotropin and thyroid hormone action during implantation and early development. Hum Reprod Update. 2014;20(6):884–904.
6. Wakim AN, Polizotto SL, Buffo MJ, Marrero MA, Burholt DR. Thyroid hormones in human follicular fluid and thyroid hormone receptors in human granulosa cells. Fertil Steril. 1993;59:1187–90.
7. Dittrich R, Beckmann MW, Oppelt PG, Hoffmann I, Lotz L, Kuwert T, Mueller A. Thyroid hormone receptors and reproduction. J Reprod Immunol. 2011;90(1):58–66.
8. Dhillon-Smith RK, Tobias A, Smith PP, Middleton LJ, Sunner KK, Baker K, Farrell-Carver S, Bender-Atik R, Agrawal R, Bhatia K, Chu JJ, Edi-Osagie E, Ewies A, Ghobara T, Gupta P, Jurkovic D, Khalaf Y, Mulbagal K, Nunes N, Overton C, Quenby S, Rai R, Raine-Fenning N, Robinson L, Ross J, Sizer A, Small R, Underwood M, Kilby MD, Daniels J, Thangaratinam S, Chan S, Boelaert K, Coomarasamy A. The prevalence of thyroid dysfunction and autoimmunity in women with history of miscarriage or subfertility. J Clin Endocrinol Metab. 2020;105(8):dgaa302.
9. Rao M, Wang H, Zhao S, Liu J, Wen Y, Wu Z, Yang Z, Su C, Su Z, Wang K, Tang L. Subclinical hypothyroidism is associated with lower ovarian reserve in women aged 35 years or older. Thyroid. 2020;30(1):95–105. https://doi.org/10.1089/thy.2019.0031.
10. Akhtar MA, Agrawal R, Brown J, Sajjad Y, Craciunas L. Thyroxine replacement for subfertile women with euthyroid autoimmune thyroid disease or subclinical hypothyroidism. Cochrane Database Syst Rev. 2019;6(6):CD011009.
11. Rao M, Zeng Z, Zhao S, Tang L. Effect of levothyroxine supplementation on pregnancy outcomes in women with subclinical hypothyroidism and thyroid autoimmunity undergoing in vitro fertilization/intracytoplasmic sperm injection: an updated meta-analysis of randomized controlled trials. Reprod Biol Endocrinol. 2018;16(1):92.
12. Poppe K, Bisschop P, Fugazzola L, Minziori G, Unuane D, Weghofer A. 2021 European thyroid association guideline on thyroid disorders prior to and during assisted reproduction. Eur Thyroid J. 2020;9:281–95.
13. Sahoo DK, Roy A, Bhanja S, Chainy GB. Hypothyroidism impairs antioxidant defence system and testicular physiology during development and maturation. Gen Comp Endocrinol. 2008;156(1):63–70.
14. Nascimento Gomes S, do Carmo Corrêa DE, de Oliveira IM, Bargi-Souza P, Degraf Cavallin M, Dobner Mariano D, Maissar Khalil N, Alves Figueiredo DL, Romano MA, de Oliveira CA, Marino Romano R. Imbalanced testicular metabolism induced by thyroid disorders: new evidences from quantitative proteome. Endocrine. 2020;67(1):209–23.
15. Romano RM, Gomes SN, Cardoso NC, Schiessl L, Romano MA, Oliveira CA. New insights for male infertility revealed by alterations in spermatic function and differential testicular expression of thyroid-related genes. Endocrine. 2017;55(2):607–17. https://doi.org/10.1007/s12020-016-0952-3.
16. Corona G, Jannini EA, Vignozzi L, Rastrelli G, Maggi M. The hormonal control of ejaculation. Nat Rev Urol. 2012;9(9):508–19. https://doi.org/10.1038/nrurol.2012.147.

17. Rao M, Yang Z, Su C, Zhao Z, Wan R, Liu J, Yao Y, Su Z, Wang K, Tang L, Zhao S. Paternal subclinical hypothyroidism affects the clinical outcomes of *in vitro* fertilization/intracytoplasmic sperm injection. Thyroid. 2021;31(1):12–22. https://doi.org/10.1089/thy.2020.0154.
18. Poppe K, Glinoer D, Van Steirteghem A, Tournaye H, Devroey P, Schiettecatte J, Velkeniers B. Thyroid dysfunction and autoimmunity in infertile women. Thyroid. 2002;12(11):997–1001.
19. Joshi JV, Bhandarkar SD, Chadha M, Balaiah D, Shah R. Menstrual irregularities and lactation failure may precede thyroid dysfunction or goitre. J Postgrad Med. 1993;39(3):137–41.
20. Mintziori G, Goulis DG, Kolibianakis EM. Thyroid function and IVF outcome: when to investigate and when to intervene? Curr Opin Obstet Gynecol. 2016;28(3):191–7.
21. Busnelli A, Paffoni A, Fedele L, Somigliana E. The impact of thyroid autoimmunity on IVF/ICSI outcome: a systematic review and meta-analysis. Hum Reprod Update. 2016;22(6):775–90. https://doi.org/10.1093/humupd/dmw019. Epub 2016 Jun 20. Erratum in: Hum Reprod Update 2016 Nov;22(6):793–794.
22. Hsieh YT, Ho JYP. Thyroid autoimmunity is associated with higher risk of premature ovarian insufficiency—a nationwide health insurance research database study. Hum Reprod. 2021;36(6):1621–9.
23. Mintziori G, Goulis DG. Endocrine causes of recurrent implantation failure. In: Recurrent implantation failure, 1st edn. Imprint CRC Press; 2019. eBook ISBN 9781315165707.

Thyroid Disorders and Hormonal Contraceptives

Samira Behboudi-Gandevani

Introduction

Contraception is the intentional prevention of conception through the use of various devices, sexual practices, chemicals, drugs, or surgical procedures. An effective contraception allows a physical relationship without fear of an unwanted pregnancy and ensures freedom to have children when desired.

The hormonal contraceptives (HCs), which contain a combination of the hormones estrogen and progestin or progestin only contraceptives, are one of the most popular form of contraception around the world (Table 1) [1]. They are highly effective for both spacing and limiting births [2], when used perfectly [3].

Combined oral contraceptives (OCs), including estrogen and a progesterone, are the most common form of HCs worldwide [4]. A dose of 35 μg ethinylestradiol (EE), a derivative of 17 beta-estradiol, has been the predominant estrogen in combined contraceptive pills because of its high oral bioavailability. As such, levonorgestrel or norethisterone have been used as the main progestin in those pills. These combination is considered the "gold standard" in OCs in relation to their safety profile [5]. Newer progestogens such as gestodene and desogestrel are structurally related to progesterone, but have greater specificity for progesterone receptors than the older progestogens. They reduce the potential for androgenic, estrogenic, and glucocorticoid effects. Drospirenone is a spironolactone analog and has a mild diuretic effect [6]. Cyproterone has anti-androgenic effects which may be beneficial in women with hyperandrogenic symptoms [7].

Generally, hormonal contraceptive could influence the hypothalamo-pituitary-ovarian axis and reduce the ovarian production of sex steroids. Combined hormonal contraceptives act primarily by preventing ovulation through the suppression of ovulation by inhibition of gonadotropin-releasing hormone (GnRH), luteinizing

S. Behboudi-Gandevani (✉)
Faculty of Nursing and Health Sciences, Nord University, Bodø, Norway
e-mail: Samira.behboudi-gandevani@nord.no

F. Azizi, F. Ramezani Tehrani (eds.), *Thyroid Diseases in Pregnancy*,
https://doi.org/10.1007/978-3-030-98777-0_17

Table 1 Female hormonal contraceptives choice

Hormonal contraceptives		Drug formulations		Instruction for use
Combined hormonal contraceptives		Estrogen	Progestin	
Oral				
Conventional	Low dose	Ethinylestradiol (35 µg or less)	One progestin: – Ethynodiol diacetate (1 mg) – Norethindrone (1 mg) – Norethindrone (0.5 mg) – Norethindrone (0.4 mg) – Norgestimate (0.25 mg) – Desogestrel (0.15 mg) – Drospirenone (3 µg) – Levonorgestrel (0.15 mg) – Norethindrone acetate (1.5 mg) – Norgestrel (0.3 mg)	The package contains 21 days of active pills and 7 days off
	High dose	Ethinylestradiol (50 µg)	One progestin: – Norethindrone (1 mg) – Norgestrel (0.5 mg) – Ethynodiol diacetate (1 mg)	The package contains 21 days of active pills and 7 days off
	Triphasic (day: 1–7, 8–14, 15–21)	Ethinylestradiol (30, 40, 30 µg) (35, 35, 35 µg) (20, 30, 35 µg)	One progestin: – Levonorgestrel (0.05, 0.075, 0.125 mg) – Norgestimate (0.18, 0.215, 0.25 mg) – Desogestrel (1.1, 0.125, 0.150 mg) – Norethindrone (1, 1, 1 mg) – Norethindrone (0.5, 0.75, 0.125 mg) – Norethindrone (0.5, 1, 0. 5 mg)	The package contains 21 days of active pills and 7 days off
Continuous dosing or extended cycle		Ethinylestradiol (35 µg)	Levonorgestrel (0.15 mg)	3-month pack contains 84 days of active pills and 7 days off

Table 1 (continued)

Hormonal contraceptives	Drug formulations		Instruction for use
Progesterone only contraceptives			
Oral, (mini-pill)	–	One progestin: – norethindrone (0.35 mg) – norgestrel (0.075 mg) – levonorgestrel (0.030 mg) – lynestrenol (0.50 mg) – ethynodiol diacetate (0.50 mg) – desogestrel (0.075 mg)	The package contains 28-daily of active pills without interruption
Injectable	–	Depot medroxyprogesterone (DMPA) – 150 mg/mL – 400 mg/mL	One shot either once every month or once every 3 months
Implant	–	Ethylene vinyl acetate (68 mg etonogestrel in each implant) (release rate: 35–45 µg/day in first year, 30–40 µg/day in second year, in 25–30 µg/day third year)	Inserted beneath the skin of the upper arm up to 3 years
Hormonal intra uterine devise	–	Levonorgestrel – 13.5 mg/device (Skyla), release rate: 14 µg/day) – 19.5 mg/device (Kyleena), release rate: 17.5 µg/day) – 52 mg/device (Liletta, Mirena), (release rate: 20 µg/day)	Inserted in the uterine up to 5 years

hormone (LH), follicle-stimulating hormone (FSH), and the mid-cycle LH surge [8]. This effect is mediated by both the progestin and estrogen component of the COs working synergistically, but estrogen suppression of FSH, which in turn prevents folliculogenesis, is likely the most important mechanism. Additionally, the estrogen component stabilizes the endometrium to maintain a regular withdrawal bleeding pattern [9]. The progestin component also renders the cervical mucus relatively impenetrable to sperm and reduces the receptivity of the endometrium to implantation [10].

It is well documented that HCs have profound interactions with thyroid function [11]. Those interactions are particularly important in women who suffer from thyroid disorders, since those diseases are very common in women of reproductive age [12–14].

This chapter focuses on the various aspects of interaction between thyroid hormones and hormonal contraceptives in order to present the clinical guide for daily practice.

Physiological Consideration

Thyroid hormones have been shown to exert a modulatory influence on female reproductive function [15]. It was reported that thyroid hormone receptors (TRs) are present in human ovarian surface epithelium and act on ovarian follicles and show some slight localization in granulosa cells of ovarian follicles [16]. As such, ovarian hormones could influence thyroid function. As such, thyroid function could be modulated by gonadal or sex steroids, primarily by altering the clearance of thyroxine-binding globulin (TBG) [17], and peripheral deiodination of thyroxine [18].

Estrogen has a well-known direct and indirect effect on thyroid economy. States of estrogen excess, either endogenous or exogenous, are associated with a rise in serum TBG concentrations [19]. This occurs through the increased sialylation of TBG, thereby slowing its clearance from the circulation by the liver and increasing its half-life [20, 21]. However, same mechanism leads to increase the levels of similar glycoproteins, mainly sex hormone binding globulin (SHBG) [22, 23]. Whether estrogen increases biosynthesis of TBG remains controversial [17].

These effects are modulated by the chemical structure of the steroid being used, its dose, and the route of administration. In this respect it is reported that, in the same therapeutic effects, transdermal administration of estradiol causes minimal changes in serum TBG concentrations, but oral administration could lead to a 50–70% increase in serum TBG [24]. Moreover, since ethinyl estradiol undergoes limited liver metabolism and remains longer in the liver, it is more potent to increase the serum concentration of binding proteins compared to estradiol or other chemical forms of estrogens [17, 25].

A rise of TBG results in a reduced clearance of thyroxine (T4) and triiodothyronine (T3) and, hence, results in a new thyroid hormone equilibrium characterized by an increase in total T3 and T4 by 20–40% and a reduced resin triiodothyronine (T3 uptake) level [26]. However, the free or bioactive fractions of thyroid hormones remain normal or only slightly affected if the patient is euthyroid, because this is the function of the circulating hormone regulated by the feedback "axis" [27–29]. In this respect, serum free T4 may transiently decrease inducing a response from the pituitary to increase TSH secretion, which, in turn, will stimulate the thyroid to produce more T4. A new steady state is reached between free and bound T4 and TSH levels remain normal [27, 30].

There are limited studies assessing the effect of progestins on thyroid function, and mostly have not demonstrated any effect of progestins on TBG concentrations [27]. Cyproterone acetate, a progestin with anti-androgenic effects, was not observed to have any effect on TBG concentrations [26, 30].

As well, only limited studies have been published on the effects of long-acting drugs containing only progesterone on thyroid function. It is reported that depot medroxyprogesterone acetate (DMPA) could significantly increase FT4 levels after the 12-month follow-up [31]. Accordingly, a randomized placebo-controlled 12-week trial found that oral micronized progesterone at the daily dose of 300 mg could decrease TSH, increase FT4, and did not have any effect on FT3 serum levels, compared to placebo [32]. This evidence suggests a greater role for progestins in influencing thyroid function.

It should be noted that these effects are generally transient and partly reversed in the hormone-free interval of 1–8 weeks; also, maximal levels of SHBG are reached at the end of the third cycle and no further rise occurs during the following cycles [32, 33].

Guide for Clinical Practice

Thyroid dysfunction is one of the most common endocrine disorders among reproductive-aged women [34], the groups of women who most commonly use effective hormonal contraception [35, 36]. Although women with no thyroid disease adapt quickly to thyroid hormonal alterations induced by gonadal steroids, those small alterations may be clinically important for women who suffer from thyroid disorders and may cause significant biochemical and clinical alterations requiring changes in the doses of thyroid medications. Likewise, there are limited studies suggesting that thyroid hormones may affect the action of estrogen and subsequently can affect the efficacy and safety of hormonal contraceptives [11, 37]. This suggests that euthyroidism is important for the effectiveness of OCs.

Meanwhile, since thyroid disorders are not contraindications to pregnancy, if pregnancy does occur, untreated thyroid dysfunctions are widely associated with increased risk of feto-maternal and neonatal morbidity among pregnant women [38–41], Therefore, it is advisable to treat the problem first and begin contraception, when pregnancy is requested. However, side effects caused by those HCs, such as weight changes, emotional lability, or changes in energy level, could be similar to symptoms of hypothyroidism, hyperthyroidism, and other types of thyroid dysfunction, and might unmask thyroid illness in previously undiagnosed subjects.

Here we provided a guide for using the hormonal contraceptives among women with thyroid dysfunction for clinical practice. However, in a the holistic approach, the steps suggested here are intended to be general guidelines that would never substitute for clinical judgment. Each patient's total clinical and psychosocial circumstances must be considered, since the physician should treat the patient and not the disease.

Hypothyroidism

In contrast to the findings in thyroid subjects, estrogen component of HCs causes clinically significant alterations in thyroid function leading to increased levothyroxine requirements in women with hypothyroidism [26]. In hypothyroid subjects, estrogen leads to an increase in serum TBG levels quantitatively similar to that observed in those with normal thyroid function [3]. This alteration in those patients leads to slow the entry of thyroxine into cells, including pituitary cells, thereby reducing thyroid hormone action in tissue. Alternatively, estrogen might lower the serum free thyroxine concentration by increasing the clearance of thyroxine. Therefore, the serum concentrations of both serum TSH levels and free thyroxine [14] decrease in those patients and cannot stimulate by thyroid gland to produce more T4. Although the alterations are small, those alterations are potentially clinically important and may need thyroxine replacement. It should be noted that this effect is dose dependent and is usually observed within 6 weeks after HCs containing estrogen initiation and reaches its peak at 12 weeks [33].

The influence of HCs containing estrogen in patients with subclinical hypothyroidism has not been clearly understood. But it might be possible that such patients become overtly hypothyroid following HCs containing estrogen usage. Based on current knowledge, there are no restrictions on the choice of HC methods in women with controlled hypothyroidism with the same guidelines that are used for healthy women. Moreover, in patients with levothyroxine treatment, it is recommended to consider up-titration of the levothyroxine dose in new HC users. In this respect, TSH and FT4 should be measured 4–8 weeks after the up-titration in order to check the adequacy of replacement. However, it is unnecessary to stop the use of hormonal contraceptive to evaluate thyroid function, but it would be prudent to assess thyroid function in those patients after withdrawal of HCs.

Hyperthyroidism

There are limited studies addressing the influence of HCs in patients with hyperthyroidism. The increase in TBG and the associated decrease in free thyroxine levels would explain the observed amelioration of Graves' hyperthyroidism with exogenous estrogen [42, 43]. Based on current knowledge, generally, there are no restrictions on the choice of hormonal contraceptive methods in women with hyperthyroidism with the same guidelines that are used for healthy women. In patients with antithyroid medications therapy, it is recommended to consider antithyroid agents dosage in new hormonal contraceptive users. In this respect, TSH and FT4 could be measured 4–8 weeks after initiation of those contraceptives to show if your thyroid medication needs a dosage adjustment. Additionally, it is unnecessary to stop the use of HCs to evaluate thyroid function, but it would be prudent to assess thyroid function in those patients after withdrawal of HCs.

Autoimmunity

Sex hormones regulate molecular mechanisms in the innate and adaptive immune systems, and control immune responses in health [44]. Hormonal contraceptives (HCs) are very potent hormones that have effects on the immune system [45]. Estrogens, in general, are considered immune-stimulatory due to enhanced cellular proliferation and antibody secretion by decreasing the CD4+/CD8+ T cell ratio and TNF-α cytotoxicity in T cells and increasing immunoglobulin secretion, B cell survival, and polyclonal activation of B cells as well as IgG and IgM production in peripheral blood mononuclear cells [46–48]. In contrast, progestins clearly have immunomodulatory and immunosuppressive effects on the immune system, by inhibition of macrophage activation, nitric oxide production, and IFN-γ production by NK cells [44, 49] and therefore counteract the pathways affected by estrogen [44]. Hormonal contraceptives also suppress pituitary gonadotropins, which have a number of additional immunomodulatory effects [50, 51]. Thus, while a specific mechanism linking HCs to autoimmune disease pathogenesis has not been elucidated, it is speculate that the administration of HCs, either combined estrogen-progestin contraceptives or progestin-only contraceptives, would modulate the immune system and may affect the predisposition of hormonal contraceptive users to autoimmune diseases [45]. Autoimmune thyroid diseases are usually accompanied by the presence of antithyroid peroxidase (TPO), anti-thyroglobulin (Tg), and antithyroid-stimulating hormone receptor (TSHR) antibodies [48]. There are some evidence showing that sex hormones may play a role in thyroid autoimmunity. In this respect, it is showed that higher circulating estradiol is related to thyroid autoimmunity in males as reflected by positive TSH receptor antibody (TRAb) [52].

However, at current time there is the lack of literature supporting the effect of HCs on autoimmune thyroid diseases. Therefore, based on indirect available evidence, generally, there are no restrictions on the choice of hormonal contraceptive methods in women with autoimmune thyroid diseases with the same guidelines that are used for healthy women. However, it is recommended to consider thyroid agents dosage in new hormonal contraceptive users. In this respect, TSH and FT4 could be measured 4–6 weeks after initiation of those contraceptives to show if your thyroid medication needs a dosage adjustment.

Summary

Hormonal contraceptives (HCs) are able to impact the thyroid gland function. Although women with no thyroid dysfunction can tolerate thyroid hormonal alterations induced by those agents, those small alterations in thyroid hormones concentrations may be clinically important for women who suffer from thyroid disorders. In such cases, serum level of thyroid hormones should be measured at least 4–8 weeks after initiation of HCs in order to check the adequacy of thyroid medications.

References

1. Hall KS, White KOC, Reame N, Westhoff C. Studying the use of oral contraception: a review of measurement approaches. J Womens Health (Larchmt). 2010;19(12):2203–10.
2. Sitruk-Ware R, Nath A, Mishell DR Jr. Contraception technology: past, present and future. Contraception. 2013;87(3):319–30.
3. Dinger J, Do Minh T, Buttmann N, Bardenheuer K. Effectiveness of oral contraceptive pills in a large U.S. cohort comparing progestogen and regimen. Obstet Gynecol. 2011;117(1):33–40.
4. Brynhildsen J. Combined hormonal contraceptives: prescribing patterns, compliance, and benefits versus risks. Ther Adv Drug Saf. 2014;5(5):201–13.
5. Benagiano G, Carrara S, Filippi V. Safety, efficacy and patient satisfaction with continuous daily administration of levonorgestrel/ethinylestradiol oral contraceptives. Patient Prefer Adherence. 2009;3:131–43.
6. Stewart M, Black K. Choosing a combined oral contraceptive pill. Aust Prescr. 2015;38(1):6–11.
7. Kelekci KH, Kelekci S, Yengel I, Gul S, Yilmaz B. Cyproterone acetate or drospirenone containing combined oral contraceptives plus spironolactone or cyproterone acetate for hirsutism: randomized comparison of three regimens. J Dermatolog Treat. 2012;23(3):177–83.
8. Bastianelli C, Farris M, Rosato E, Brosens I, Benagiano G. Pharmacodynamics of combined estrogen-progestin oral contraceptives 3. Inhibition of ovulation. Expert Rev Clin Pharmacol. 2018;11(11):1085–98.
9. Sober SP, Schreiber CA. Controversies in family planning: are all oral contraceptive formulations created equal? Contraception. 2011;83(5):394–6.
10. Erkkola R, Landgren BM. Role of progestins in contraception. Acta Obstet Gynecol Scand. 2005;84(3):207–16.
11. Torre F, Calogero AE, Condorelli RA, Cannarella R, Aversa A, La Vignera S. Effects of oral contraceptives on thyroid function and vice versa. J Endocrinol Invest. 2020;43(9):1181–8.
12. Garmendia Madariaga A, Santos Palacios S, Guillén-Grima F, Galofré JC. The incidence and prevalence of thyroid dysfunction in Europe: a meta-analysis. J Clin Endocrinol Metab. 2014;99(3):923–31.
13. Poppe K, Velkeniers B, Glinoer D. Thyroid disease and female reproduction. Clin Endocrinol. 2007;66(3):309–21.
14. Panth P, Guerin G, DiMarco NM. A review of iodine status of women of reproductive age in the USA. Biol Trace Elem Res. 2019;188(1):208–20.
15. Mintziori G, Anagnostis P, Toulis KA, Goulis DG. Thyroid diseases and female reproduction. Minerva Med. 2012;103(1):47–62.
16. Aghajanova L, Lindeberg M, Carlsson IB, Stavreus-Evers A, Zhang P, Scott JE, et al. Receptors for thyroid-stimulating hormone and thyroid hormones in human ovarian tissue. Reprod Biomed Online. 2009;18(3):337–47.
17. Tahboub R, Arafah BM. Sex steroids and the thyroid. Best Pract Res Clin Endocrinol Metab. 2009;23(6):769–80.
18. Kester MH, van Dijk CH, Tibboel D, Hood AM, Rose NJ, Meinl W, et al. Sulfation of thyroid hormone by estrogen sulfotransferase. J Clin Endocrinol Metab. 1999;84(7):2577–80.
19. Santin AP, Furlanetto TW. Role of estrogen in thyroid function and growth regulation. J Thyroid Res. 2011;2011:875125.
20. Sänger N, Stahlberg S, Manthey T, Mittmann K, Mellinger U, Lange E, et al. Effects of an oral contraceptive containing 30 mcg ethinyl estradiol and 2 mg dienogest on thyroid hormones and androgen parameters: conventional vs. extended-cycle use. Contraception. 2008;77(6):420–5.
21. Coussa A, Hasan HA, Barber TM. Impact of contraception and IVF hormones on metabolic, endocrine, and inflammatory status. J Assist Reprod Genet. 2020;37(6):1267–72.
22. Sitruk-Ware R, Plu-Bureau G, Menard J, Conard J, Kumar S, Thalabard JC, et al. Effects of oral and transvaginal ethinyl estradiol on hemostatic factors and hepatic proteins in a randomized, crossover study. J Clin Endocrinol Metab. 2007;92(6):2074–9.

23. Shifren JL, Rifai N, Desindes S, McIlwain M, Doros G, Mazer NA. A comparison of the short-term effects of oral conjugated equine estrogens versus transdermal estradiol on C-reactive protein, other serum markers of inflammation, and other hepatic proteins in naturally menopausal women. J Clin Endocrinol Metab. 2008;93(5):1702–10.
24. Shifren JL, Desindes S, McIlwain M, Doros G, Mazer NA. A randomized, open-label, crossover study comparing the effects of oral versus transdermal estrogen therapy on serum androgens, thyroid hormones, and adrenal hormones in naturally menopausal women. Menopause. 2007;14(6):985–94.
25. Dickson RB, Eisenfeld AJ. 17 alpha-ethinyl estradiol is more potent than estradiol in receptor interactions with isolated hepatic parenchymal cells. Endocrinology. 1981;108(4):1511–8.
26. Arafah BM. Increased need for thyroxine in women with hypothyroidism during estrogen therapy. N Engl J Med. 2001;344(23):1743–9.
27. Wiegratz I, Kutschera E, Lee JH, Moore C, Mellinger U, Winkler UH, et al. Effect of four oral contraceptives on thyroid hormones, adrenal and blood pressure parameters. Contraception. 2003;67(5):361–6.
28. Loriaux DL, Wild RA. Contraceptive choices for women with endocrine complications. Am J Obstet Gynecol. 1993;168(6 Pt 2):2021–6.
29. Ågren UM, Anttila M, Mäenpää-Liukko K, Rantala ML, Rautiainen H, Sommer WF, et al. Effects of a monophasic combined oral contraceptive containing nomegestrol acetate and 17β-oestradiol in comparison to one containing levonorgestrel and ethinylestradiol on markers of endocrine function. Eur J Contracept Reprod Health Care. 2011;16(6):458–67.
30. Bisschop PH, Toorians AW, Endert E, Wiersinga WM, Gooren LJ, Fliers E. The effects of sex-steroid administration on the pituitary-thyroid axis in transsexuals. Eur J Endocrinol. 2006;155(1):11–6.
31. Quintino-Moro A, Zantut-Wittmann DE, Silva Dos Santos PN, Melhado-Kimura V, da Silva CA, Bahamondes L, et al. Thyroid function during the first year of use of the injectable contraceptive depot medroxyprogesterone acetate. Eur J Contracept Reprod Health Care. 2019;24(2):102–8.
32. Sathi P, Kalyan S, Hitchcock CL, Pudek M, Prior JC. Progesterone therapy increases free thyroxine levels—data from a randomized placebo-controlled 12-week hot flush trial. Clin Endocrinol. 2013;79(2):282–7.
33. Alexopoulou O, Beguin C, De Nayer P, Maiter D. Clinical and hormonal characteristics of central hypothyroidism at diagnosis and during follow-up in adult patients. Eur J Endocrinol. 2004;150(1):1–8.
34. Li H, Li J. Thyroid disorders in women. Minerva Med. 2015;106(2):109–14.
35. Behboudi-Gandevani S, Ramezani Tehrani F, Cheraghi L, Noroozzadeh M, Farahmand M, Azizi F. Trends of contraception use among married reproductive age women: Tehran lipid and glucose cohort study 2002-2011. Sex Reprod Healthc. 2017;12:116–22.
36. Jarosz AC, Jamnik J, El-Sohemy A. Hormonal contraceptive use and prevalence of premenstrual symptoms in a multiethnic Canadian population. BMC Womens Health. 2017;17(1):87.
37. Vasudevan N, Ogawa S, Pfaff D. Estrogen and thyroid hormone receptor interactions: physiological flexibility by molecular specificity. Physiol Rev. 2002;82(4):923–44.
38. Zhou M, Wang M, Li J, Luo X, Lei M. Effects of thyroid diseases on pregnancy outcomes. Exp Ther Med. 2019;18(3):1807–15.
39. Ramezani Tehrani F, Nazarpour S, Behboudi-Gandevani S. Isolated maternal hypothyroxinemia and adverse pregnancy outcomes: a systematic review. J Gynecol Obstet Hum Reprod. 2021;50(7):102057.
40. Ge GM, Leung MTY, Man KKC, Leung WC, Ip P, Li GHY, et al. Maternal thyroid dysfunction during pregnancy and the risk of adverse outcomes in the offspring: a systematic review and meta-analysis. J Clin Endocrinol Metab. 2020;105(12):dgaa555.
41. Sun X, Hou N, Wang H, Ma L, Sun J, Liu Y. A meta-analysis of pregnancy outcomes with levothyroxine treatment in euthyroid women with thyroid autoimmunity. J Clin Endocrinol Metab. 2020;105(4):dgz217.

42. Knudsen N, Bülow I, Laurberg P, Perrild H, Ovesen L, Jørgensen T. Low goitre prevalence among users of oral contraceptives in a population sample of 3712 women. Clin Endocrinol. 2002;57(1):71–6.
43. Furlanetto TW, Nguyen LQ, Jameson JL. Estradiol increases proliferation and down-regulates the sodium/iodide symporter gene in FRTL-5 cells. Endocrinology. 1999;140(12):5705–11.
44. Tan IJ, Peeva E, Zandman-Goddard G. Hormonal modulation of the immune system—a spotlight on the role of progestogens. Autoimmun Rev. 2015;14(6):536–42.
45. Williams WV. Hormonal contraception and the development of autoimmunity: a review of the literature. Linacre Q. 2017;84(3):275–95.
46. Cutolo M, Brizzolara R, Atzeni F, Capellino S, Straub RH, Puttini PC. The immunomodulatory effects of estrogens: clinical relevance in immune-mediated rheumatic diseases. Ann N Y Acad Sci. 2010;1193:36–42.
47. Moulton VR. Sex hormones in acquired immunity and autoimmune disease. Front Immunol. 2018;9:2279.
48. Fröhlich E, Wahl R. Thyroid autoimmunity: role of anti-thyroid antibodies in thyroid and extra-thyroidal diseases. Front Immunol. 2017;8:521.
49. Ngo ST, Steyn FJ, McCombe PA. Gender differences in autoimmune disease. Front Neuroendocrinol. 2014;35(3):347–69.
50. Michel KG, Huijbregts RPH, Gleason JL, Richter HE, Hel Z. Effect of hormonal contraception on the function of plasmacytoid dendritic cells and distribution of immune cell populations in the female reproductive tract. J Acquir Immune Defic Syndr. 2015;68(5):511–8.
51. Soria-Jasso LE, Cariño-Cortés R, Muñoz-Pérez VM, Pérez-Hernández E, Pérez-Hernández N, Fernández-Martínez E. Beneficial and deleterious effects of female sex hormones, Oral contraceptives, and phytoestrogens by immunomodulation on the liver. Int J Mol Sci. 2019;20(19):4694.
52. Chailurkit LO, Aekplakorn W, Ongphiphadhanakul B. The relationship between circulating estradiol and thyroid autoimmunity in males. Eur J Endocrinol. 2014;170(1):63–7.

GPSR Compliance

The European Union's (EU) General Product Safety Regulation (GPSR) is a set of rules that requires consumer products to be safe and our obligations to ensure this.

If you have any concerns about our products, you can contact us on ProductSafety@springernature.com

In case Publisher is established outside the EU, the EU authorized representative is:

Springer Nature Customer Service Center GmbH
Europaplatz 3
69115 Heidelberg, Germany

Batch number: 10732090

Printed by Printforce, the Netherlands